# The EACVI
# Echo Handbook

# European Society of Cardiology publications

**The ESC Textbook of Cardiovascular Medicine (Second Edition)**
Edited by A. John Camm, Thomas F. Lüscher, and Patrick W. Serruys

**The EAE Textbook of Echocardiography**
Editor-in-Chief: Leda Galiuto, with Co-Editors: Luigi Badano, Kevin Fox, Rosa Sicari, and Jose Luis Zamorano

**The ESC Textbook of Intensive and Acute Cardiovascular Care (Second Edition)**
Edited by Marco Tubaro, Pascal Vranckx, Susanna Price, and Christiaan Vrints

**The ESC Textbook of Cardiovascular Imaging (Second Edition)**
Edited by Jose Luis Zamorano, Jeroen Bax, Juhani Knuuti, Patrizio Lancellotti, Luigi Badano, and Udo Sechtem

**The ESC Textbook of Preventive Cardiology**
Edited by Stephan Gielen, Guy De Backer, Massimo Piepoli, and David Wood

**The EHRA Book of Pacemaker, ICD, and CRT Troubleshooting:** *Case-based learning with multiple choice questions*
Edited by Haran Burri, Jean-Claude Deharo, and Carsten Israel

**The EACVI Echo Handbook**
Edited by Patrizio Lancellotti and Bernard Cosyns

*Forthcoming*

**The ESC Handbook of Preventive Cardiology:** *Putting prevention into practice*
Edited by Catriona Jennings, Ian Graham, and Stephan Gielen

**The EACVI Textbook of Echocardiography 2e**
Edited by Patrizio Lancellotti, Jose Luis Zamorano, Gilbert Habib, and Luigi Badano

# The EACVI
# Echo Handbook

Edited by

## Patrizio Lancellotti

University of Liege, Hospital Sart Tilman, Belgium

## Bernard Cosyns

Free University of Brussels, Belgium

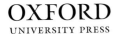

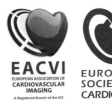

EACVI
EUROPEAN ASSOCIATION OF
CARDIOVASCULAR
IMAGING
A Registered Branch of the ESC

EUROPEAN
SOCIETY OF
CARDIOLOGY®

# OXFORD

## UNIVERSITY PRESS

Great Clarendon Street, Oxford, OX2 6DP,
United Kingdom

Oxford University Press is a department of the University of Oxford.
It furthers the University's objective of excellence in research, scholarship,
and education by publishing worldwide. Oxford is a registered trade mark of
Oxford University Press in the UK and in certain other countries

Published in the United States of America by Oxford University Press
198 Madison Avenue, New York, NY 10016, United States of America

British Library Cataloguing in Publication Data

Data available

Library of Congress Control Number: 2015941609

ISBN 978-0-19-871362-3

Printed in Great Britain by
Bell & Bain Ltd., Glasgow

# Foreword

Echocardiography has been in use for over 50 years yet it continues to evolve at a surprisingly rapid rate. Echocardiography has become the first-line imaging in the diagnostic work-up and monitoring of most cardiac diseases. Providing a high-quality book that encompasses what anyone in the field of echocardiography wants and needs to know has been our aim.

The *EACVI Echo Handbook* does not intend to be a cut-down version of an echocardiography textbook. It presents the information a busy clinician needs to review or to consult while performing or reporting an echo or making clinical decisions based on echo findings and reports the most practical information required at the bedside.

A formidable team of internationally prominent clinicians have contributed to the various chapters according to their areas of expertise. Most have published or participated in the publication of the EACVI echocardiography recommendations. The *Handbook* thus heavily relies on the EACVI recommendations and the updated EACVI Core Curriculum.

The *EACVI Echo Handbook* provides a wide range of clinicians with a foundation for the practice of the skills necessary for assessing patients using echocardiography. This book belongs on the desk of all sonographers, trainees in cardiology, cardiologists as well as other clinicians such as intensivists, anaesthesiologists, and students interested in echocardiography. It is laid out in a very logical sequence starting with how to set up the echomachine to optimize an examination and how to perform and interpret an echocardiogram accurately. The subsequent chapters are disease-focused and provide in-depth overviews of all relevant information needed in daily practice. A future digital edition is planned as a companion to the present printed edition, allowing users to access online videos to illustrate most of the topics addressed, to track favourites, keep a history of navigation, and to retrieve information even more rapidly.

The *EACVI Echo Handbook* is a valuable resource that deserves a place in your echo reporting room.

Patrizio Lancellotti and
Bernard Cosyns

# Contents

# Contributors

## Editors

Bernard Cosyns
Patrizio Lancellotti

## Section editors

Erwan Donal
Madalina Garbi
Ruxandra Jurcut
Pierre Monney
Jadranka Separovic Hanzevacki

## Contributors

Nuno Cardim
Jan D'hooge
Raluca Dulgheru
Thor Edvardsen
Arturo Evangelista
Frank Flachskampf
Maurizio Galderisi
Luna Gargani
Gilbert Habib
Lieven Herbots

Andre La Gerche
Patrizio Lancellotti
David Messika-Zeitoun
Owen Miller
Denisa Muraru
Bernard Paelinck
Agnes Pasquet
Kelly Peacock
Mauro Pepi
Luc Pierard

Edyta Plonska
Bogdan Popescu
Kathryn Rice
Raphael Rosenhek
Raymond Roudaut
Roxy Senior
Rosa Sicari
Alex Stefanidis
Philippe Unger
Jens Uwe Voigt

# Abbreviations

| | |
|---|---|
| 2D | two dimensional |
| 2DE | two-dimensional echocardiography |
| 3CV | three-chamber view |
| 3D | three dimensional |
| 3DE | three-dimensional echocardiography |
| 4CV | four-chamber view |
| 5CV | five-chamber view |
| A2C | apical two-chambers |
| AA | ascending aorta |
| AAS | acute aortic syndrome |
| AD | aortic dissection |
| AF | atrial fibrillation |
| AL | area–length |
| ALI | acute lung injury |
| ALC | anterolateral commissure |
| ALS | advanced life support |
| AMI | acute myocardial infarction |
| AML | anterior mitral leaflet |
| Ao | aorta |
| AP | apical |
| APS | antiphospholipid syndrome |

| | |
|---|---|
| AR | aortic regurgitation |
| ARDS | acute respiratory distress syndrome |
| ARVC | arryhthmogenic right ventricular cardiomyopathy |
| AS | aortic stenosis |
| ASD | atrial septal defect |
| AV | aortic valve |
| AVA | aortic valve area |
| AVSD | atrioventricular septal defects |
| BAV | bicuspid aortic valve |
| BNP | brain natriuretic peptide |
| BSA | body surface area |
| C | compaction |
| CCTGA | congenitally corrected transposition of the great arteries |
| CD | coaptation distance |
| CDRIE | cardiac device-related IE |
| CMR | cardiac magnetic resonance |
| CO | cardiac output |
| COPD | chronic obstructive pulmonary disease |
| CT | cardiac transplantation |
| CT | computed tomography |
| CTD | connective tissue disease |
| CV | chamber view |
| CW | continuous wave |
| DA | descending aorta |
| DCM | dilated cardiomyopathy |
| DDD | daily defined dose |

| | |
|---|---|
| DI | dimensionless index |
| DMI | digital media initiative |
| DSE | dobutamine stress echocardiography |
| DTI | Doppler tissue imaging |
| DVI | diastolic velocity integral |
| EDV | end-diastolic volume |
| EF | ejection fraction |
| E-FAST | extended focused assessed sonography in trauma |
| EOA | effective orifice area |
| ER | emergency room |
| EROA | effective regurgitant orifice area |
| ESV | end-systolic volume |
| ET | ejection time |
| FAST | focused assessed sonography in trauma |
| FATE | focused assessed transthoracic echocardiography |
| FEEL | focused echo evaluation in life support |
| FL | false lumina |
| FS | fractional shortening |
| GCA | giant cell arteritis |
| GLS | global longitudinal strain |
| GV | great vessels |
| HCM | hypertrophic cardiomyopathy |
| HOCM | hypertrophic obstructive cardiomyopathy |
| IAS | interatrial septum |
| ICU | intensive care unit |
| IDCM | idiopathic dilated cardiomyopathy |

| | |
|---|---|
| IMH | intramural haematoma |
| IVA | isovolumic acceleration time |
| IVC | inferior vena cava |
| IVRT | isovolumic relaxation time |
| IVS | interventricular septum morphology |
| LA | left atrial/atrium |
| LAA | left atrial abnormality |
| LAD | left anterior descending |
| LAX | long axis |
| LBBB | left bundle branch block |
| LCC | left coronary cusp |
| LCX | left circumflex coronary artery |
| LPA | left pulmonary artery |
| LUQ | left upper quadrant |
| LV | left ventricle/ventricular |
| LVAD | LV assisted device |
| LVEDV | left ventricular end-diastolic volume |
| LVEF | left ventricular ejection fraction |
| LVNC | left ventricular non-compaction |
| LVO | left ventricular opacification |
| LVOT | left ventricular outflow tract |
| MCTD | mixed connective tissue disease |
| MI | mechanical index |
| MPA | main pulmonary artery |
| MPG | mean pressure gradient |
| MPI | myocardial performance index |

| | |
|---|---|
| MPR | multi-planar reconstruction |
| MR | mitral regurgitation |
| MRI | magnetic resonance imaging |
| MS | mitral stenosis |
| MV | mitral valve |
| MV | myocardial velocity |
| MVI | myocardial velocity imaging |
| NC | non-compaction |
| NCC | non-coronary cusp |
| NYHA | New York Heart Association |
| OR | operating room |
| PA | pulmonary artery |
| PACU | post-anaesthesia care unit |
| PAH | pulmonary arterial hypertension |
| PASP | pulmonary arterial systolic pressure |
| PAT | paroxysmal atrial tachycardia |
| PAU | penetrating aortic ulcer |
| PDA | patent ductus arteriosus |
| PE | pulmonary embolism |
| PEEP | positive end-expiratory pressure |
| PET | positron emission tomography |
| PFO | patent foramen ovale |
| PH | pulmonary hypertension |
| PHT | pressure half-time |
| PISA | proximal isovelocity surface area |
| PLA | posterolateral angle |

| | |
|---|---|
| PLAX | parasternal long-axis view |
| PMC | percutaneous mitral commissurotomy |
| PMC | posteromedial commissure |
| PML | posterior mitral leaflet |
| PNX | pneumothorax |
| PPG | maximum pressure gradient |
| PR | pulmonary regurgitation |
| PrV | prosthetic valve |
| PrVIE | prosthetic valve IE |
| PS | parasternal |
| PSA | pseudoaneurysm |
| PSAP | pulmonary arterial systolic arterial pressure |
| PSS | post systolic shortening |
| PSSA | Pennsylvania System of School Assessment |
| PSAX | parasternal short-axis view |
| PTLAX | parasternal long-axis |
| PTSAX | parasternal short-axis |
| PV | pulmonary valve |
| PVH | pulmonary venous hypertension |
| PW | posterior wall |
| PW | pulsed wave |
| RA | rheumatoid arthritis |
| RAA | right atrial appendage |
| RCA | right coronary artery |
| RCC | right coronary cusp |
| RCM | restrictive cardiomyopathy |

| | |
|---|---|
| RPA | right pulmonary artery |
| RUPV | right upper pulmonary vein |
| RUQ | right upper quadrant |
| RV | right ventricle/ventricular |
| RVA | right ventricular apical |
| RVEDP | right ventricular end-diastolic pressure |
| RVEF | right ventricular ejection fraction |
| RVFAC | right ventricular fractional area change |
| RVOT | right ventricle outflow tract |
| RVSP | right ventricular systolic pressure |
| RWT | relative wall thickness |
| SAM | systolic anterior motion |
| SAX | short axis |
| SC | subcostal |
| SEC | spontaneous echo contrast |
| SLE | systemic lupus erythematosus |
| SNR | signal-to-noise ratio |
| SPECT | single photon emission cardiac tomography |
| SR | sinus rhythm |
| SSc | systemic sclerosis |
| SSN | suprasternal notch |
| SV | stroke volume |
| SVC | superior vena cava |
| SW | septal wall |
| T1/2 | pressure half-time |
| TA | tenting area |

| | |
|---|---|
| TAD | tricuspid annulus diameter |
| TAPSE | tricuspid annular plane systolic excursion |
| TAV | tricuspid aortic valve |
| TAVI | tricuspid aortic valve implantation |
| TD | tumour dose |
| TE | truncated ellipsoid |
| TEVAR | thoracic endovascular aortic repair |
| TGA | transposition of the great arteries |
| TIA | transient ischaemic attack |
| TL | true lumina |
| TOE | transoesophageal echocardiography |
| TR | tricuspid regurgitation |
| TS | tricuspid stenosis |
| TTE | transthoracic echocardiography |
| TV | tricuspid valve |
| TVA | tricuspid valve area |
| TVI | time velocity interval |
| ULP | ulcer-like projection |
| US | ultrasonic |
| VAD | ventricle assisted device |
| VC | vena contracta |
| Vp | velocity propagation |
| VPS | views per segment |
| VSD | ventricular septal defects |
| WM | wall motion |

# CHAPTER 1

# Examination

# 1.1 How to set up the echo machine to optimize your examination

## Preparing for the TTE examination

- Make sure the patient is comfortable/relaxed in a left decubitus position, with the left arm up to open up intercostal spaces and breathing quietly to minimize translation of the heart
- The echo-room should be:
  - darkened: avoid sunlight for optimal contrast
  - silent: auditory feedback allows optimizing Doppler sample positions
- A time-aligned ECG of good quality is mandatory for timing of cardiac events
- Select the appropriate probe according to the patient size
- Start with cardiac pre-settings (Fig. 1.1.1AB)

**Important note:**

The ultrasound machine needs maintenance for optimal performance

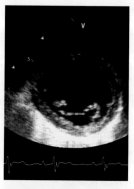

**Fig. 1.1.1A** Cardiac

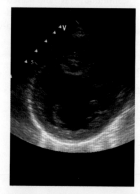

**Fig. 1.1.1B** Abdominal

# Acoustic power

## Controls acoustic energy output

- More energy → better signal → better image quality (i.e. better signal-to-noise ratio: SNR) (Fig. 1.1.2AB, see also Box 1.1.1)
- Expressed in decibel [dB] relative to the maximal energy output available on the system (100% output = 0dB; 50% reduction = −6dB)
- Too much acoustic energy can result in tissue damage due to:
  - Heating: monitored through the 'thermal index' (TI should remain below 2)
  - Cavitation (i.e. formation of small gas bubbles with subsequent bubble collapse associated with high pressures/temperatures locally): monitored through the 'mechanical index' (MI should remain below 1.9)

**Box 1.1.1** Recommendation

Although higher acoustic power increases SNR, it also increases the likelihood of bio-effects. Therefore, only increase transmit power if the default setting results in low SNR

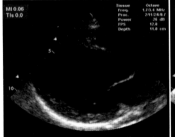 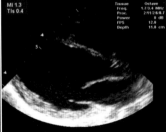

**Fig. 1.1.2A** Low acoustic      **Fig. 1.1.2B** High acoustic

# Gain

**Controls overall amplification of the echo signals**

More gain

→ amplifies the echo signal

→ equally amplifies the noise

→ SNR remains identical! (Figs 1.1.3 and 1.1.4, **see also** Box 1.1.2)

| Box 1.1.2 Recommendation |
| --- |
| Use a gain setting that provides images with the desired brightness/appearance |

# Depth gain compensation

**Depth-specific amplification of the echo signals to compensate for attenuation**

→ Automatic: amplifies signals from deeper structures

→ Manual: allows correction of the automatic compensation (Figs 1.1.5ABC, see also Box 1.1.3)

| Box 1.1.3 Recommendation |
| --- |
| Start each examination with the sliders in their neutral (i.e. centre) position |

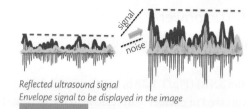

*Reflected ultrasound signal*
*Envelope signal to be displayed in the image*

**Fig. 1.1.3** Effect of gain SNR

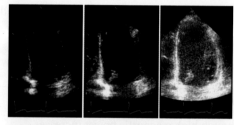

**Fig. 1.1.4** Effects of increased gain on 2D image

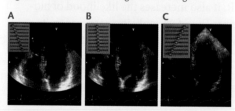

**Fig. 1.1.5** Manual adjustment of depth gain settings. 5A: slider to the right, 5B: neutral, 5C: slider to the left

# Transmit frequency

**Controls transmit frequency of the transducer (see Box 1.1.4)**

Lower frequency (Fig. 1.1.6)

→ Worse spatial resolution

→ Better penetration

Lowering transmit frequency will activate harmonic imaging (Fig.1.1.7)

→ Worse spatial resolution along the image line

→ Better SNR (i.e. less noise)

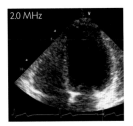 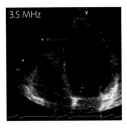

**Fig. 1.1.6** Effects of changing transmit frequency
**Note**: Changing the frequency away from the centre frequency of the probe lowers spatial resolution

---

**Box 1.1.4  Recommendation**

♦ Use harmonic mode as default setting

♦ Keep the transmit frequency equal to the centre frequency of the probe unless:

1. Penetration is insufficient and no other probe is available

2. Switching between fundamental and harmonic imaging is required

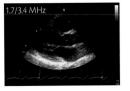 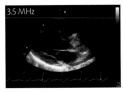

**Fig. 1.1.7** Effects of lowering transmit frequency
**Note:** Harmonic imaging increases SNR but reduces intrinsic spatial resolution along the image line. This is particularly relevant when studying small/thin structures (i.e. valve leaflets)

# Focal position

**Controls the depth at which the ultrasonic (US) beam is focused**

Around this region spatial (lateral) resolution is optimal (Fig. 1.1.8, see also Box 1.1.5)

# Frame rate

**Controls the trade-off between number of lines in a single frame and the number of frames created per second (see also Box 1.1.6)**

Higher frame rate will result in less lines in the image and thus worse spatial (lateral) resolution (Fig. 1.1.10)

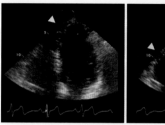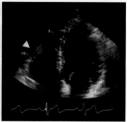

**Fig. 1.1.8** Position of the focal point
**Note**: The position of the focal point is indicated alongside the sector image (arrow point)

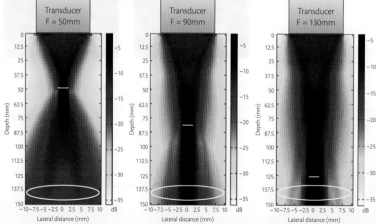

> ### Box 1.1.5 Recommendation
>
> Place the focal point *near the deepest structure of interest* (Fig. 1.1.9, right panel)

**Fig. 1.1.9** Simulated pressure field of a cardiac transducer
White horizontal bar = beam width in focal zone when focus point at 50 mm (i.e. left panel) Mark the difference in beam width at larger depth with changing focal position (white circles)
*Focus point deeper: less effective focusing, lateral resolution decreases*
*Beyond this focus point, beam widens, lateral resolution worsens*

**Box 1.1.6** Recommendation

Keep frame rate at its default value unless modifications are required for specific processing methodologies (i.e. speckle tracking analysis)

## Continuous-wave and pulsed-wave Doppler

**High-quality/reliable Doppler recordings require:**

1. Proper alignment of the image (i.e. Doppler) line with the flow direction (< 20° off-axis) (Fig. 1.1.11, see also Box 1.1.7)

**Box 1.1.7** Recommendation

Reposition and angulate the probe under colour Doppler guidance to obtain optimal alignment

2. Proper velocity scale (also referred to as Nyquist velocity/ PRF) (Fig. 1.1.12AB)
   - Scale too low: aliasing
   - Scale too high: sub-optimal velocity resolution (i.e. smallest difference between two different velocities that can be measured is larger)

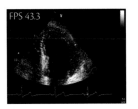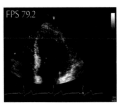

**Fig. 1.1.10** Frame rate and spatial resolution

Adequate           Not optimal

**Fig. 1.1.11** Doppler recording

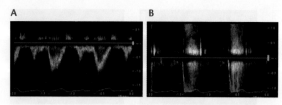

**Fig. 1.1.12** Doppler velocity scale. A: Adequate, B: Too low (i.e. aliasing)

# Continuous-wave and pulsed-wave Doppler

## Sample position

Controls the position of the sample volume (Fig. 1.1.13ABC, see also Box 1.1.8)

## Sample volume

Controls the size of the sample volume (Fig. 1.1.14ABC)

**Box 1.1.8** Recommendation

Sample volume should be positioned at the tips of the (open) valve leaflets (for MV inflow)

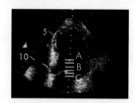

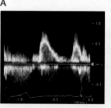
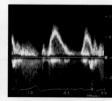
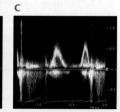

**Fig. 1.1.13** Sample position. A: Too high, B: Appropriate C: Too low

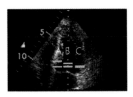

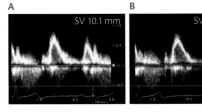

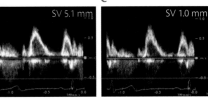

**Fig. 1.1.14** Sample size. A: Too large, B: Appropriate, C: Too small
- Small sample volume: good spatial resolution at lower velocity resolution
- Large sample volume: good velocity resolution at lower spatial resolution

# Continuous-wave and pulsed-wave Doppler: settings

## Wall filter

Controls the threshold for velocities displayed in the velocity spectrum (Fig. 1.1.15ABC, Box 1.1.9)

## Sweep speed

Controls the refresh rate of the velocity spectrum (Fig. 1.1.16AB, Box 1.1.10)

**Box 1.1.9** Recommendation

Wall filter should be as low as possible while avoiding pollution by myocardial velocities

**Box 1.1.10** Recommendation

Always use a sweep speed of 100 mm/s unless looking for inter-beat variations

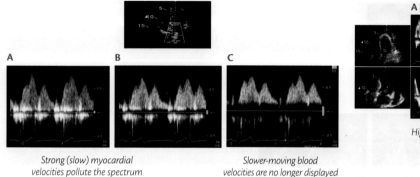

Fig. 1.1.15 Wall filter. A: Too low, B: Appropriate, C: Too high

*Strong (slow) myocardial velocities pollute the spectrum*

*Slower-moving blood velocities are no longer displayed*

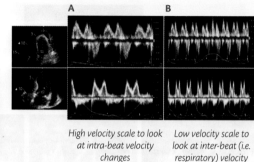

*High velocity scale to look at intra-beat velocity changes*

*Low velocity scale to look at inter-beat (i.e. respiratory) velocity changes*

Fig. 1.1.16 Sweep speed. A: 100 mm/s, B: 33 mm/s

# Colour-flow mapping

## Velocity scale

Controls the range of velocities displayed in the colour box (Fig. 1.1.17, Box 1.1.11)

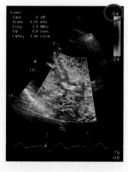

Fig. 1.1.17 Velocity scale
**Aliasing**
- Blue: motion away from transducer
- Red: motion towards the transducer
- Green: velocity out of range (i.e. aliasing)/ large spatial variance (i.e. turbulence)

| Box 1.1.11 Recommendation |
| --- |
| Velocity scale should be as low as possible without aliasing |

## Colour gain

Controls amplification of the colour Doppler signals
(see Box 1.1.12)

> **Box 1.1.12** Recommendation
>
> Should be as high as possible, without noise appearance

## Size of colour box

Directly impacts frame rate (Fig. 1.1.18AB, Box 1.1.13)

> **Box 1.1.13** Recommendation
>
> Colour box should be as small as possible, to optimize
> temporal and spatial resolution

# Advanced techniques

### Myocardial velocity imaging (MVI) (Fig. 1.1.19)

1. Proper alignment of the image line with the wall motion direction
2. Proper velocity scale (Nyquist velocity/PRF)
3. Small sector angles for higher frame rates (optimal > 115 fps)

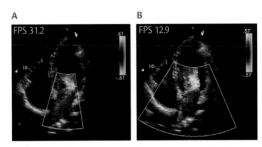

**Fig. 1.1.18** Colour box size. A: Adequate, B: Not optimal

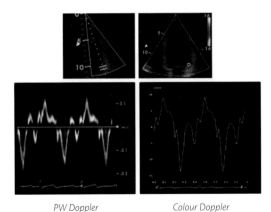

*PW Doppler*      *Colour Doppler*

**Fig. 1.1.19** Myocardial velocity imaging

4. Adjust sample position, sample size, wall filter, and sweep speed
5. High-quality ECG required for optimal timings all apply for myocardial PW and colour Doppler analyses *(as for blood pool Doppler)*

## Speckle tracking—2D strain (rate) imaging (Fig. 1.1.20)

1. Optimize gain settings and focus position
2. Centre the region of interest
3. Adjust depth and region of interest size for optimal spatial resolution *(MV annulus at the bottom of the image for LV regional function analysis)*
4. Adjust frame rates since specific analysis software often requires specific frame rate settings (optimal 50–90 fps)
5. High-quality ECG required for automated tracking

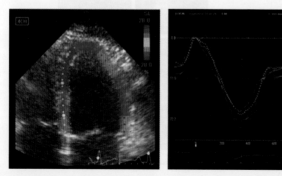

**Fig. 1.1.20** 2D–speckle tracking imaging

## 3D imaging (Fig. 1.1.21)

1. Transducer position: a good acoustic window is essential for optimal 3D visualization (difficult because of larger probe size)
2. Use 2D guidance for centring of the region of interest
3. Image acquisition during breath hold or quiet respiration
4. Adjust volume size to optimize volume rate (real time vs stitched images for post-processing)
5. Adjust gain and avoid drop-out artefacts
6. Crop, translate, and rotate the 3D volume to visualize the structure of interest

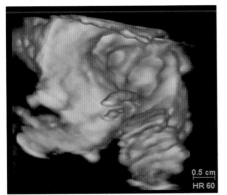 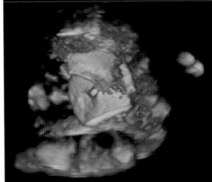

**Fig. 1.1.21** 3D imaging

# CHAPTER 2

# The Standard Transthoracic Echo Examination

## 2.1 2D echocardiography and M-mode echocardiography

### 2D echocardiography

- **Provides real-time tomographic views of the heart in motion**
- Represents the starting point of an echo examination because:
  - it allows morphology and function assessment
  - it guides the use of all other imaging modes (M-mode, Doppler, 3D)
- ECG-gated video clips of cardiac cycles can be acquired and stored for later review
- ECG-gated frozen still-frames allow measurements and calculations
  - during the examination: *online*
  - following the examination: *offline*

### M-mode echocardiography

- Provides a display of motion-related changes in time along one single scan line
- High temporal resolution
- Current use:
  - motion tracking and timing of events
  - measurements: *only if* the scan line is perpendicular to the measured structure

# Windows

## Parasternal (left parasternal) window

Patient in left lateral decubitus position. Transducer in the 3rd to 4th left intercostal space near the sternum (Fig. 2.1.1)

## Subcostal window

Patient in supine position flexing knees to relax abdominal muscles. Transducer in upper mid-epigastric position (Fig. 2.1.2)

## Apical window

Patient in left lateral decubitus position. Transducer usually in 5th intercostal space at median axillary line pointing towards the left to obtain four-chamber view (CV) (Fig. 2.1.3)

## Suprasternal window

Patient in supine position with chin pointing up. Transducer in suprasternal fossa (Fig. 2.1.4) pointing up for the **long-axis view** which is the most used

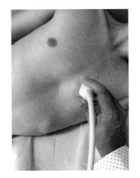

**Fig. 2.1.1** Patient in left lateral decubitus position

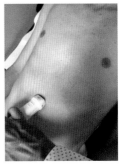

**Fig. 2.1.2** Patient in supine position

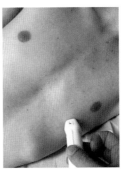

**Fig. 2.1.3** Patient in left lateral decubitus position

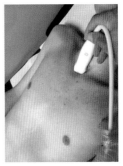

**Fig. 2.1.4** Patient in supine position with chin pointing up

## Right parasternal window

Patient in right lateral decubitus. Used mainly in aortic stenosis to assess the aortic transvalvular velocity with a CW Doppler-only transducer (Fig. 2.1.5A) or with a 2D transducer (Fig. 2.1.5B)

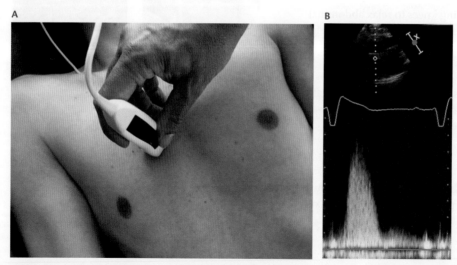

**Fig. 2.1.5** Right parasternal approach

# Views

## Parasternal long-axis view (PTLAX) (Fig. 2.1.6)—transducer points towards right shoulder

- If you see LV apex in PTLAX it usually means foreshortened left ventricle (LV)
- LV M-mode—derived from PTLAX to align cursor perpendicular to walls correctly (Fig. 2.1.7A)
- PTLAX M-mode tracing at the aortic valve (AV) plane (Fig. 2.1.7B), of the mitral valve (MV) (Fig. 2.1.7C)
- Apical M-mode tracing of the tricuspid annular plane systolic excursion (TAPSE) (Fig. 2.1.7D)

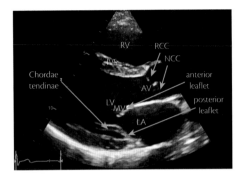

**Fig. 2.1.6** PTLAX
AV: aortic valve; LA: left atrium; NCC: non-coronary cusp; RCC: right coronary cusp

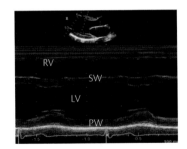

**Fig. 2.1.7A** M-mode tracing at AV
PW: posterior wall; RV: right ventricle, SW: septal wall

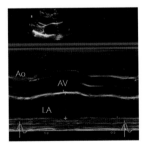

**Fig. 2.1.7B** M-mode tracing at AV
Ao: aorta

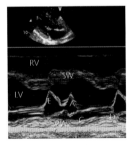

**Fig. 2.1.7C** M-mode tracing at MV
EACD: anterior leaflet motion

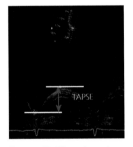

**Fig. 2.1.7D** M-mode tracing of TAPSE

## Parasternal short-axis view (PTSAX)

- **at mitral valve (MV) level** (Fig. 2.1.8A)—rotate transducer 90º clockwise from PTLAX, tilt towards LV apex
- **at papillary muscle (PM) level** (Fig. 2.1.8B)—further tilt towards LV apex from PTSAX at MV level
- **at LV apex level** (Fig. 2.1.8C)—further tilt towards LV apex from PTSAX at PM level
- **at great vessels (GV) level** (Fig. 2.1.8D)—rotate 90º clockwise from PTLAX, tilt away from LV apex
- **Right ventricular (RV) outflow view** (Fig. 2.1.9A)—from great vessels PTSAX tilt transducer superiorly
- **RV inflow view** (Fig. 2.1.9B)—from PTLAX tilt superiorly

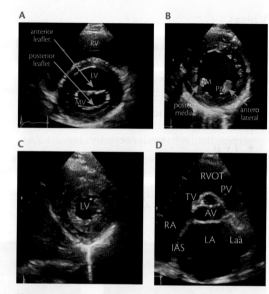

**Fig. 2.1.8** PTSAX
A: at MV level, B: at PM level, C: at apex level, D: at GV level

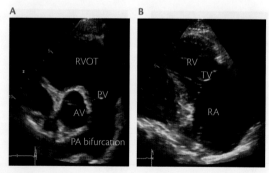

**Fig. 2.1.9** Right ventricular (RV) outflow view (A) and RV inflow view (B)

## Apical 4-chamber view (4CV)

- ◆ A standard apical window gives an upright image (Fig. 2.1.10, centre) compared with a too-medial window (Fig. 2.1.10, left) and a too-lateral window (Fig. 2.1.10, right)
- ◆ Use the lowest intercostal space showing 4CV to avoid LV foreshortening (rounded instead of bullet-shaped LV apex) (Fig. 2.1.11)
  - ◆ TV is more apical than MV
  - ◆ TV septal and anterior leaflets are seen
  - ◆ Posterior part of IVS is seen
  - ◆ Posterior tilt reveals the coronary sinus

## Apical 5-chamber view (5CV) (Fig. 2.1.12A)

- ◆ Tilt transducer anteriorly from 4CV to visualize AV for LVOT and AV flow assessment
- ◆ More anterior part of the IVS is seen
- ◆ LV cavity may be distorted

## Apical 2-chamber view (2CV) (Fig. 2.1.12B)

- ◆ Rotate transducer counter-clockwise 60°–90° from 4CV
- ◆ May display the MV bi-commissural view

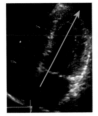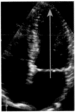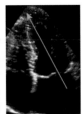

**Fig. 2.1.10** Standard apical window

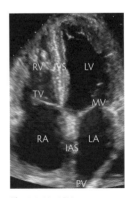

**Fig. 2.1.11** 4CV

### Apical 3-chamber view (3CV) (Fig. 2.1.12C)

◆ Rotate transducer counter-clockwise further 30°–60° from 2CV to obtain the 'apical long-axis view'
◆ Contrary to the PTLAX, the apical LAX visualizes the LV apex/apical antero-septum
◆ May provide better Doppler alignment than 5CV

### Apical RV 4-chamber view (RV 4CV) (Fig. 2.1.12D)

◆ Modify 4CV to see entire RV and to measure RV
◆ Derive TV annulus M-mode to measure TAPSE from RV 4CV lateral annulus zoom

### Subcostal 4-chamber view (4CV)

◆ Transducer pointing to the left (Fig. 2.1.13)
◆ Used mainly for shunt (ASD/VSD) diagnosis

### Subcostal short-axis view (SAX)

◆ Transducer rotated 90° from subcostal 4CV
◆ Mainly great arteries SAX used (Fig. 2.1.14) to measure RVOT diameter and velocity

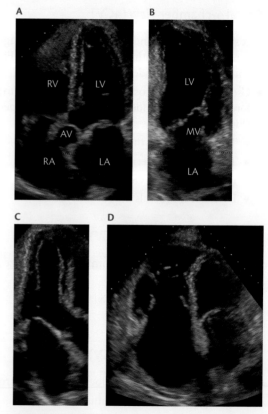

**Fig. 2.1.12** Apical views

## Inferior vena cava (IVC) view

♦ Transducer tilted to the right
♦ Used to measure IVC diameter in expiration (Fig. 2.1.15A) and inspiration (Fig. 2.1.15B)
♦ M-mode can be derived to assess IVC-diameter respiratory variation (Fig. 2.1.15C)

## Suprasternal long-axis view

♦ Used to visualize the aortic arch and descending aorta (Fig. 2.1.16)

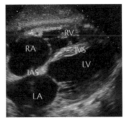

**Fig. 2.1.13** Subcostal 4-chamber view

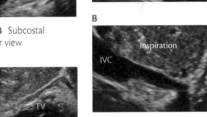

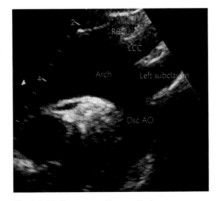

**Fig. 2.1.16** Suprasternal long-axis view

**Fig. 2.1.14** Subcostal short-axis view

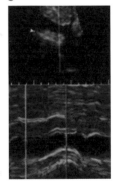

**Fig. 2.1.15** IVC view

## 2.2  Doppler echocardiography

### Doppler echocardiography

**Provides information regarding blood flow:**

- **direction** - towards the transducer
  - colour flow coded red (Fig. 2.2.1 LV inflow)
  - spectral display above baseline (Fig. 2.2.2 LV inflow)
  - away from the transducer
  - colour flow coded blue (Fig. 2.2.3 LV outflow)
  - spectral display below baseline (Fig. 2.2.4 LV outflow)
- **velocity** = spectral display distance from baseline
- **amplitude** = spectral display signal brightness

**Allows assessment of valves, haemodynamics, and coronary flow reserve through:**

- calculation of valve gradient (stenosis) and functional area (stenosis, regurgitation)
- calculation of SV (stroke volume), CO (cardiac output), dP/dt, intracardiac pressures, intracardiac shunt, and coronary flow reserve (CFR)
- colour Doppler lesion detection: convergence zone (stenosis, regurgitation) or regurgitant jet
- estimation of LV filling pressure/diastolic function

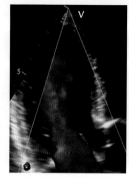

**Fig. 2.2.1**  LV inflow

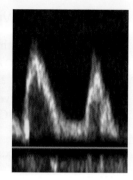

**Fig. 2.2.2**  LV inflow

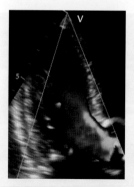

**Fig. 2.2.3**  LV outflow

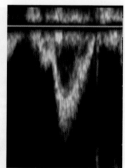

**Fig. 2.2.4**  LV outflow

# Modalities

## Continuous-wave Doppler (CW)

- can assess high-velocity flow (Figs 2.2.5 and 2.2.6)
- has no spatial resolution
→ use to measure high velocities

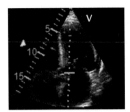

**Fig. 2.2.5** CW cursor

## Pulsed-wave Doppler (PW)

- cannot assess high velocity flow aliasing (misreads flow direction and velocity) (Fig. 2.2.7, PW in HOCM)
- high PRF (multiple sample volumes) can assess higher velocities (Fig. 2.2.8)
- has spatial resolution within the sample volume
→ use to detect flow origin/measure low velocities

## Colour-flow Doppler

- multiple PW sample volumes along multiple scan lines
- real-time 2D/M-mode superimposed colour-coded flow map
→ use to detect time flow (Fig. 2.2.9)/abnormal flow (Fig. 2.2.10)/align PW–CW with flow (see also Box 2.2.1)

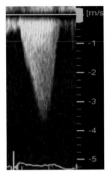

**Fig. 2.2.6** CW in hypertrophic obstructive cardiomyopathy (HOCM)

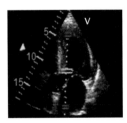

**Fig. 2.2.8** High PRF

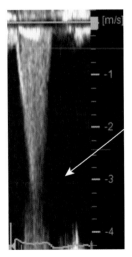

**Fig. 2.2.7** PW in HOCM

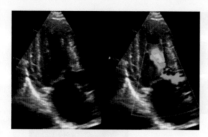

**Fig. 2.2.9** Colour turbulence: LVOT flow acceleration (HOCM)

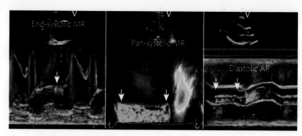

**Fig. 2.2.10** Colour-flow Doppler: Abnormal flow

---

**Box 2.2.1  Tips for measurements**

- maximize spectral displays to minimize error by reducing the scale (too low-scale results in aliasing or poor definition of peak velocity)

- shifting the baseline and increasing the sweep speed to 100 mm/s

- average over five cardiac cycles in atrial fibrillation excluding extreme cycle length

## PW/CW assessment of valves

### Assessment of valve stenosis

**Assessment of aortic (AS) and pulmonary (PS) valve stenosis**

- **Transvalvular velocity (m/s)/gradient (mmHg)**
  - Record the highest velocity (best aligned) (use multiple windows)
    - *AS: apical, suprasternal, right parasternal*

- ◆ *PS:* left parasternal, subcostal
- ◆ Use imaging transducer if the valve opening is well seen and the velocity is < 3 m/s
- ◆ Use dedicated **CW** transducer for better alignment and higher signal-to-noise ratio
- ◆ Use high wall filters/low gain/greyscale
- ◆ Trace the dense velocity curve—avoid noise/fine linear signals (Fig. 2.2.11)
- ◆ Measure the **peak velocity** and the machine will derive:
- → **peak gradient** ($4V^2$—simplified Bernoulli equation)
- → the simplified Bernoulli equation ignores the proximal velocity
  - → not valid if the proximal velocity is > 1.5 m/s or the valvular velocity is < 3 m/s
  - → use the Bernoulli equation: $4 (V_{transvalvular}^2 - V_{proximal}^2)$
  - → Bernoulli equation not valid for mean gradient → use peak gradient in these cases
- → pressure recovery
  - → higher gradients, mainly if small ascending aorta (no post-stenotic dilatation)
  - → significantly higher gradients if the ascending aorta is < 30 mm
- ◆ Trace velocity curve (Fig. 2.2.12) and the machine will derive:
  - → **TVI** (velocity time interval)
  - → **mean gradient** (instantaneous gradients average)—used in **AS**

### Effective (functional) valve area (cm²)

- ◆ Calculated based on continuity equation (smaller than the anatomic valve area)
- → SV through valve = SV before valve - for example:
  - → $SV_{AV} = SV_{LVOT} \rightarrow CSA_{AV} \times TTI_{AV} = CSA_{LVOT} \times TVI_{LVOT}$
  - → $AVA = [\Pi(D/2)^2 \times TVI_{LVOT}]/TVI_{AV}$ (the LVOT area is assumed to be circular)

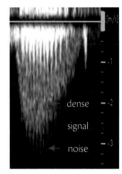

dense
signal
← noise

**Fig. 2.2.11** Dense velocity curve

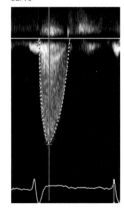

**Fig. 2.2.12** Trace velocity curve

- LVOT diameter (D) measurement error would be squared
  - → zoom to measure accurately (Fig. 2.2.13)
  - → measure on TOE if the TTE window is poor
- LVOT velocity (Fig. 2.2.14) assumed to be the same throughout the LVOT area
  - → not valid in case of subaortic flow acceleration or AR
  - → use dedicated **PW** transducer (sample volume above acceleration zone)
- Peak velocity can be used instead of TVI (simplified continuity equation)
  - → more variable results (assumes similar TVI:peak velocities ratio)

**Mitral (MS) and tricuspid (TS) stenosis assessment**

- **Transvalvular velocity (m/s)/gradient (mmHg)**
  - ◆ record the highest velocity (best aligned)
  - ◆ use apical window for MS/apical or parasternal window for TS
  - ◆ use colour flow to guide Doppler alignment (Fig. 2.2.15)
  - ◆ use **CW/PW** Doppler at or just after leaflet tips
  - ◆ PW may help clear trace in case of superimposed AR on CW (Fig. 2.2.16)
  - ◆ MS: E > A in sinus rhythm (Fig. 2.2.17)—no significant MS (pseudostenosis): E < A

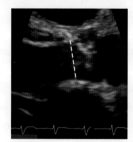

**Fig. 2.2.13** LVOT diameter measurement

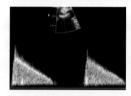

**Fig. 2.2.15** Guiding Doppler alignment

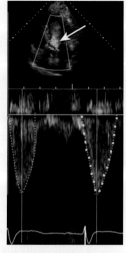

**Fig. 2.2.14** LVOT velocity

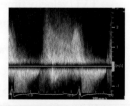

**Fig. 2.2.16** PW Doppler

- measure peak velocity (used in TS) and the machine will derive:

→ peak gradient ($4V^2$—simplified Bernoulli equation)—no use in MS

- Trace velocity curve (Fig. 2.2.18) and the machine will derive:

  → VTI (velocity time interval)

  → Mean gradient (instantaneous gradients average)—use in MS/TS

- Pressure half-time (PHT/T1/2)

  - Trace E-wave mid-diastolic deceleration slope (Fig. 2.2.19A)—machine will derive

  → PHT (ms)

  → Valve area ($cm^2$)—validated mainly for the mitral valve (MVA)

  MVA = 220/PHT (220 = empirically determined constant)

  *Not valid*: immediately post valvotomy
  in case of very low atrial compliance
  in coexistent aortic regurgitation
  in case of LV diastolic dysfunction (calcific MS in elderly)

## Continuity equation based valve-area calculation

- If no atrial fibrillation + no MR/AR for **MVA** and no TR/AR for **TVA**

- **MVA** (or **TVA**) = $[\Pi(D/2)^2 \times TVI]_{LVOT} : TVI_{MV}$ (or TV)

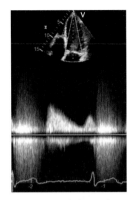

**Fig. 2.2.17** Mitral stenosis assessment

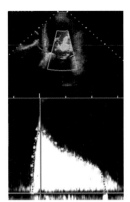

**Fig. 2.2.18** Trace velocity curve

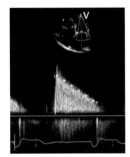

**Fig. 2.2.19A** Trace E-wave mid-diastolic deceleration slope

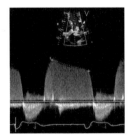

**Fig. 2.2.19B** Trace well aligned

## Assessment of valve regurgitation

### Any valvular regurgitation

- Not aligned Doppler/eccentric regurgitation → poor envelope definition → tracing error
- **Doppler volumetric method**
  - **R Vol** = **SV** regurgitant valve – **SV** normal valve (R Vol = regurgitant volume, SV = stroke volume)
  - **RF%** = (**R Vol/SV** regurgitant valve) × 100 (RF% = regurgitant fraction)

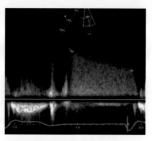

**Fig. 2.2.20** Trace well aligned

### Aortic (AR)/Pulmonary (PR) regurgitation assessment

- **Pressure half-time (PHT/T1/2)**
  - Trace well-aligned (5CV or 3CV) AR CW signal (Fig. 2.2.19B)—the machine derives **PHT** (ms)
  - Shorter (abrupt deceleration slope) in more severe AR
- **Deceleration time**
  - Trace well-aligned (parasternal or subcostal view) PR CW signal (Fig. 2.2.20)
  - Rapid deceleration is not specific but compatible with severe regurgitation
- **Diastolic flow reversal in descending aorta**
  - PW below left subclavian artery (in suprasternal view)
  - Measure end-diastolic velocity at R wave and trace TVI (Fig. 2.2.21)

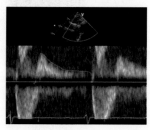

**Fig. 2.2.21** Diastolic flow reversal

### Mitral (MR) and tricuspid (TR) regurgitation assessment

- CW Doppler envelope

- Complete envelope (Fig. 2.2.22)/dense signal → more severe regurgitation
- Incomplete envelope (Fig. 2.2.23)/weak signal → less severe regurgitation (! misinterpretation in eccentric regurgitation/non-aligned Doppler)
- MR/TR velocity amplitude is not a measure of MR/TR severity
- Free-flow (massive) TR: narrow envelope with low velocity reminding AS envelope (Fig. 2.2.24)

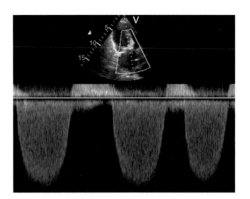

**Fig. 2.2.22** Mitral and tricuspid regurgitation assessment: complete envelope

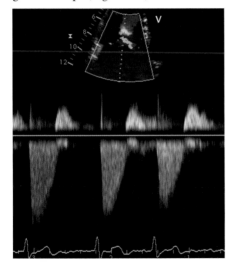

**Fig. 2.2.24** Free flow (massive) TR

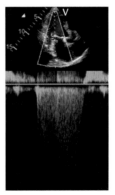

**Fig. 2.2.23** Mitral and tricuspid regurgitation assessment: incomplete envelope

# Colour-flow Doppler assessment of valves

## Assessment of valve stenosis

### Aortic/Pulmonary stenosis (AS/PS) assessment

- Detects stenosis based on flow acceleration/flow convergence
- Helps differentiate valvular/subvalvular/supravalvular stenosis (Fig. 2.2.25ABCD)

### Mitral (MS) and tricuspid (TS) stenosis assessment

- Detects stenosis based on flow acceleration/flow convergence (Figs 2.2.26–2.2.28AB)
- Allows MVA calculation with proximal isovelocity surface area (PISA) method:

    **MVA** = Π (r²) (Valiasing)/(**Peak V**mitral × α/180°)

    **r** = PISA radius, α = MV leaflets opening angle

    **MVA** = functional (effective) mitral valve area

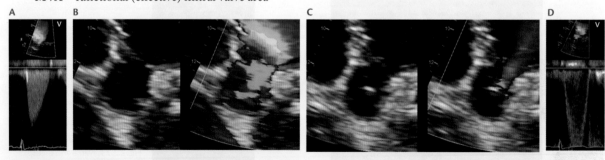

**Fig. 2.2.25** ABCD: CW records high-velocity suggesting aortic stenosis (A). Colour Doppler identifies the level of stenosis (B) as being subvalvular (flow convergence before the valve). The AR jet origin marks the position of the valve (C). PW detects flow-acceleration origin (D) but cannot measure velocity (too high)

- Can use colour M-mode for **r** measurement timing at **Peak Vmitral**

## Assessment of valve regurgitation

### Any valvular regurgitation

- Detects regurgitation
- Allows assessment of all three components of the regurgitant jet (flow convergence zone, vena contracta, jet turbulence)

### Aortic (AR) and pulmonary (PR) regurgitation assessment

- Inspection of the regurgitant jet
  - colour jet area and length (Fig. 2.2.29)
    - depends on LV/RV compliance (end-diastolic pressure) and driving pressure

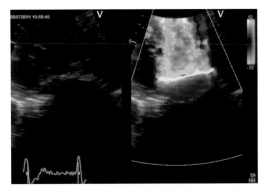

**Fig. 2.2.26** No suspicion from 2D image but convergence in colour flow suggests a degree of MS

A        B

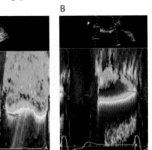

**Figs 2.2.28** PISA radius variation throughout diastole in MS colour M-mode. A: in sinus rhythm (early diastolic and post atrial contraction peak). B: in atrial fibrillation

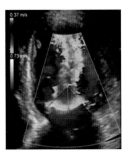

**Fig. 2.2.27** PISA radius and MV leaflets opening angle measured on colour-flow Doppler to calculate MVA

- ◆ weak correlation with regurgitation severity → not valid quantification method
- ◆ duration of regurgitation (early diastolic or throughout diastole)
- ◆ 2D or colour M-mode timing (Fig. 2.2.30)
- ◆ Jet width
  - ◆ jet width percent of outflow tract (Fig. 2.2.31)
  - ◆ mainly used in PR but also useful in AR
  - ◆ measure at the RVOT (LVOT) – PV (AV) junction
- ◆ Vena contracta
  - ◆ The smaller diameter of the regurgitant jet below the convergence zone
  - ◆ Validated for AR—parasternal window preferred because it uses axial resolution (Fig. 2.2.32)
  - ◆ Current image resolution allows accurate lateral measurements
    - ◆ AR vena contracta measurement in apical 5CV or 3CV (Fig. 2.2.33)
    - ◆ PR vena contracta measurement
  - ◆ Measure in zoom image to reduce error
  - ◆ Use colour scale 50–60 cm/s with no colour baseline shift

## PISA method of regurgitation quantification

- ◆ Can be used in AR/not validated in PR

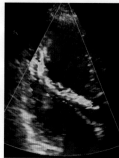
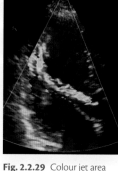

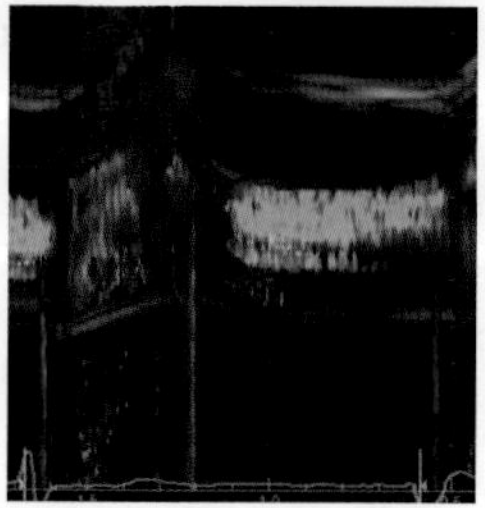

**Fig. 2.2.30** 2D or colour M-mode timing

**Fig. 2.2.29** Colour jet area and length

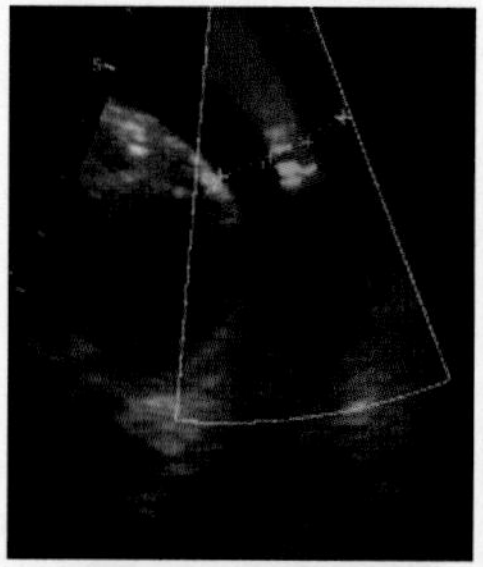

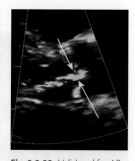

**Fig. 2.2.31** Jet width percent of outflow tract

**Fig. 2.2.32** Validated for AR

- Measure in zoom image to reduce error (Fig. 2.2.34)
- Preferably use:
  - apical window for central jet
  - parasternal window for eccentric jet
- Shift baseline in the direction of the jet to get well-defined PISA
- Measure radius (**r**) from regurgitant orifice to first aliasing velocity surface
- Calculate **EROA** (effective regurgitant orifice area) and **R Vol** (regurgitant volume)
  - **EROA** = flow rate/peak velocity ($cm^2$)
  - Flow rate = $2\Pi r^2 \times$ aliasing velocity
  - **R Vol** = EROA $\times$ TVI (ml)
- Not valid in:
  - aneurysmal dilatation of the aortic root (obtuse flow-convergence angle)
  - confined convergence zone (cusp perforation, commissural regurgitation)
- Diastolic flow reversal in the descending aorta
  - Colour Doppler visualization of flow reversal
  - Colour M-mode timing of flow reversal—throughout diastole in severe AR (Fig. 2.2.35)

### Mitral (MR) and tricuspid (TR) regurgitation assessment

- Inspection of the regurgitant jet
  - Colour jet area and jet reached depth within the atrium
    - can vary in between apical views (Fig. 2.2.36ABC)
    - depends on colour Doppler settings

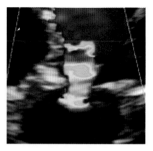

**Fig. 2.2.33** AR vena contracta measurement

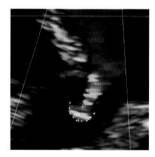

**Fig. 2.2.34** PISA method

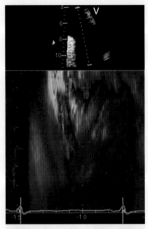

**Fig. 2.2.35** Colour M-mode timing of flow reversal

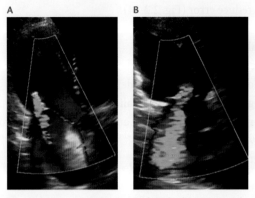
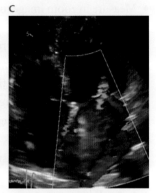

**Fig. 2.2.36** Eccentric MR jet in 3CV (A), 2CV (B), and 4CV (C)

- ◆ lower with higher atrial pressure and usually but not always in eccentric jets (Fig. 2.2.37)
- ◆ not recommended for regurgitation quantification
- ◆ Regurgitation timing/variation throughout systole
  - ◆ colour M-mode
  - ◆ examples of variation throughout systole:
    - → enhancement in late systole → prolapse (Fig. 2.2.38)
    - → enhancement in early systole → rheumatic (Fig. 2.2.39)

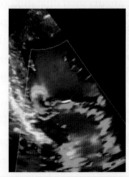

**Fig. 2.2.37** Inspection of the regurgitant jet

- ◆ Vena contracta
  - ◆ The smaller diameter of the regurgitant jet below the convergence zone
  - ◆ Measure in 4CV (MR/TR) or parasternal long-axis (MR)
  - ◆ Measure in zoom image to reduce error and use narrow colour sector (Fig. 2.2.40)
  - ◆ Average two orthogonal planes/two to three cardiac cycles
- ◆ PISA method of regurgitation quantification
  - ◆ Recommended in MR/some evidence in TR (Fig. 2.2.41)
  - ◆ Measure in zoom image to reduce error (Fig. 2.2.42)
  - ◆ Use 4CV (preferably) or view with better-defined PISA
  - ◆ Take off 'variance' and shift baseline below 40 cm/s for well defined PISA
  - ◆ Measure radius from regurgitant orifice to first aliasing velocity surface

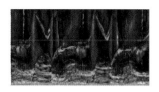

**Fig. 2.2.38** Regurgitation timing

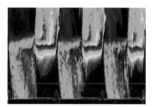

**Fig. 2.2.39** Regurgitation timing

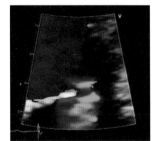

**Fig. 2.2.40** Vena contracta

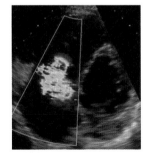

**Fig. 2.2.41** Large TR convergence zone and vena contracta but short truncated jet area

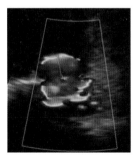

**Fig. 2.2.42** PISA method of regurgitation quantification

- ◆ Calculate **EROA** (flow rate/peak velocity) and **R Vol** (EROA × VTI)
- ◆ Assumptions:
  - ◆ Hemispheric PISA
    - → PISA method not valid with flow constraint PISA distortion (Fig. 2.2.43)
  - ◆ Constant PISA radius throughout systole
    - → PISA method overestimates end-systolic MR due to prolapse
- ◆ Systolic flow reversal in the hepatic veins
  - ◆ Colour Doppler visualization of flow reversal in hepatic veins zoom
  - ◆ Colour M-mode timing—systolic flow reversal suggests severe TR (Fig. 2.2.44)

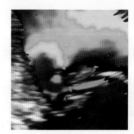

**Fig. 2.2.43** PISA method

## Non-invasive haemodynamic assessment

### Intracardiac flows

**LV outflow**

- ◆ Apical 5CV or 3CV
- ◆ PW sample volume just on LV side of AV—laminar flow (Fig. 2.2.45)
- ◆ Sample volume far from AV sub-estimates velocity (Fig. 2.2.46)

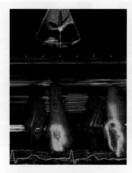

**Fig. 2.2.44** Colour M-mode timing

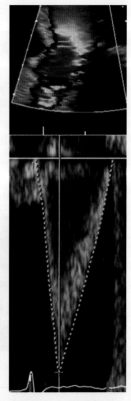

**Fig. 2.2.45** PW sample volume

- Use low wall-filter settings
- Trace the dense modal velocity to derive TVI
- Normal values (Table 2.2.1)

### RV outflow

- Parasternal short-axis view
- PW sample volume just on RV side of the pulmonary valve (laminar flow) (Fig. 2.2.47)
- Normal values (Table 2.2.2)

### LV inflow

- Apical 4CV
- E and A velocity varies: higher E towards LV apex/higher A towards LA

**Table 2.2.1** Normal LV outflow values

| Max velocity (m/s) | Ejection time (ms) | Acceleration time (ms) | Acceleration (m/s²) | TVI (cm) |
|---|---|---|---|---|
| 0.88 (0.47–1.29) | 286 (240–332) | 84 (48–10) | 11 (5–17) | 20–25 |

**Table 2.2.2** Normal RV outflow values

| Max velocity (m/s) | Ejection time (ms) | Acceleration time (ms) | Acceleration (m/s²) | TVI (cm) |
|---|---|---|---|---|
| 0.72 (0.36–1.08) | 281 (212–350) | 118 (70–166) | 6.1 (3–9) | – |

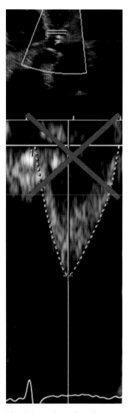

**Fig. 2.2.46** Sample volume

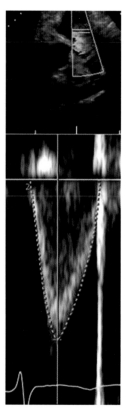

**Fig. 2.2.47** PW sample volume

- PW sample volume at MV leaflet tips (Fig. 2.2.48A) for flow profile (E, A, E/A)
- PW sample volume at MV ring level (Fig. 2.2.48B) for flow quantification and A duration
- CW (Fig. 2.2.48C) for flow quantification (TVI) and gradient
- Normal values (Table 2.2.3)

**Pulmonary venous flow**

- Apical 4CV
- PW 2–3 mm sample volume 0.5 cm within right upper pulmonary vein (RUPV)
- Flow profile: systolic **S**, diastolic **D**, atrial reversal **AR** waves (Fig. 2.2.49A)
- S/D ratio increases with age (see Fig. 2.2.49B—flow profile in elderly patient)

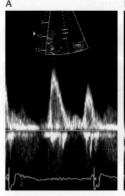
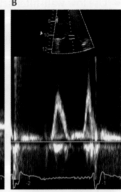
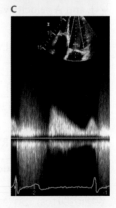

**Figs 2.2.48** PW sample volume at MV leaflet tips (A). PW sample volume at MV ring level (B). CW for flow quantification and gradient (C)

**Table 2.2.3** Normal LV inflow values

| Measurement | Age group (y) | | | |
|---|---|---|---|---|
| | 16–20 | 21–40 | 41–60 | > 60 |
| IVRT (ms) | 50 ± 9 (32–68) | 67 ± 8 (51–83) | 74 ± 7 (60–88) | 87 ± 7 (73–101) |
| E/A ratio | 1.88 ± 0.45 (0.98–2.78) | 1.53 ± 0.40 (0.73–2.33) | 1.28 ± 0.25 (0.78–1.78) | 0.96 ± 0.18 (0.6–1.32) |
| EDT (ms) | 142 ± 19 (104–180) | 166 ± 14 (138–194) | 181 ± 19 (143–219) | 200 ± 29 (142–258) |
| A duration (ms) | 113 ± 17 (79–147) | 127 ± 13 (101–153) | 133 ± 13 (107–159) | 138 ± 19 (100–176) |

**Table 2.2.4** Normal PV flow values

| Measurement | Age group (y) | | | |
|---|---|---|---|---|
| | **16–20** | **21–40** | **41–60** | **>60** |
| PV S/D ratio | 0.82 ± 0.18 (0.46–1.18) | 0.98 ± 0.32 (0.34–1.62) | 1.21 ± 0.2 (0.81–1.61) | 1.39 ± 0.47 (0.45–2.33) |
| PV Ar (cm/s) | 16 ± 10 (1–36) | 21 ± 8 (5–2.37) | 23 ± 3 (17–29) | 25 ± 9 (11–39) |
| PV Ar duration (ms) | 66 ± 39 (1–144) | 96 ± 33 (30–162) | 112 ± 15 (82–142) | 113 ± 30 (53–173) |

- S-wave blunted in significant MR (Fig. 2.2.49CD) and negative in severe MR
- Normal values (Table 2.2.4)

### Descending aorta flow

- Suprasternal view (Fig. 2.2.50A)
- PW sample volume below the origin of the left subclavian artery (Fig. 2.2.50B)
- CW in aortic coarctation (high flow velocity)
- Normal values (Table 2.2.5)

**Table 2.2.5** Normal descending aorta flow values

| Max velocity (m/s) | Ejection time (ms) | Acceleration time (ms) | Acceleration (m/s²) |
|---|---|---|---|
| 1.07 | 261 | 91 | 12 |
| (0.59–1.75) | (202–302) | (70–122) | (5–19) |

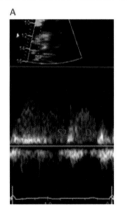
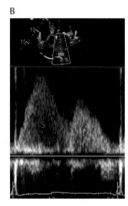

**Figs 2.2.49AB** (A) Flow profile. Flow profile in elderly patient (B)

## Hepatic veins flow

- ◆ Subcostal view
- ◆ Flow profile (Fig. 2.2.51)
    - ◆ forward systolic **S** and diastolic **D** waves
    - ◆ +/– reverse ventricular **v** and atrial **a** waves
- ◆ In severe TR there is systolic flow reversal (Fig. 2.2.52)
- ◆ Respirometer: flow timing in restriction/constriction/tamponade

## Superior vena cava (SVC) flow

- ◆ Suprasternal and right supraclavicular view (Fig. 2.2.53)
- ◆ Flow profile (Fig. 2.2.54)
    - ◆ forward systolic **S** and diastolic **D** waves

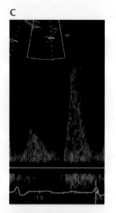
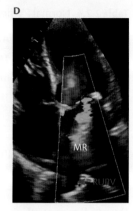

**Figs 2.2.49CD** S wave blunted in significant MR (C)

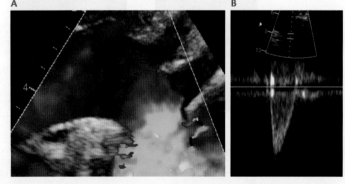

**Figs 2.2.50** (A) Descending aorta flow—suprasternal view. (B) PW sample volume below the origin of the left subclavian artery

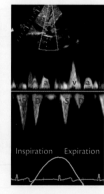

**Fig. 2.2.51** Hepatic veins flow

- ◆ +/– reverse ventricular **v** and atrial **a** waves
- ◆ Normal **S/D ≥ 1 ≤ 2**

## Flow-related calculations

- ◆ **Stroke volume (SV)**
  - ◆ Cross-sectional area (CSA) × time velocity integral (TVI) $[\Pi \times (D/2)^2] \times$ **TVI** (D = the diameter of the respective area which is assumed circular)

- ◆ **Cardiac output (CO)**
  - ◆ SV × heart rate

- ◆ **Shunt calculation**
  - ◆ Pulmonary (Qp) to systemic (Qs) flow ratio (**Qp:Qs**)
  - ◆ $Qs = SVLV = [\Pi \times (DLVOT/2)^2] \times TVI_{LVOT}$

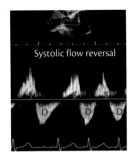

**Fig. 2.2.52** Hepatic veins flow

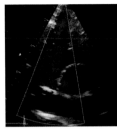

**Fig. 2.2.53** Superior vena cava flow

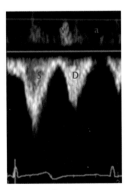

**Fig. 2.2.54** Superior vena cava flow

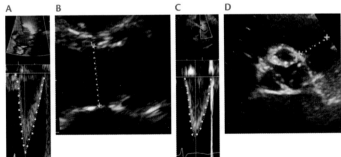

**Fig. 2.2.55** Shunt calculation. Trace LVOT velocity to measure TVI (A). Measure DLVOT in systole on zoom image (B). Trace RVOT velocity to measure TVI (C). Measure DRVOT in systole on zoom image (D)

- ◆ trace LVOT velocity to measure TVI (Fig. 2.2.55A)
- ◆ measure DLVOT in systole on zoom image (Fig. 2.2.55B)
- ◆ Qp = SVRV = [Π × (DRVOT/2)²] x TVI$_{RVOT}$
  - ◆ trace RVOT velocity to measure TVI (Fig. 2.2.55C)
  - ◆ measure DRVOT in systole on zoom image (Fig. 2.2.55D)

**Intracardiac pressures**

- ◆ **Right atrial pressure (RAP)**
  - ◆ Estimated from the IVC diameter and its respiratory variation (Table 2.2.6)
  - ◆ Measure IVC diameter in expiration and inspiration on 2D or M-mode
  - ◆ The respirometer may help estimate the respiratory IVC diameter variation (Fig. 2.2.56)
- ◆ **RV systolic pressure (RVSP)/PA systolic pressure (PASP)**
  - ◆ In the absence of pulmonary stenosis RVSP = PASP

**Table 2.2.6** IVC diameter and RAP estimation

| IVC diameter (cm) | Reduction with inspiration | RAP (mmHg) |
|---|---|---|
| < 1.5 | Collapse | 0–5 |
| 1.5–2.5 | > 50% | 5–10 |
| 1.5–2.5 | < 50% | 10–15 |
| > 2.5 | < 50% | 15–20 |
| > 2.5 | no change | > 20 |

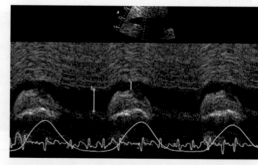

**Fig. 2.2.56** Right atrial pressure

- The RVSP (PASP) is calculated using the TR velocity (Fig. 2.2.57)
  - $4 (VTR)^2 + RAP$ (VTR = TR maximal velocity)
- The calculation is not valid if there is:
  - severe (free) TR
  - tricuspid stenosis or tricuspid prosthetic valve
  - RV systolic dysfunction (e.g. RV infarct)
- If there is no TR it does not mean that there is no pulmonary hypertension
- In the presence of a VSD: $RVSP = SBP - 4(VVSD)^2$
  - $SBP$ = systolic blood pressure $VVSD$ = VSD LV→RV flow velocity

## Pulmonary artery diastolic pressure (PADP)

- Is calculated using the PR velocity (Fig. 2.2.58)
- $4 (VendPR)^2 + RAP$ (VendPR = PR end-diastolic velocity)

## Pulmonary artery mean pressure (PAMP)

- Is calculated using the PR velocity (Fig. 2.2.58)
- $4 (VearlyPR)^2 + RAP$ (VearlyPR = PR early-diastolic velocity)

## LV diastolic pressure (LVDP)

- Can be calculated using the aortic regurgitation (AR) velocity (Fig. 2.2.59)

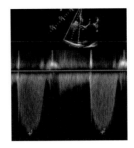
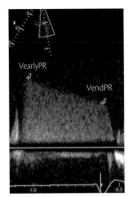

**Fig. 2.2.57** RV systolic pressure/PA systolic pressure

**Fig. 2.2.58** Pulmonary artery diastolic pressure

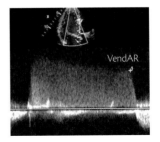

**Fig. 2.2.59** LV diastolic pressure

- **DBP – 4(VendAR)$^2$** (DBP = diastolic blood pressure/VendAR = AR end-diastolic velocity)
- Can be estimated from the LV inflow pattern

**Estimation of myocardial contractility based on dP/dt**

- From CW Doppler envelope of mitral regurgitation (MR)
- Measure time from 1 m/s to 3 m/s MR velocity (Fig. 2.2.60) (time from 4 mmHg to 36 mmHg–32 mmHg pressure difference)
- **dP/dt (mmHg/s) = 32 mmHg/time (s)**
- Normal values > 1200 mmHg/s
- Load-independent parameter
- dP/dt is not a measure of MR severity

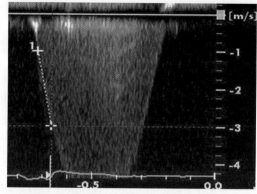

**Fig. 2.2.60** Estimation of myocardial contractility

## Coronary flow—assessment of coronary flow reserve (CFR)

**Coronary flow more likely accessible:**

- **Left anterior descending artery (LAD) flow** (95% feasibility)
  - use high-frequency imaging and low-aliasing velocity colour Doppler to detect flow
  - modified apical 3CV: distal-mid LAD aligned with antero-septum (Fig. 2.2.61AB)

- ◆ modified (medial) 4CV: distal LAD between LV and RV apex (Fig. 2.2.61CD)
- ◆ **Posterior descending artery (PDA) flow** (60% feasibility)
  - ◆ modified apical 3CV/2CV: PDA aligned with infero-posterior wall (Fig. 2.2.62AB)
  - ◆ coronary flow profile:
    - ◆ flow mainly diastolic
    - ◆ lower systolic and higher diastolic velocity (Fig. 2.2.63)
    - ◆ only diastolic velocity (Fig. 2.2.64)
- ◆ reversed flow in septal branches (Fig. 2.2.65ABC) or collateral flow in blocked vessel

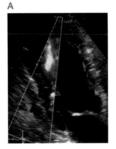
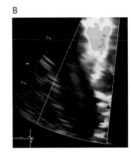

**Fig. 2.2.62** Posterior descending artery

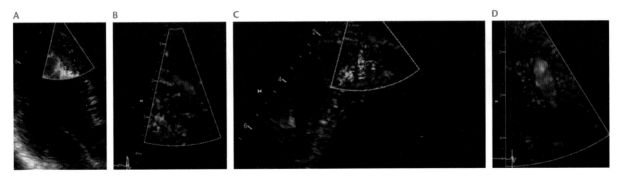

**Fig. 2.2.61** Left anterior descending artery flow

- ◆ coronary flow reserve (CFR)
  - ◆ coronary vasodilatation obtained infusing:
    - ◆ adenosine (149 mcg/kg/min)
    - ◆ dipyridamole (0.84 mg/kg/min)
  - ◆ CFR = vasodilatation to baseline peak diastolic velocity ratio
  - ◆ abnormal CFR ≤ 2

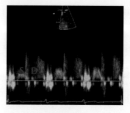

**Fig. 2.2.63** Posterior descending artery

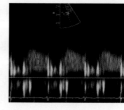

**Fig. 2.2.64** Posterior descending artery

A

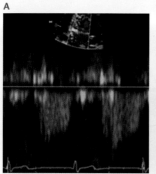

B

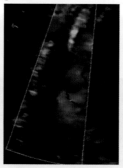

C

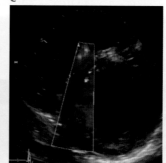

**Fig. 2.2.65** Posterior descending artery

# 2.3 Functional echocardiography

## General considerations

**Functional imaging by modern echocardiography offers a variety of methods to assess regional and global myocardial function beyond classic dimension, volume, and ejection fraction measurements**

Information on myocardial function is extracted from echo images using either a tissue Doppler or a speckle-tracking approach. Both approaches are valid and useful but differ in their strengths and weaknesses, the optimal machine settings for image acquisition, the way of post-processing, and the obtained parameters

Four basic parameters are extracted:

- Velocity
- Motion (displacement)
- Strain rate (rate of deformation) (Table 2.3.3)
- Strain (deformation) (see Tables 2.3.4, 2.3.5, 2.3.6)

All echocardiographic function parameters are load-dependent. When interpreting functional imaging parameters, factors influencing regional myocardial fibre load, such as chamber geometry, wall curvature, and thickness or cavity pressure, must be considered

# Basic parameters

- Velocity
  - Gradient base–apex (Fig. 2.3.1)
  - Tethering effect (artefact) (Fig. 2.3.2)
- Motion (displacement)
- Strain rate (rate of deformation)
- Strain (deformation) (Fig. 2.3.3)

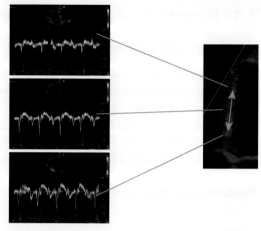

**Fig. 2.3.1** Velocity

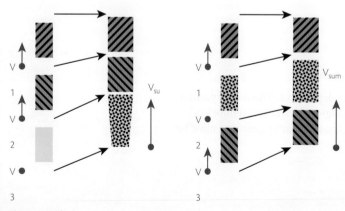

**Fig. 2.3.2** Velocity

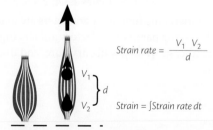

$$Strain\ rate = \frac{V_1 - V_2}{d}$$

$$Strain = \int Strain\ rate\ dt$$

**Fig. 2.3.3** Strain (deformation)

# Tissue Doppler—principles (Figs. 2.3.4AB and 2.3.5AB)

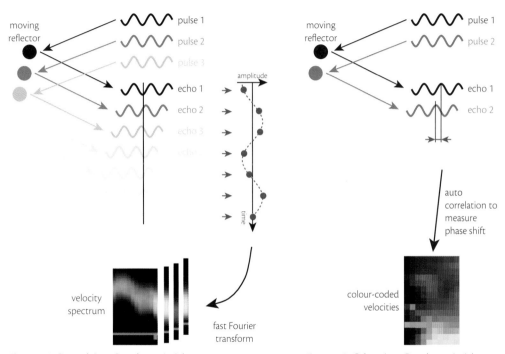

**Fig. 2.3.4A** Spectral tissue Doppler—principle

**Fig. 2.3.4B** Colour tissue Doppler—principle

Both pulsed-wave spectral tissue Doppler and colour tissue Doppler evaluate the phase shift between several ultrasound pulses. The result is either displayed as velocity spectrum or colour coded in the image

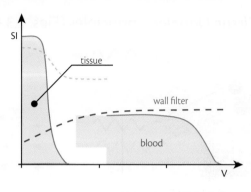

**Fig. 2.3.5A** Wall filter

Velocity signals from the tissue and the blood pool can be distinguished using a so-called wall filter. Blood has low signal intensity and moves fast, while tissue has a high signal intensity and moves at an order of magnitude slower

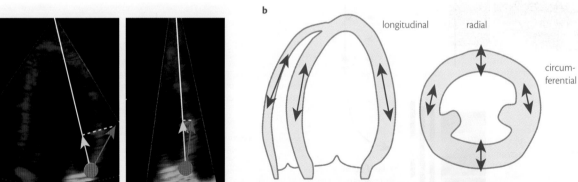

**Fig. 2.3.5B** Motion direction

Tissue Doppler measures velocities along the ultrasound beam which must therefore be carefully aligned with the wall (a). Only certain motion directions can be measured, depending on the window used (b). See also Table 2.3.2

# Tissue Doppler

## Data acquisition (Fig. 2.3.6AB)

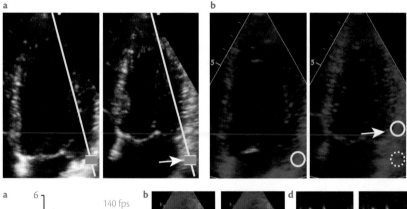

**Fig. 2.3.6A** Sample volume position
In contrast to spectral Doppler, where sample volumes are set during acquisition (a), colour Doppler post-processing allows the retrospective choice of sample volume position and even its tracking (b)

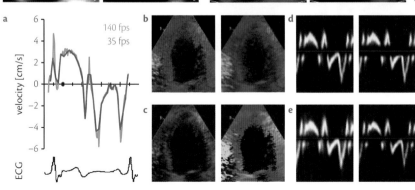

**Fig. 2.3.6B** Acquisition settings
High acquisition frame rate is important for high temporal resolution of the colour Doppler data. Note the blunting of the peaks (a). Other settings are comparable to blood Doppler: tissue priority (b), transparency (c), low velocity reject, (d) and threshold (e)

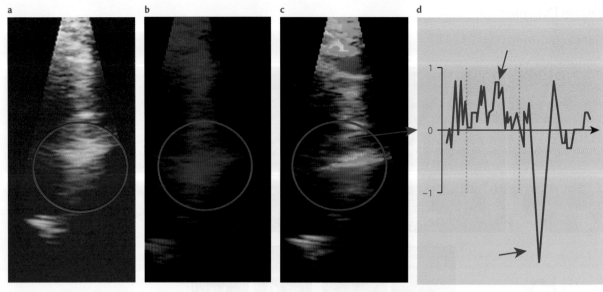

**Fig. 2.3.7A**  Reverberation artefacts

Reverberation artefacts appear as horizontal, bright stationary echoes (a) and disturb both tissue Doppler and speckle tracking analysis. They are hardly visible in a tissue Doppler display (b), but during strain rate post-processing, they result in a zone of inverted signals (c,d) which can be best recognized in (c)

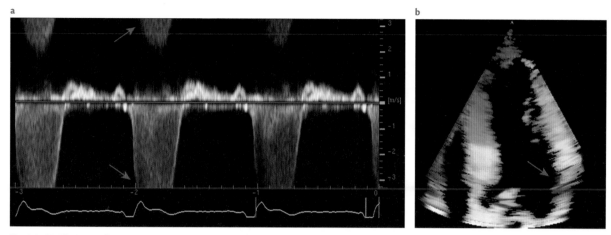

**Fig. 2.3.7B** Aliasing artefacts

Aliasing occurs when the velocity range is set too low. In spectral Doppler, the spectrum appears cut while the peak appears on the other side of the scale (a). In colour tissue Doppler, data quality during strain/strain rate post-processing will be affected. Acquisitions should be carefully reviewed for sharp yellow–blue colour changes (b) by slowly scrolling though the loop

## Post-processing (Figs. 2.3.8ABCD and 2.3.9AB)

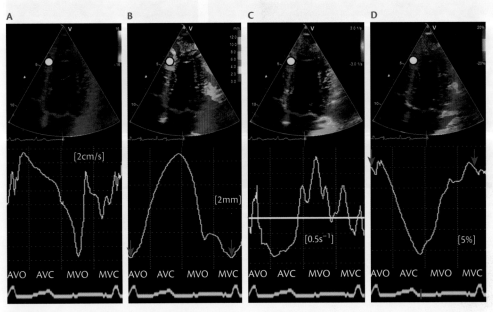

**Fig. 2.3.8** Basic parameters of function imaging

The figures show velocity (A), motion (B), strain rate (C), and strain (D) images with typical septal curves (yellow dot). Since cardiac function is cyclic, the definition of baseline in motion and strain curves is arbitrary. In most applications, zero is defined at end-diastole, usually derived from the ECG trigger signal (red arrows)

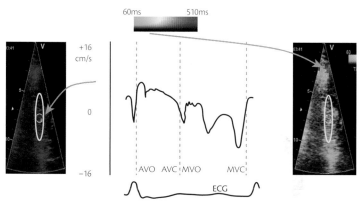

**Fig. 2.3.9A** Tissue synchronicity imaging
Velocity data can also be colour coded for timing of events.
While regular colour tissue Doppler codes the velocity, tissue
synchronicity imaging codes the timing of the occurrence
of the systolic velocity peak. This type of display is intended
to visualize regional dyssynchrony. However, peak velocities
do not necessarily describe the timing of regional shortening
correctly

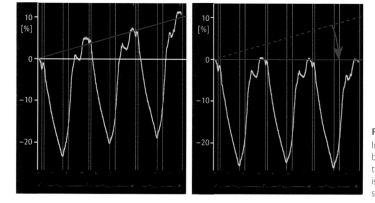

**Fig. 2.3.9B** Baseline drift compensation
In both tissue Doppler and speckle tracking, a drift of the
baseline may be observed in motion and strain data for different
technical reasons. To compensate for this, a linear correction
is commonly applied (red arrow). With this, each cardiac cycle
starts at the defined baseline

# Speckle tracking

## Principles (Fig. 2.3.10AB)

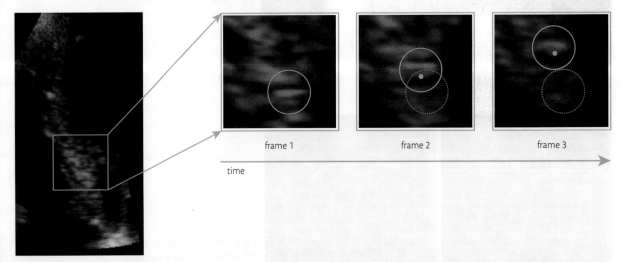

frame 1          frame 2          frame 3

time

**Fig. 2.3.10A**  Tracking features in the image
In speckle tracking, complex image analysis software identifies features of the image (i.e. bright speckles, as indicated by the green dot) and follows them over time from frame to frame. Analysing the displacement of several speckles over time allows to calculate motion, velocity, strain, and strain rate

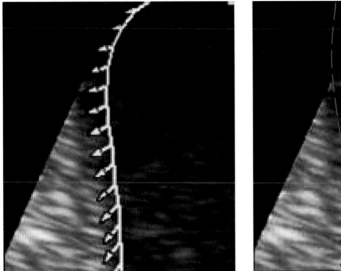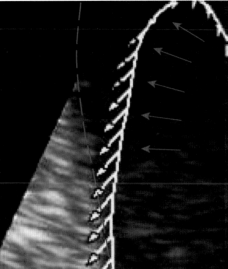

**Fig. 2.3.10B** Careful visual verification of the tracking result
Speckle tracking relies on following a certain image feature from frame to frame. This principle depends strongly on good image quality and may fail. A careful visual verification of the tracking result is always mandatory. Segments, in which tracking lines (points do not follow the myocardium (red arrows)) must be excluded from further analysis

# Post-processing (Fig. 2.3.11AB)

a

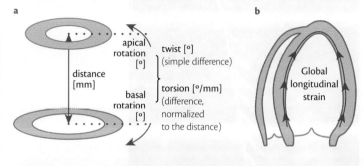

apical
rotation
[°]

twist [°]
(simple difference)

distance
[mm]

basal
rotation
[°]

torsion [°/mm]
(difference,
normalized
to the distance)

b

Global
longitudinal
strain

**Fig. 2.3.11A**  Twist, torsion, and global longitudinal strain
(a) Speckle tracking allows to calculate twist and torsion.
(b) Global longitudinal strain is defined as the deformation of
the myocardium parallel with the endocardium. Measuring may
be done mid-wall or subendocardially.

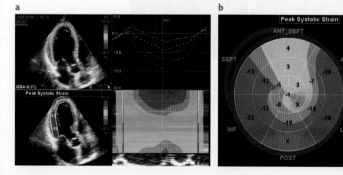

**Fig. 2.3.11B**  Display options
Speckle tracking offers a lot of post-processing options. Similar
to tissue Doppler, colour coding, curve displays, and curved
M-modes are available (a). In addition, colour-coded bull's
eye displays offer a good overview over regional ventricular
function (b).

# Data analysis and measurements (Figs. 2.3.12AB and 2.3.13AB)

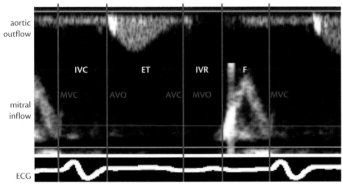

**Fig. 2.3.12A** Timing of cardiac events
A correct data analysis requires certainty about timing. In particular, aortic valve closure (AVC) as marker of end-systole is relevant for many measurements. In regular heart rhythm, blood Doppler traces of the aortic and mitral valve may be used as reliable indicators.

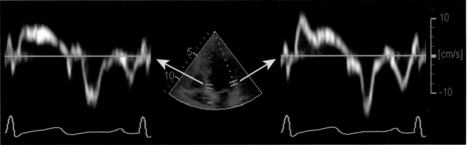

**Fig. 2.3.12B** Regional differences
Function data may differ by region. Septal data usually have lower values and a round shape in systole (Table 2.3.1). Lateral data show higher peaks and have a double peak in systole. Valve timing should be used to differentiate peaks from different time intervals.

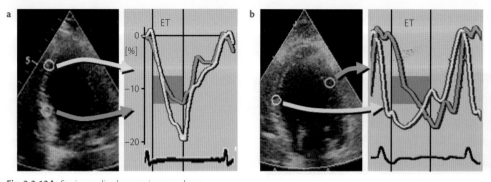

**Fig. 2.3.13A** Strain amplitude vs strain curve shape

In principle, deformation data may differ in amplitude (a) or in shape (b). The latter is a strong indicator of regional function inhomogeneity as it occurs in scar tissue, ischaemic regions or in a dyssynchronous LV.

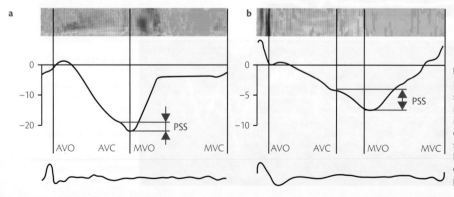

**Fig. 2.3.13B** Post-systolic shortening
Post systolic shortening (PSS) is a sensitive indicator of regional function inhomogeneity. It appears in scar and indicates ischaemia during a stress echo. Minor PSS with normal systolic shortening may be physiologic (a). Reduced systolic function and PSS of > 25% of the curve amplitude is pathologic (b).

# Reference Values

**Table 2.3.1** Longitudinal tissue Doppler velocities (cm/s)

| Wall | Level | Systole | e'-wave | a'-wave |
|------|-------|---------|---------|---------|
| LV septal | apical | 3.2 ± 0.9 | 4.3 ± 1.9 | 2.7 ± 1.1 |
| | medial | 5.4 ± 0.9 | 9.9 ± 2.9 | 6.2 ± 1.5 |
| | basal | 7.8 ± 1.1 | 11.2 ± 1.9 | 7.8 ± 2.0 |
| LV lateral | apical | 6.0 ± 2.3 | 5.5 ± 2.7 | 3.0 ± 2.4 |
| | medial | 9.8 ± 2.3 | 12.0 ± 3.3 | 5.7 ± 2.4 |
| | basal | 10.2 ± 2.1 | 14.9 ± 3.5 | 6.6 ± 2.4 |
| LV inferior | apical | 4.0 ± 1.7 | 5.2 ± 2.4 | 2.9 ± 1.8 |
| | medial | 6.6 ± 0.7 | 9.1 ± 2.7 | 6.4 ± 1.8 |
| | basal | 8.7 ± 1.3 | 12.4 ± 3.8 | 7.9 ± 2.5 |
| LV anterior | apical | 4.0 ± 1.5 | 3.9 ± 1.1 | 2.0 ± 1.5 |
| | medial | 7.7 ± 2.2 | 10.4 ± 3.0 | 5.5 ± 1.7 |
| | basal | 9.0 ± 1.6 | 12.8 ± 3.0 | 6.5 ± 1.6 |
| RV free wall | apical | 7.0 ± 1.9 | 8.1 ± 3.4 | 5.6 ± 2.4 |
| | medial | 9.6 ± 2.1 | 10.6 ± 2.6 | 9.7 ± 3.3 |
| | basal | 12.2 ± 2.6 | 12.9 ± 3.5 | 11.6 ± 4.1 |

**Table 2.3.2** Radial and circumferential velocities (cm/s)

| | Radial | | | | Circumferential | |
|--------|-------------|-------------|-------------|-------------|-------------|-------------|
| | anteroseptal | anterior | posterior | inferior | septal | lateral |
| Medial | 1.94 ± 2.15 | 2.66 ± 1.89 | 4.78 ± 1.53 | 4.93 ± 1.45 | 3.31 ± 1.99 | 1.94 ± 2.15 |
| Basal | 1.92 ± 2.32 | 2.64 ± 1.85 | 4.65 ± 1.51 | 4.85 ± 1.37 | 3.25 ± 2.02 | 4.16 ± 1.24 |

**Table 2.3.3**  Regional strain rate (1/s)

| LV wall | Level | Systole | e'-wave | a'-wave |
|---------|-------|---------|---------|---------|
| lateral | apical | −1.93 ± 0.70 | 2.23 ± 1.09 | 0.61 ± 0.14 |
| | medial | −1.25 ± 0.40 | 2.45 ± 0.29 | 1.30 ± 1.17 |
| | basal | −1.23 ± 0.30 | 2.16 ± 0.95 | 1.12 ± 0.57 |
| septal | apical | −0.98 ± 0.31 | 2.12 ± 0.52 | 0.70 ± 0.26 |
| | medial | −1.33 ± 0.19 | 2.01 ± 0.33 | 1.22 ± 0.63 |
| | basal | −1.15 ± 0.18 | 2.02 ± 0.30 | 1.27 ± 0.44 |
| anteroseptal | apical | −1.04 ± 0.45 | 1.86 ± 0.71 | 0.91 ± 0.17 |
| | medial | −1.43 ± 0.27 | 2.11 ± 0.80 | 1.28 ± 0.46 |
| | basal | −1.22 ± 0.22 | 1.54 ± 0.38 | 1.11 ± 0.59 |
| posterior | apical | −1.32 ± 0.40 | 2.04 ± 0.94 | 0.97 ± 0.86 |
| | medial | −1.13 ± 0.51 | 1.86 ± 0.65 | 1.05 ± 0.70 |
| | basal | −1.54 ± 0.39 | 2.67 ± 0.74 | 0.78 ± 0.47 |
| anterior | apical | −1.32 ± 0.89 | 1.42 ± 0.74 | 0.91 ± 0.52 |
| | medial | −1.17 ± 0.42 | 1.95 ± 0.49 | 0.99 ± 0.67 |
| | basal | −1.51 ± 0.33 | 1.97 ± 0.53 | 1.60 ± 0.58 |
| inferior | apical | −1.34 ± 0.26 | 1.55 ± 0.85 | 0.97 ± 0.77 |
| | medial | −1-32 ± 0.60 | 1.66 ± 0.31 | 1.31 ± 0.77 |
| | basal | −1.14 ± 0.15 | 1.90 ± 0.46 | 1.00 ± 0.45 |

**Table 2.3.4** Regional strain

| Study | Method | n | Age (y) | Mean strain (%) | Septal (%) | Lateral (%) | Inferior (%) | Anterior (%) |
|---|---|---|---|---|---|---|---|---|
| Edvardsen et al. | DTI | 33 | 41 + 13 | 19 + 4 | | | | |
| Basal | | | | | 17 + 3 | 18 + 4 | 20 + 4 | 19 + 4 |
| Apical | | | | | 19 + 4 | 17 + 3 | 21 + 2 | 18 + 5 |
| Kowalski et al. | DTI | 40 | 29 + 5 | 17 + 5 | | | | |
| Basal | | | | | 21 + 5 | 13 + 4 | 15 + 5 | 17 + 6 |
| Midventricular | | | | | 21 + 5 | 14 + 4 | 16 + 5 | 17 + 6 |
| Apical | | | | | 23 + 4 | 15 + 5 | 18 + 5 | 18 + 6 |
| Sun et al. | DTI | 100 | 43 + 15 | 18 + 5 | | | | |
| Basal | | | | | 18 + 5 | 18 + 7 | 15 + 6 | 22 + 8 |
| Midventricular | | | | | 18 + 1 | 19 + 5 | 14 + 5 | 18 + 6 |
| Apical | | | | | 19 + 6 | 18 + 6 | 24 + 5 | 13 + 6 |
| Marwick et al. | 2D STE | 242 | 51 + 12 | 19 + 5 | | | | |
| Basal | | | | | 14 + 4 | 18 + 5 | 17 + 4 | 20 + 4 |
| Midventricular | | | | | 19 + 3 | 18 + 3 | 20 + 4 | 19 + 3 |
| Apical | | | | | 22 + 5 | 19 + 5 | 23 + 5 | 19 + 5 |

**Table 2.3.5**  Global strain

| Parameter | Mean | Range | 95% CI |
| --- | --- | --- | --- |
| GLS | −19.7% | (−15.9%, −22.1%) | (−18.9%, −20.4%) |
| GCS | −23.3% | (−20.9%, −27.8%) | (−24.6%, −22.1%) |
| GRS | +47.3% | (+35.1%, +59.0%) | (+43.6%, +51.0%) |

**Table 2.3.6**  Normal LV strain values according to vendors' specific equipment and software

| Vendor | Software | n | Mean | SD | LLN |
| --- | --- | --- | --- | --- | --- |
| Varying | Meta-analysis | 2597 | −19.7% | − | n/a |
| GE | EchoPac BT 12 | 247 | −21.5% | 2.0% | −18% |
| | EchoPac BT 12 | 207 | −21.2% | 1.6% | −18% |
| | EchoPac BT 12 | 131 | −21.2% | 2.4% | −17% |
| | EchoPac 110.1.3 | 133 | −21.3% | 2.1% | −17% |
| Philips | Qlab 7.1 | 330 | −18.9% | 2.5% | −14% |
| Toshiba | UltraExtend | 337 | −19.9% | 2.4% | −15% |
| Siemens | VVI | 116 | −19.8% | 4.6% | −11% |
| | VVI | 82 | −17.3% | 2.3% | −13% |
| Esaote | Mylab 50 | 30 | −19.5% | 3.1% | −13% |

# Suggested reading

1. Mor-Avi V, Lang RM, Badano LP, et al. Current and evolving echocardiographic techniques for the quantitative evaluation of cardiac mechanics: ASE/EAE consensus statement on methodology and indications endorsed by the Japanese Society of Echocardiography. *Eur J Echocardiogr* 2011;12:167–205.
2. Garcia-Fernandez MA, Azavedo J, Moreno M. Relation between transversal and longitudinal planes in the calculation of left ventricular myocardial isovolumic relaxation time using pulsed Doppler tissue imaging. *J Am Soc Echo* 1997;10:438.
3. Kukulski T, Voigt JU, Wilkenshoff UM, et al. A comparison of regional myocardial velocity information derived by pulsed and color Doppler techniques: an in vitro and in vivo study. *Echocardiography* 2000;17:639–51.
4. Voigt JU, Arnold MF, Karlsson M, et al. Assessment of regional longitudinal myocardial strain rate derived from Doppler myocardial imaging indices in normal and infarcted myocardium. *J Am Soc Echo* 2000 13:588–598
5. Yingchoncharoen T, Agarwal S, Popović ZB, et al. Normal ranges of left ventricular strain: a meta-analysis. *J Am Soc Echocardiogr* 2013;26:185–91.
6. Lang R, Badano LP, Mor-Avi V, et al. Recommendations for Cardiac Chamber Quantification by Echocardiography: An Update from the American Society of Echocardiography and the European Association of Cardiovascular Imaging. *Eur Heart J Cardiovasc Imag*, 2015;28(1):1–39.

# 2.4 3D echocardiography

## 3D echocardiography

**Provides real-time or near real-time three-dimensional images of the heart in motion**

- ◆ Allows inspection and display of cardiac structures from all perspectives based on cropping and rendering ('electronic dissection' of the heart in motion)
- ◆ Temporal resolution (volume rate or frame rate)/spatial resolution (line density) trade-off
- ◆ Specific artefacts:
  - ◆ **Stitching artefact**
    - ◆ obvious demarcation of sub-volumes in multi-cycles acquisition (Fig. 2.4.1)
    - ◆ how to avoid:
      - ◆ ask the patient to hold their breath on inspiration
      - ◆ use real-time 3D (Fig. 2.4.2 real-time 3D in the same patient as in Fig. 2.4.1)
      - ◆ wait for a more regular RR interval in case of arrhythmia
  - ◆ **Dropout artefact**
    - ◆ false solutions of continuity due to low gain (Fig. 2.4.3)
    - ◆ how to avoid → use higher gain than for 2D (Fig. 2.4.4)

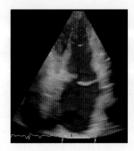

**Fig. 2.4.1** Stitching artefact

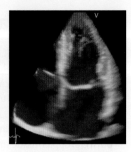

**Fig. 2.4.2** Stitching artefact

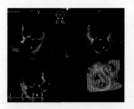

**Fig. 2.4.3** Dropout artefact

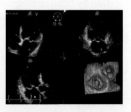

**Fig. 2.4.4** Dropout artefact

# Modalities of image acquisition and display

## Image acquisition

- **Simultaneous multi-plane**
  - uses 3D probe to provide simultaneously live 2D images from two or three planes
- **Real-time (live) 3D**
  - image acquired within one cardiac cycle and available during acquisition
    - → no stitching artefact (due to motion, breathing, or arrhythmia)
    - → lower temporal/spatial resolution
- **ECG gated multi-beat 3D imaging**
  - image acquired over two to seven cardiac cycles and available after stitching
    - → higher temporal/spatial resolution
    - → stitching artefact (acquire during breath hold, avoid RR variation)

## Image display

- **Full volume**
  - external view of the complete 3D dataset acquired (Fig. 2.4.5)
- **Cropped volume**
  - dataset 'dissected' to reveal cardiac structures of interest/to allow internal view
  - cropped

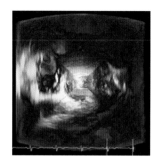

**Fig. 2.4.5** External view of the complete 3D dataset acquired

→ on-line → better spatial/temporal resolution but possible information loss

→ off-line → retains information (full volume can be restored)

◆ cropped:
  ◆ using standard cropping planes to reveal views similar with standard 2D views
    ◆ <u>Example</u>: volume cropped on LV PTSAX plane (Fig. 2.4.6)
  ◆ using adjustable cropping planes to reveal structures or colour flow
    ◆ <u>Example</u>: TR jet 'dissected' from surrounding tissue data (Fig. 2.4.7)
◆ current echo machines display the volume reversibly cropped on PTSAX or 4CV plane

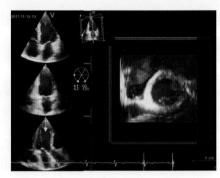

**Fig. 2.4.6** Volume cropped on LV PTSAX plane

## Processed volume

◆ **Volume rendered**
  ◆ processed to enhance 3D appearance/anatomy-like appearance
    ◆ <u>Example</u>: volume rendered cropped LV 3D (Fig. 2.4.8)
    ◆ <u>Example</u>: anatomy like MV:LV view (Fig. 2.4.9), LA view (Fig. 2.4.10)

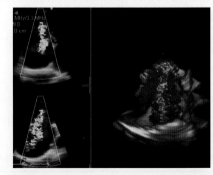

**Fig. 2.4.7** TR jet 'dissected' from surrounding tissue data

## Surface rendered

- ◆ display of surface traced during analysis
  - ◆ <u>Example</u>: endocardial surface rendering of LV (Fig. 2.4.11) and RV diastole (Fig. 2.4.12) and systole (Fig. 2.4.13)

## 2D sliced

- ◆ display of 2D slices derived from the 3D volume
- ◆ adjustable level and orientation of slicing plane
  - ◆ <u>Example</u>: LV 2D slices (Fig. 2.4.14) 4CV, 2CV, 3CV, and 9 SAX views
  - ◆ <u>Example</u>: colour Doppler slices (Fig. 2.4.15) to measure MR EROA

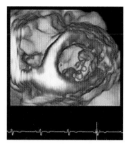

**Fig. 2.4.8** Volume rendered cropped LV 3D

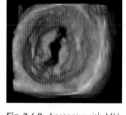

**Fig. 2.4.9** Anatomy with MV: LV view

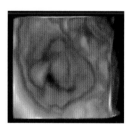

**Fig. 2.4.10** LA view

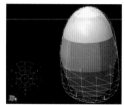

**Fig. 2.4.11** Endocardial surface rendering of LV

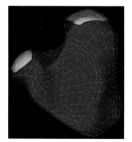

**Fig. 2.4.12** RV diastole

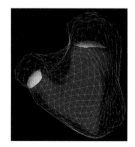

**Fig. 2.4.13** RV systole

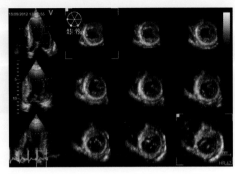

**Fig. 2.4.14** LV 2D slices, 4CV, 2CV, 3CV and 9 SAX views

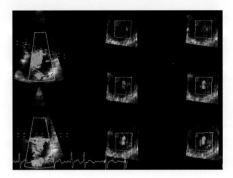

**Fig. 2.4.15** Colour Doppler slices to measure MR EROA

## Modalities: how and when?

### Simultaneous multi-plane

- multi-plane (biplane and tri-plane)/X-plane (biplane)
- the first image is the reference image—the second and third image are derived images
- the level of reference/derived image plane intersection can be adjusted
  - Example: biplane (X-plane) to locate MV flail scallop. LAX derived from PTSAX at level of central scallops P2–A2 (Fig. 2.4.16) and medial scallops P3–A3 (Fig. 2.4.17). Flail posterior scallop P2

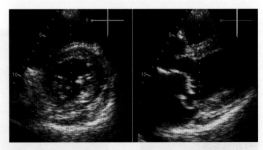

**Fig. 2.4.16** LAX derived from PTSAX at level of central scallops P2-A2

- the rotation angle of the derived image(s) plane can be adjusted
  - Example: LV tri-plane standard (Fig. 2.4.18)/adjusted rotation angle (Fig. 2.4.19) for better 3CV
- multi-plane colour Doppler/DTI—assessment during the same cardiac cycle
  - Example: tri-plane DTI in AF (Fig. 2.4.20) and colour Doppler in eccentric MR (Fig. 2.4.21)

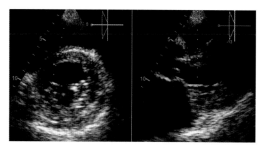

**Fig. 2.4.17** Medial scallops P3-A3

### Real-time (live) 3D

- the sector size can be adjusted but the higher the sector size the lower the frame rate
- the frame rate can be adjusted but the higher the frame rate the lower the line density

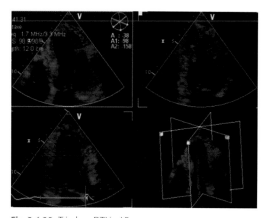

**Fig. 2.4.20** Tri-plane DTI in AF

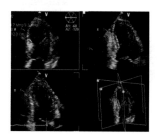

**Fig. 2.4.18** LV tri-plane standard

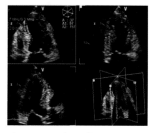

**Fig. 2.4.19** Adjusted rotation angle for better 3CV

- real-time 3D is used for 3D TOE guidance of procedures
- real-time 3D modes available depending on echo machine characteristics:

**Narrow-sector**

- encompasses only a limited part of the heart
  → cannot encompass the entire LV (Fig. 2.4.22)
  → can be used to assess valves
- <u>Example</u>: MV LV view (Fig. 2.4.23) and LA (surgical) view (Fig. 2.4.24)
- has relatively high temporal/spatial resolution

**Wide-sector**

- wide-angle/one cardiac cycle (one heart beat) full volume (Fig. 2.4.25)
  → can be used in case of arrhythmia to avoid stitching artefact
- <u>Example</u>: LV in patient with AF (Fig. 2.4.26)
- can have acceptable temporal/spatial resolution

**Zoom**

- focused wide-sector
  → can be used to assess valves

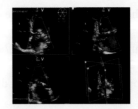
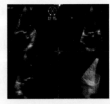

**Fig. 2.4.21** Colour Doppler in eccentric MR

**Fig. 2.4.22** Narrow sector

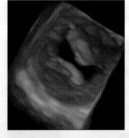
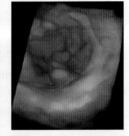

**Fig. 2.4.23** Narrow sector

**Fig. 2.4.24** Narrow sector

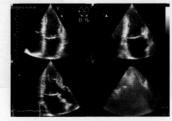

**Fig. 2.4.25** Wide sector

- ◆ <u>Example</u>: MV zoom surgical view in patient with AF (Fig. 2.4.27)
- ◆ reduce sector width to improve temporal/spatial resolution

## Colour Doppler

- ◆ smaller sector size than for narrow-sector 3D
- → can be used to detect the origin of flow—the abnormal orifice
- ◆ <u>Example</u>: LV inflow—colour-flow aliasing due to MS (Fig. 2.4.28)
- ◆ reduce sector width to a minimum for acceptable temporal resolution

## ECG gated multi-beat 3D imaging

- ◆ we can select the number of beats (**n**) to stitch (from two to seven)
- ◆ the image is split in **n** sub-volumes
- ◆ almost real-time

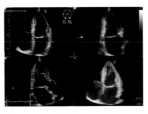

**Fig. 2.4.26** Wide sector

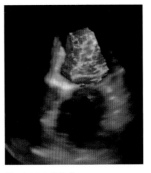

**Fig. 2.4.28** LV inflow

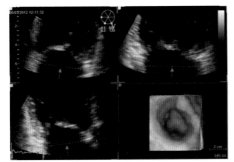

**Fig. 2.4.27** MV zoom surgical view in patient with AF

◆ each sub-volume is acquired in one beat → the full volume is acquired in **n** beats

◆ after **n** beats the image appears 'real-time' → 'almost real-time'

◆ we can display the dataset as full-volume pyramid (Fig. 2.4.29) or cropped volume (Fig. 2.4.30ABC) together with derived 2D images (**A**) or alone (**BC**)

◆ we can crop the volume in any plane and at any level

◆ <u>Example</u>: MV level PTSAX (Fig. 2.4.30A), PM level PTSAX (Fig. 2.4.30B), 4CV (Fig. 2.4.30C)

◆ a marker on the ECG (Figs. 2.4.29–30ABC) reveals ECG gated multi-beat acquisition

◆ has higher frame rate

→ can use for LV function analysis for good frame rate despite wide sector

→ can trade in frame rate for better line density (image quality) in assessment of valves

→ can use for colour Doppler assessment to ensure better volume rate

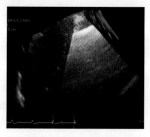

**Fig. 2.4.29** ECG gated multi-beat 3D imaging

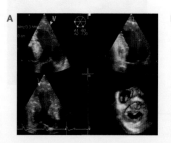
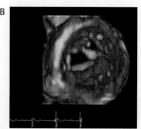
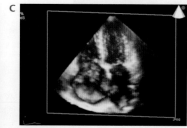

**Fig. 2.4.30** ECG gated multi-beat 3D imaging

- ◆ <u>Example</u>: multi-beat TR colour Doppler (Fig. 2.4.31) and 3D-guided 2D slices (multi-planar reconstruction, MPR) reveals TR in 4CV and perpendicular view and allows vena contracta area (EROA) measurement in transverse plane at the level of the vena contracta (Fig. 2.4.32)

## Windows and views

**All echo windows can be used to acquire 3D datasets**

- ◆ Conventional views can be obtained by cropping and rendering 3D volumes
    - ◆ <u>Example</u>: apical 4CV, 2CV, and 3CV (Fig. 2.4.33) obtained by cropping and rendering from apical full-volume dataset (Fig. 2.4.34)

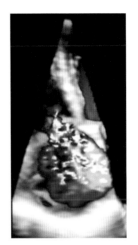

**Fig. 2.4.31** Multi-beat TR colour Doppler

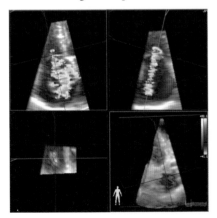

**Fig. 2.4.32** Transverse plane at the level of the vena contracta

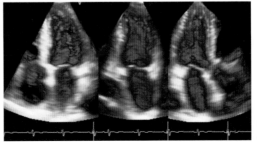

**Fig. 2.4.33** Apical 4CV, 2CV and 3CV

- ◆ <u>Example</u>: RV 4CV, outflow, and inflow views (Fig. 2.4.35) from apical 3D dataset
- ◆ Conventional views can be also obtained by using the desired view as reference for 3D dataset acquisition, positioning the 3D transducer similarly with the 2D transducer for the same view
  - ◆ <u>Example</u>: parasternal views obtained in real time: PTLAX (Fig. 2.4.36A), PTSAX at the level of the great arteries (Fig. 2.4.36B), of the mitral valve (Fig. 2.4.36C), of the papillary muscles (Fig. 2.4.36D), and of the cardiac apex (Fig. 2.4.36E)

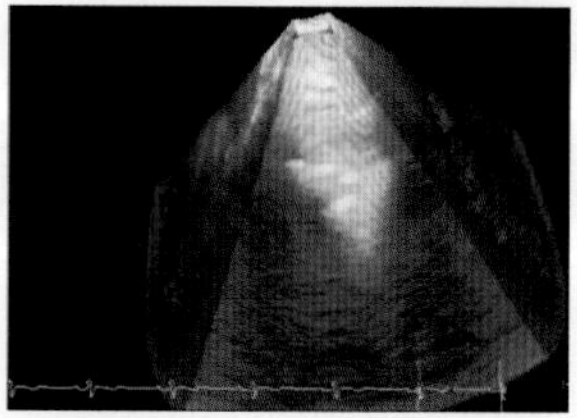

## The 3D echocardiographic examination

### Focused examination

- ◆ Complete 2D examination and 3D examination focused only on the clinical question
  - ◆ <u>Example</u>: 3D dataset for LV systolic function assessment (Fig. 2.4.37) needs low depth imaging (LV only) and multi-beat acquisition (higher frame rate)

**Fig. 2.4.34** Cropping and rendering from apical full volume dataset

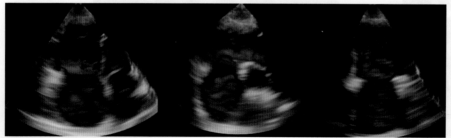

**Fig. 2.4.35** Apical 3D dataset

◆ Example: 3D dataset for MS assessment with MV 3D-guided 2D planimetry using multi-slice (Fig. 2.4.38) or multi-planar reconstruction for measurement plane orthogonal alignment at the leaflet tips. One-beat (real-time) acquisition can be used in AF. Zoom can be used for better resolution

◆ Example: 3D dataset for morphological valve assessment needs optimization of image resolution by trading in frame rate if possible and using zoom (real-time or multi-beat). Volume rendering and cropping plane adjustment better reveal morphology. Example of TV assessment in diastole (Fig. 2.4.39) and in systole (Fig. 2.4.40)

## Complete examination

◆ multiple 3D datasets from all windows

◆ real-time +/− multi-beat acquisition +/− zoom in both modes

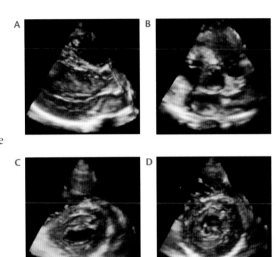

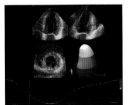

**Fig. 2.4.37** 3D dataset for LV systolic function assessment

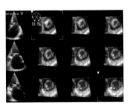

**Fig. 2.4.38** 3D dataset for MS assessment

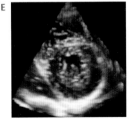

**Fig. 2.4.36** Parasternal views obtained in real time. PTLAX (A). PTSAX at the level of the great arteries (B). The mitral valve (C). Papillary muscles (D). Cardiac apex (E)

- based on cropping plane adjustment, cropping can generate:
  - conventional views
  - anatomic views
    - <u>Example</u>: base of the heart view (Fig. 2.4.41)
- a whole heart full volume can be obtained and used to analyse all structures
- for better image quality (frame rate/line density) consider specific 3D datasets for each structure (Table 2.4.1)

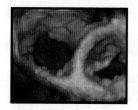

**Fig. 2.4.39** Example of TV assessment in diastole

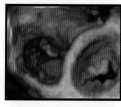

**Fig. 2.4.40** Example of TV assessment in systole

**Table 2.4.1** Adapted from Recommendations for image acquisition and display using 3D echocardiography

| LV/RV | MV | TV |
|---|---|---|
| **Apical dataset** (4CV/modified 4CV for RV) real-time (wide-angle) multi-beat | **Apical dataset +/– colour** (4CV) real-time (narrow-angle)/zoom real-time multi-beat/zoom multi-beat | **Apical dataset +/– colour** (modified 4CV as for RV) real-time (narrow-angle)/zoom real-time multi-beat/zoom multi-beat |
| | **Parasternal dataset +/– colour** (PTLAX) real-time (narrow-angle)/zoom real-time multi-beat/zoom multi-beat | **Parasternal dataset +/– colour** (RV inflow) real-time (narrow-angle)/zoom real-time multi-beat/zoom multi-beat |
| **IAS/IVS** | **AV** | **PV** |
| **Apical dataset** (4CV) real-time (narrow-angle)/zoom real-time multi-beat/zoom multi-beat | **Parasternal dataset +/– colour** (PTLAX) real-time (narrow-angle)/zoom real-time multi-beat/zoom multi-beat | **Parasternal dataset +/– colour** (RVOT view) real-time (narrow-angle)/zoom real-time multi-beat/zoom multi-beat |

# LV segmentation

- ◆ See standard LV segmentation in Chapter 2.1
- ◆ Assessment of myocardial segments/regional wall motion is performed on 2D images obtained with the 3D probe (one plane or multi-plane imaging), or on 2D images derived from 3D datasets
- ◆ 3D echocardiography allows correct myocardial segmentation through:
  - ◆ cutting planes alignment to avoid foreshortening → better visualization of apical segments
  - ◆ cutting planes alignment perpendicular to LV walls → better LV SAX images at multiple levels
  - ◆ recognition of spatial orientation of cutting planes → better prediction of myocardial territories
- ◆ When using simultaneous multi-plane imaging → adjust imaging planes to obtain correct standard 2D views for LV segmentation (Figs. 2.4.18 and 2.4.19)
- ◆ When parasternal views are poor → derive LV SAX from apical 3D dataset (Fig. 2.4.14)
- ◆ When using 3D-derived 2D views → adjust cutting planes orientation to obtain correct standard 2D views, to assess myocardial segments in all coronary territories or to reveal pathology

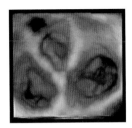

**Fig. 2.4.41** Base of the heart view

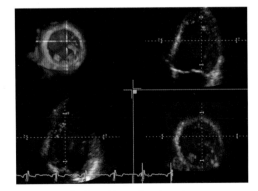

**Fig. 2.4.42** 4CV view with anterior orientation

- ◆ <u>Example</u>: 4CV view with anterior orientation of the cutting plane (Fig. 2.4.42) reveals anterolateral wall (LAD/diagonal territory) while 4CV with posterior orientation of the cutting plane (Fig. 2.4.43) reveals posterolateral wall (LCx territory). 3D allows recognition of cutting plane orientation, while if the 4CV is obtained with a 2D transducer the plane orientation is not defined

- ◆ <u>Example</u>: LV 3D wall-motion analysis: automatic 2D slicing (Fig. 2.4.44) can be manually adjusted. Alignment with LV long axis avoids foreshortening (Fig. 2.4.45). Automatic slicing (like opening a book) displays the inferior wall on the right side of 2CV (Figs. 2.4.44 and 2.4.45). Plane rotation 180° brings the inferior wall on the left side of 2CV and improves orientation guided by the SAX view (Fig. 2.4.46). Planes rotation generates any views: 4CV and 3CV

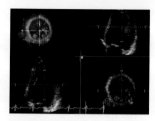

**Fig. 2.4.43** 4CV with posterior orientation

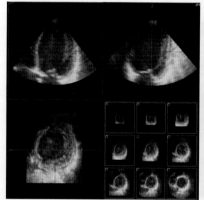

**Fig. 2.4.44** LV 3D wall motion analysis

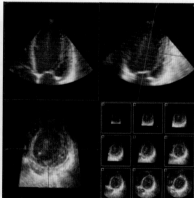

**Fig. 2.4.45** Alignment with LV long axis

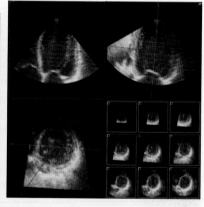

**Fig. 2.4.46** Improving orientation guided by the SAX view

(Fig. 2.4.47), or 2CV and 3CV (Fig. 2.4.48). Cutting plane anterior translation reveals the anterior part of the lateral wall obtaining 5CV (Fig. 2.4.49)

## Measurements and chamber quantification

### Linear dimensions and areas

- ◆ Measured on 3D-guided 2D or on volumetric rendered images
- ◆ 3D-guided 2D measurements are better aligned than 2D measurements
  - ◆ <u>Example</u>: for MV area 3D-guided 2D planimetry the cutting planes are aligned perpendicular to the funnel at the level of the leaflet tips (Fig. 2.4.50). The level and orientation of the 2D parasternal MV SAX is not precisely determined.

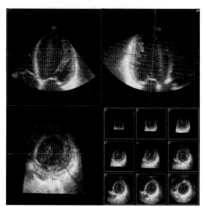

**Fig. 2.4.47** 4CV and 3CV views

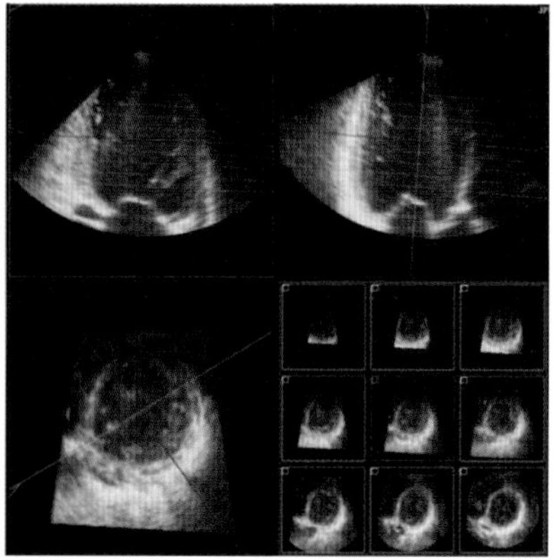

**Fig. 2.4.48** 2CV and 3CV views

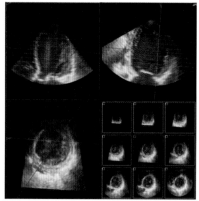

**Fig. 2.4.49** Obtaining 5CV

- ◆ <u>Example</u>: for LVOT area 3D-guided 2D planimetry the cutting plane is aligned perpendicular to the LVOT long axis (Fig. 2.4.51)
- ◆ Measurements performed on volume-rendered images are not accurate because they are highly dependent on image processing
  - ◆ <u>Example</u>: IVS dimension measured on volume-rendered 3D PTSAX: small change in image processing results in ~30% higher measurement value (Fig. 2.4.52AB)

## Volumes, ejection fraction, and mass

- ◆ LV volumes (EDV, ESV, SV) and EF (Fig. 2.4.53)
  - ◆ use low depth and check that LV cavity fits in at end-diastole
  - ◆ use preferably multi-beat 3D for better frame rate
  - ◆ low frame rate overestimates ESV so underestimates EF
  - ◆ align LV long axis and correct semi-automatic endocardial borders

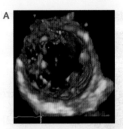

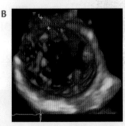

**Fig. 2.4.52** IVS dimension measured on volume-rendered 3D PTSAX: small change in image processing results in ~30% higher measurement value

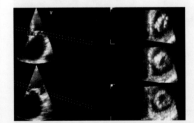

**Fig. 2.4.50** MV area: 3D-guided 2D planimetry

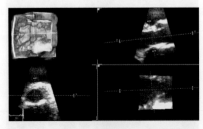

**Fig. 2.4.51** LVOT area: 3D-guided 2D planimetry

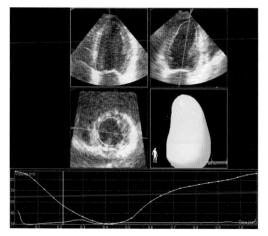

**Fig. 2.4.53** LV volumes (EDV, ESV, SV) and EF

| | | |
|---|---|---|
| Volume | | |
| EDV | 239.7 | ml |
| ESV | 89.5 | ml |
| SV | 150.2 | ml |
| EF | 62.7 | % |

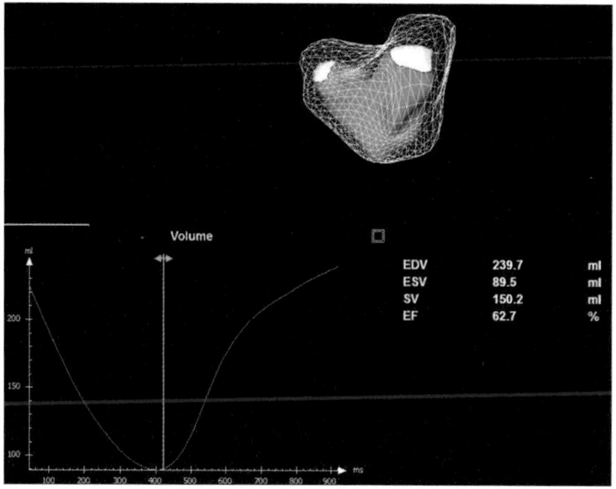

**Fig. 2.4.54** RV volumes (EDV, ESV, SV) and EF

- ◆ trace LV cavity including trabeculations within the cavity
- ◆ EF is calculated both using operator selected end-diastole and end-systole and using the larger and smaller volumes
- ◆ RV volumes (EDV, ESV, SV) and EF (Fig. 2.4.54)
  - ◆ RV wraps around LV so do not restrict sector width to RV in 4CV
  - ◆ use low depth and check that the RV cavity fits in at end-diastole
  - ◆ use multi-beat for higher frame rate
  - ◆ correct semi-automatic endocardial borders
  - ◆ the image quality is not always appropriate

- LV mass (Fig. 2.4.55)
  - the entire LV has to fit in at the end-diastole (challenging for large LV)
  - higher sector width results in lower frame rate
  - recognizing and tracing the epicardial surface is challenging
  - correct semi-automatic endocardial and epicardial borders

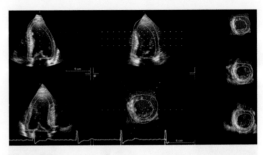

**Fig. 2.4.55** LV mass

## Size of septal defects

- 3D-guided 2D measurements or measurements on volume-rendered images
- mainly on 3D TOE → be aware of interatrial septum (thin structure) dropout artefacts

## LV dyssynchrony

- assessment performed at the same time with LV volumes and EF (Fig. 2.4.56)
- challenging to fit in large LV (heart failure) → fit in LV cavity only
- 17 myocardial segments (16 + apical cap) → 17 segmental sub-volumes
- segmental volume change curves should reach minimum volume simultaneously

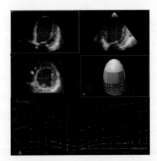

**Fig. 2.4.56** LV dyssynchrony

- dyssynchrony → segmental time to minimum volume dispersion
- segmental time to minimum volume standard deviation → dyssynchrony index

**Mitral valve annulus size and shape**

- measurements performed mainly on 3D TOE
- annulus diameters/circumference/area

# Reference values

- 3D echo-derived reference values for LV volumes and mass per gender and body size are not established
  → LV volumes are underestimated compared with CMR
  → LV mass is overestimated compared with CMR
- 3D echo RV volumes reference values differ between men and women (EDV 79 ml/m² for men and 71 ml/m² for women, and ESV at 32 ml/m² for men and 28 ml/m² for women)
  → adjusting to lean body mass eliminates the difference
  → RV volumes are underestimated compared with CMR

# Suggested reading

1. Lang R, Badano LP, Tsang W, et al. EAE/ASE Recommendations for Image Acquisition and Display Using Three-Dimensional Echocardiography. *Eur Heart J Cardiovascular Imaging* 2012;13:1–46.

## 2.5 Left ventricular opacification with contrast echocardiography

### General considerations

- **Contrast agents comprise microbubbles that consist of an outer shell and an inner gas** (Fig. 2.5.1, Table 2.5.1)
- The diameter of these microbubbles is usually less than 8 µm allowing their passage through the pulmonary capillaries and therefore their injection into a peripheral vein
- Microbubbles oscillate when exposed to ultrasound waves
- Non-linear oscillation produces harmonic signals at multiple frequencies of the fundamental frequency signal, which greatly improves image quality
- Act as red blood cell tracers—remain entirely intravascular at all times
- Entirely different from iodine-based contrast used in angiography/CT and gadolinium-based contrast used in CMR
- Used in rest and stress echocardiography to improve image quality, allowing accurate assessment of cardiac structure and function

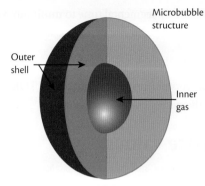

**Fig. 2.5.1** Structure of a contrast microsphere

**Table 2.5.1** Types of contrast agents

| | SONOVUE | OPTISON | LUMINITY |
|---|---|---|---|
| **Outer shell** | Predominantly phospholipid | Human albumin | Predominantly phospholipid |
| **Inner gas** | Sulphur hexafluoride | Perfluoropropane | Perfluoropropane |
| **Mean bubble size** | 2–8 μm | 3.0–4.5 μm | 1.1–2.5 μm |
| **Storage** | No special precautions | Refrigerator (2–8˚C) | Refrigerator (2–8˚C) |
| **Approved in EU** | Yes | Yes | Yes |
| **Approved in USA** | No | Yes | Yes |
| **Manufacturer** | Bracco | GE Healthcare | Bristol-Myers Squibb |
| **Preparation** | Use MiniSpike™ transfer system to inject 5 ml saline into vial containing sulphur hexafluoride. Shake gently for 20–30 s | Invert and gently rotate Optison vial for approx 3 minutes to resuspend microspheres | Must be 'activated' using specific Vialmix™ device, which shakes/agitates contrast to produce homogenous suspension |
| **Administration** | **0.2-0.4 ml bolus injection.** Maximum suggested dose is 3 ml. Bracco also produce a specific oscillating pump for continuous intravenous infusion | **0.1-0.3 ml bolus injection.** Maximum suggested dose is 3 ml, as little experience with higher doses in clinical practice. | **10 μL/kg body weight** slow dose bolus injection over 30 seconds. |
| **Reported side effects** | Headache; nausea; chest pain; injection site reaction; paraesthaesia; vasodilation | Headache; nausea and/or vomiting; warm sensation or flushing; dizziness | Headache; flushing; back pain |

# Understanding contrast imaging

- Frequency at which sound waves leave the transducer is the *fundamental frequency*
- With tissue, fundamental frequency produces an equal and opposite vibration (**linear response**)
- Microbubbles can expand (**rarefaction**) to a greater degree than they can contract (**compression**), and unequal oscillation is observed (**non-linear response**). These non-linear signals may also be produced by tissues, only at high **mechanical index (MI)**
- Microbubbles reflect sound waves not only at the fundamental frequency but also at higher harmonic frequencies
- Microbubble contrast agents interact with ultrasound in three ways depending upon the MI (Fig. 2.5.2)
- Standard 2D-echocardiography (using MI of 1.0–1.4) would destroy the outer shells of the microspheres, resulting in bubble implosion
- Thus, a lower MI (MI of 0.1–0.5) is required for contrast echocardiography

# Indications for contrast echocardiography

Ultrasound contrast can be used for left ventricular opacification (LVO) in both rest and stress echocardiography studies.

### Rest echocardiography

In patients with suboptimal image quality, contrast is indicated:

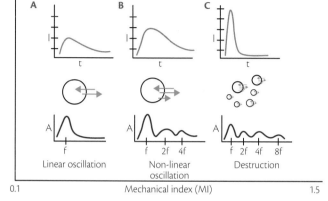

**Fig. 2.5.2** Contrast–ultrasound interaction

**A. Low acoustic power (MI < 0.1)**
Linear oscillation occurs
Compression and rarefaction equal in amplitude and no enhanced signal is generated

**B. Intermediate acoustic power (MI 0.1–0.5)**
Non-linear oscillation occurs
(rarefaction > compression)
Ultrasound waves created at harmonic frequencies different from fundamental frequency

**C. High acoustic power (MI > 0.5)**
Microbubble destruction with transient emission of high intensity signals, very rich in non-linear components. Only used for perfusion assessment

- to enable improved endocardial visualization and assessment of LV structure and function when ≥ 2 adjacent segments are NOT seen on unenhanced images (Fig. 2.5.3)
- to have accurate and reproducible measurements of LV volumes and ejection fraction by 2D-echocardiography (Fig. 2.5.4)
- to confirm or exclude the following echocardiographic diagnosis, when unenhanced images are suboptimal for definitive diagnosis:
  - apical hypertrophic cardiomyopathy (Fig. 2.5.5)
  - ventricular non-compaction (Fig. 2.5.6)

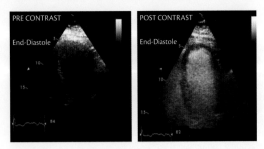

**Fig. 2.5.3** Contrast cardiography

- ◆ apical thrombus (Fig. 2.5.7)
- ◆ ventricular pseudoaneurysm

## Stress echocardiography

When the endocardial borders of ≥ 2 adjacent segments are NOT seen in order to:

- ◆ obtain diagnostic assessment of segmental wall thickening at rest and at peak stress
- ◆ increase the proportion of diagnostic studies
- ◆ increase confidence of interpreting physician

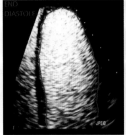
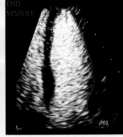

**Fig. 2.5.4** End-diastolic (left) and end-systolic (right) volumes can be quantitated by tracing the endocardial borders (red lines), clearly seen after contrast administration

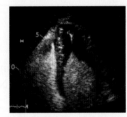

**Fig. 2.5.5** Example of apical hypertrophic cardiomyopathy

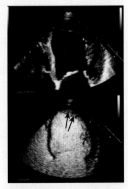

**Fig. 2.5.6** Example of left ventricular non-compaction

# Contraindications for contrast echocardiography

## All contrast agents

◆ Known hypersensitivity/allergy to contrast agent or constituent chemical

## SonoVue

◆ Known allergy to sulphur-containing products or drugs (i.e. Septrin)
◆ Recent (< 7 days) acute coronary syndrome
◆ NYHA Class III—IV heart failure
◆ Severe pulmonary hypertension (PA systolic pressure > 90 mmHg)

# Contrast administration protocols

Two methods of IV contrast administration: bolus injection vs continuous infusion (Table 2.5.2). For LV opacification performed during resting echocardiography, bolus injection is adequate for the majority of patients. Continuous infusion generally could be reserved for patients with apical or extensive

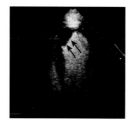

**Fig. 2.5.7** Example of thrombus

**Table 2.5.2** Advantages and disadvantages of bolus vs continuous infusion

|  | Advantages | Disadvantages |
|---|---|---|
| **Bolus injection** | Simple to perform Rapid opacification | Short duration of contrast effect Contrast attenuation artefacts Usually second operator needed |
| **Continuous infusion** | Longer opacification duration Homogenous contrast effect Simple to adjust dose to each individual Reproducible (e.g. for serial studies) | More complicated (infusion pump) OGen uses higher contrast dose |

wall-motion abnormalities, in whom swirling artefact may be more common and infusion would most likely produce better image quality.

## Rest echocardiography: bolus injection protocol

Prepare the contrast agent as per provided instructions.

- Obtain intravenous access: a large antecubital fossa vein will yield superior opacification to a small vein in the lower arm
- Change the imaging settings of the machine by pressing a contrast pre-set button. MI should then change from > 1.0 to between 0.2–0.4
- Use a three-way tap for injection. Inject using the port in line with the cannula, not the side port or the port on top of the cannula, to reduce bubble destruction (Fig. 2.5.8)
- Inject 0.2–0.4 ml contrast slowly (over 3–5 seconds) and then give a slow 2 ml saline flush. Giving the contrast or flush too quickly increases risk of attenuation artefact
- Repeated doses can be given up to a suggested maximum of 3 ml

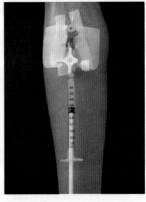

**Fig. 2.5.8** Site of injection

## Rest echocardiography: continuous infusion (see Boxes 2.5.1, 2.5.2)

| Box 2.5.1 SonoVue, using the VueJect pump |
| --- |
| ◆ Turn on VueJect pump (1–2 min for initialization) |
| ◆ Aspirate SonoVue into the specific 20 ml syringe |
| ◆ Insert syringe into pump and close lid—90 seconds of mixing occurs before pump is ready for use |
| ◆ Press 'Purge' button to flush the line |
| ◆ The infusion rate can be controlled via the touchpad and increased/decreased as necessary |
| ◆ **Begin infusion at 1.0 ml/min**. Once contrast appears in the left heart, this often needs to be reduced to 0.8 ml/min (or less) to prevent shadowing (attenuation) artefact |

| Box 2.5.2 Optison and Luminity |
| --- |
| ◆ No specific infusion pumps are available |
| ◆ Optison/Luminity can simply be dissolved in saline or glucose and infused using a standard intravenous giving set |
| ◆ The recommended dose is via an intravenous infusion of **1.3 ml contrast added to 50 ml of 0.9% NaCl or 5% glucose** solution for injection |
| ◆ The rate of infusion should **be initiated at 4.0 ml/min**, but titrated as necessary to achieve optimal image enhancement, not to exceed 10 ml/min |

## Stress echocardiography

### Treadmill exercise stress and bicycle exercise stress

◆ 0.4–0.5 ml bolus injection 15–30 s prior to terminating exercise and flush with 2 ml saline

◆ A second injection is usually not necessary but can be given if required

### Dobutamine stress

- Both dobutamine and SonoVue can be infused simultaneously through one cannula using a three-way tap (Fig. 2.5.9)
- For **bolus technique**, give 0.3 ml bolus injection once 85% THR achieved or if other end point achieved (e.g. limiting chest pain, etc.)
- For **infusion technique**, restart pump as soon as 85% THR achieved: effective LV opacification will be achieved within 15–30 seconds
- Technical note for viability studies: at low and intermediate dose, injecting contrast via the three-way tap will inadvertently deliver a small bolus of dobutamine and often cause an undesired rise in heart rate. Inject via the top of the cannula (Fig. 2.5.10) for the low and intermediate stages

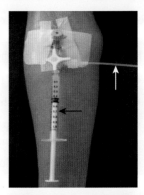

**Fig. 2.5.9** Three-way tap cannula

### Dipyridamole stress

- If only wall motion is being assessed, either bolus injection or continuous infusion can be used. After dipyridamole has been administered, imaging should commence within 30 s. Thus, bolus injection should be given 20–30 s after dipyridamole or, for infusion, the pump should be recommenced as soon as dipyridamole has been given

## Artefacts in contrast echocardiography

### Attenuation (Fig. 2.5.11AB)

**Problem**: Excessive microbubble concentration in the heart. Ultrasound signal completely absorbed in near field, usually producing shadowing in the far field.

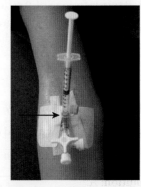

**Fig. 2.5.10** Top of the cannula

**Solution**: Wait for contrast washout. Alternatively, use slower injection/lower dose of bolus injection, or continuous infusion.

## Swirling (Fig. 2.5.11CDE)

**Problem**: Excessive bubble destruction in the apex (near field)—could be due to high mechanical index (MI), high frame rate, too low contrast concentration, or apical akinesia with sluggish flow. Results in large apical contrast artefacts and suboptimal opacification and endocardial border visualization.

**Solution**: Reduce MI (Fig. 2.5.11F), inject larger contrast dose, move focus towards apex.

## Blooming

**Problem**: Spread of contrast beyond tissue of origin. Thus, cavity signals may be confused with myocardial perfusion.

**Solution**: Slower rate of bolus injection or use continuous infusion.

## Thoracic cage/linear artefacts (Figs. 2.5.11GH)

**Problem**: Suboptimal myocardial visualization due to shadowing from ribs, lung tissue or movement of heart in and out of scan plane.

**Solution**: Adjust transducer position, breath-hold during imaging.

# Safety of ultrasound contrast

- Contrast is safe in vast majority of patients (safety data from studies including millions of patients)
- Equally safe during rest and stress echocardiography
- Studies have shown no difference in mortality or serious adverse events between patients that did and did not receive contrast

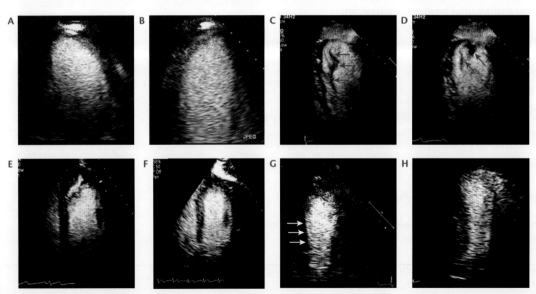

**Fig. 2.5.11** Artefacts in contrast echocardiography

## Mild side-effects

Headache, weakness, fatigue, palpitations, nausea, dizziness, dry mouth, taste or smell perversion, dyspnoea, chest pain, back pain, urticaria, pruritus, or rash

## Serious reactions (very rare)

Angioedema, hypoxaemia, cyanosis, hypotension, anaphylactoid and anaphylactic reactions. Frequency 1 in 10 000 cases (see Boxes 2.5.3, 2.5.4)

# Managing contrast reactions in practice

♦ Ensure resuscitation equipment readily available prior to contrast echocardiography
♦ At least one person (doctor/nurse/sonographer) trained in advanced life support (ALS)
♦ Ensure drug allergies/intolerances verified prior to beginning of stress test

| Box 2.5.3 Symptoms/signs of a serious contrast reaction |
| --- |
| ♦ Breathing difficulties |
| ♦ Facial/tongue swelling |
| ♦ Dizziness |
| ♦ Fall in blood pressure |

| Box 2.5.4 If a serious reaction occurs |
| --- |
| ♦ Alert medical emergency/cardiac arrest team |
| ♦ High-flow oxygen |
| ♦ Further large-bore intravenous access |
| ♦ Intravenous fluid |
| ♦ Intravenous hydrocortisone and anti-histamine |
| ♦ Intramuscular adrenaline |

# Suggested reading

1. Senior R, Becher H, Monaghan M, et al. Contrast echocardiography: evidence-based recommendations by European Association of Echocardiography. *Eur J Echocardiogr* 2009; 10:194–212.
2. Mulvagh SL, Rakowski H, Vannan MA, et al. American Society of Echocardiography Consensus Statement on the Clinical Applications of Ultrasonic Contrast Agents in Echocardiography. *J Am Soc Echocardiogr* 2008; 21:1179–201.
3. Chahal NS and Senior R. Clinical applications of left ventricular opacification. *J Am Coll Cardiol Img* 2010; 3:188–96.

# 2.6 The storage and report on transthoracic echocardiography (TTE) (Tables 2.6.1, 2.6.2, 2.6.3, 2.6.4)

**Table 2.6.1** Minimal basic dataset to acquire and store

| | Projections | 2D[a] | M-mode[a,b] | Doppler[a] | | | |
|---|---|---|---|---|---|---|---|
| | | | | Colour | Spectral | | DTI |
| | | | | | PW | CW | |
| 1 | Parasternal LAX view of the LV | ■ | LV and Ao/LA | ■ | | | |
| 2 | Parasternal RV inflow tract view | ■ | | ■ | | Tricuspid if TR jet present | |
| 3 | Parasternal RVOT view | ■ | | ■ | | | |
| 4 | Parasternal SAX view Aortic valve level | ■ | | ■ | RVOT | Tricuspid if TR jet present<br>Pulmonary if PS suspected | |
| 5 | Parasternal SAX view Mitral valve level | ■ | | | | | |

| | Projections | 2D[a] | M-mode[a,b] | Doppler[a] | | | |
|---|---|---|---|---|---|---|---|
| | | | | Colour | Spectral | | DTI |
| | | | | | PW | CW | |
| 6 | Parasternal SAX view Mid-papillary level | | LV | | | | |
| 7 | Parasternal SAX view at apex | | | | | | |
| 8 | Apical four-chamber view | | | | Mitral and pulmonary veins | Mitral if MS suspected | Septal and lateral mitral annular velocities |
| 9 | Apical modified four-chamber view for RV | | TAPSE | | | Tricuspid if TR jet present | Tricuspid annulus |
| 10 | Apical five-chamber view | | | | LVOT | Aortic valve | |
| 11 | Apical two-chamber view | | | | | | |
| 12 | Apical LAX view | | | | | | |
| 13 | Subcostal four-chamber view | | | | | | |

| | Projections | 2D[a] | M-mode[a,b] | Doppler[a] | | | |
|---|---|---|---|---|---|---|---|
| | | | | Colour | Spectral | | DTI |
| | | | | | PW | CW | |
| 14 | Subcostal-IVC collapse during inspiration or sniff | ■ | IVC diameter and sniff test | | | | |
| 15 | Suprasternal LAX view of the aortic arch | ■ | | | | Aortic isthmus | |

■ **Mandatory acquisitions**    ■ **Conditional acquisitions**

[a.] 2D and colour Doppler views are acquired as loops (2–3 beats) whereas PwD/CwD/TDI spectra as well as M-mode tracings are acquired as still frames (sweep speed 50–100 cm/s).

[b.] Measurements only if adequately aligned, otherwise only for detection of very rapid events like septal flash, RV-LV interdependence, SAM of the mitral valve.

**2D**, two-dimensional echocardiography; **Ao**, aorta; **CW**, continuous-wave Doppler; **DTI**, Doppler tissue imaging; **IVC**, inferior vena cava; **LA**, left atrium; **LAX**, long axis; **LV**, left ventricle; **LVOT**, left ventricular outflow tract; **MS**, mitral stenosis; **PS**, pulmonary stenosis; **PW**, pulsed-wave Doppler; **RV**, right ventricle; **RVOT**, right ventricular outflow tract; **SAX**, short axis; **TAPSE**, tricuspid annular plane systolic excursion; **TR**, tricuspid regurgitation.

**Table 2.6.2** 3D dataset acquisition and display

| VIEW \ STRUCTURE | Aortic valve | Left ventricle | Right ventricle* | Pulm. valve | Mitral valve | Inter-atrial septum | Inter-ventr. septum | Tricuspid valve |
|---|---|---|---|---|---|---|---|---|
| **Parasternal long-axis view** | ■■ NZ | | | | ■■ NZ | | | |
| **Parasternal RV inflow tract view** | | | | | | | | ■■ NZ |
| **Parasternal RV outflow tract view** | | | | ■■ NZ | | | | |
| **Apical four-chamber view** | | ■ NZ | ■ NZ | | ■■ NZ | ■ NZ | ■ NZ | ■■ NZ |

*The image must be tilted to position the RV in the centre of the image for proper acquisition

| | | | |
|---|---|---|---|
| N | Narrow-angle acquisition | ■ | Loop without colour |
| Z | Zoomed acquisition | ■ | Loop with colour |

**Table 2.6.3  Recommendations for reporting TTE**

| HOSPITAL NAME | First Name | | Study ordered | dd-mm-yyyy | Height | 167 cm | Rhythm | AF |
|---|---|---|---|---|---|---|---|---|
| DEPARTMENT | Last Name | | Study performed | dd-mm-yyyy | Weight | 75 kg | Heart rate | 90 bpm |
| | Date of birth | dd-mm-yyyy | Image Quality | Good | BSA | 1.7 m² | Blood pressure | 120/80 |
| Referring physician | Patient ID | | Indication | New-onset shortness of breath | | | | |
| ☑ Inpatient  ☐ Outpatient | Gender | F | | | | | | |

**2D & 3D measurements**
(M-mode, M; 2D; 3D; circle selected acquisition technique)

## LEFT VENTRICLE

| | | |
|---|---|---|
| Septum thickness (end-diastole) (M/2D) | 6–11 mm | 10 |
| Posterior wall thickness (end-diastole) (M/2D) | 6–11 mm | 8 |
| Internal dimension (end-diastole) (M/2D) | 37–53 mm | 65 |
| | 21–29 mm/m² | 38 |
| Internal dimension (end-systole) (M/2D) | 22–38 mm | 50 |
| | 12–21 mm/m² | 29 |
| Fractional shortening (%) | 26–44 | 23 |
| Relative wall thickness (%) | <45% | 25 |
| End-diastolic volume (2D/3D) | 59–141 mL | 170 |
| | 34–71 mL/m² | 100 |

**Regional LV Function**

1: Normal          3: Akinetic
2: Hypokinetic     4: Dyskinetic

## ATRIA and AORTA

### Left atrium (LA)

| | | |
|---|---|---|
| Antero-posterior diameter (M/2D) | 27–41 mm | 50 |
| | 15–23 mm/m² | 29 |
| Area | ≤ 23 cm² | 29 |
| Volume (2D/3D) | 29–70 mL | 100 |
| | 17–37 mL/m² | 59 |

**Table 2.6.3 Recommendations for reporting TTE** (*continued*)

| LEFT VENTRICLE | | | | RIGHT VENTRICLE | | | ATRIA and AORTA | | |
|---|---|---|---|---|---|---|---|---|---|
| | | | | | | | **Right atrium (RA)** | | |
| End–systolic volume (2D/3D) | | 19–54 mL | 120 | **RIGHT VENTRICLE** | | | Minor axis – 4 chamber | 27–46 mm | 29 |
| | | 11–27 mL/m² | 71 | | | | | 15–24 mm/m² | 17 |
| Ejection fraction (2D/3D) | | 56–72 % | 29 | Mid–internal dimension (4–ch) (end–diastole) | 20–38 mm | 32 | Area | ≤ 20 cm² | 21 |
| Hypertrophy (M/2D/3D) | Men | 49–115 g/m² (Normal) | | RV subcostal wall thickness | <5 mm | 3 | IVC diameters (mm) Expiration/sniff | 13 | 5 |
| | | 116–131 g/m² (Mild) | | RV area (end–diastole) | 11–24 cm² | 27 | Estimated RA pressure (mmHg) | | 3 |
| | | 132–148 g/m² (Moderate) | | RV area (end–systole) | 5–13 cm² | 14 | | | |
| | | ≥149 g/m² (Severe) | | RV area change (%) | 36–64% | 48 | **Aorta (Ao)** | | |
| | Women | 43–95 g/m² (Normal) | | RV ejection fraction (3D) | 44–69% | 50 | Ao annulus (M/2D/3D) | 17–24 mm | |
| | | 96–108 g/m² (Mild) ✓ | | TAPSE | 16–30 mm | 16 | Sinus of Valsalva level (m/2D/3D) | 21–38 mm | 24 |
| | | 109–121 g/m² (Moderate) | | Tricuspid annulus S′ DTI | 10–19 cm/s | 15 | Sinotubular junction (M/2D/3D) | 19–36 mm | |
| | | ≥122 g/m² (Severe) | | RVOT diameter (distal) | 16–27 mm | 21 | Ascending aorta (M/2D/3D) | 20–35 mm | 23 |

## Table 2.6.4 Recommendations for reporting TTE—continued

**Doppler measurement and valve assessment**

DIASTOLIC FUNCTION EVALUATION

| | | | | | | |
|---|---|---|---|---|---|---|
| E wave velocity (cm/s) | 100 | Valsalva | IVRT (ms) | 90 | e' lateral DTI (cm/s) | 6 |
| E Deceleration time (ms) | 160 | | QRS to onset of E wave (ms) | 320 | e' septum DTI (cm/s) | 5 |
| A wave velocity (cm/s) | | Valsalva | QRS to onset of e' wave (ms) | 330 | E/A ratio | Valsalva |
| A wave duration (ms) | | | Time e' – E (ms) | 10 | E/e' ratio | 18 |
| PV Ar wave duration (ms) | | | IVRT/Time e' – E | 9 | | |

| MITRAL VALVE (MV) | | | | AORTIC VALVE (AV) | | | | | |
|---|---|---|---|---|---|---|---|---|---|
| MV Area (cm²) | Planimetry (2D/3D) | Regurgitation (0–4+) | ++ | | ☑ Tricuspid<br>☐ Bicuspid | | LVOT diameter (mm) | 18 | Regurgitation (0 – 4+) |
| | PHT | Vena contracta (mm) | 3 | | Aortic valve area (cm²) | | Ao V flow vel. (m/s) | 1.1 | Vena contracta (mm) |
| Mean gradient (mmHg) | | ERO (cm²) | 0.07 | | Max gradient (mmHg) | | Ao V VTI (cm) | | ERO (cm²) |
| PHT (ms) | | Regurgitant volume (ml) | 12 | | Mean gradient (mmHg) | | LVOT flow vel. (m/s) | 1 | Regurgitant vol (ml) |
| Wilkins score (1–6) | | R PISA (mm) | 4 | V Aliasing   34 | Stroke volume (ml) | 40 | LVOT VTI (cm) | 16 | Ao diastolic vel. (cm/s) |

**Table 2.6.4 Recommendations for reporting TTE** *(continued)*

| Doppler measurement and valve assessment | | | | | | |
|---|---|---|---|---|---|---|
| TRICUSPID VALVE (TV) | | | PULMONARY VALVE (PV) | | | |
| Mean diastolic gradient (mmHg) | Peak regurgitant velocity (m/s) | 2,2 | Peak velocity (m/s) | 0.9 | Regurgitation (0 – 4+) | |
| | RV-RA peak systolic gradient (mmHg) | 19 | Peak systolic gradient (mmHg) | | Early-diastolic PR velocity (cm/s) | |
| Regurgitation (0 – 4+) + | RV systolic pressure (mmHg) | 22 | RVOT VTI (cm) | | End-diastolic PR velocity (cm/s) | |

**COMMENTS**

Open-text field or descriptive statements should elucidate the main findings of the study. This part of the report is crucial and answers the clinical queries, highlights the important findings and compares the data of the index study with previous ones. Major limitations or particular conditions (clinical, haemodynamics, etc.) prone to influencing the results should be reported. Additional data that cannot be included in the above tables (e.g. pericardium description etc.) are also prescribed in this section. The list of items to comment on could be:

**Left ventricle:** size, mass, global and regional systolic function, dynamic obstruction, mass, thrombus, dyssynchrony

**LV filling pressures :** normal, elevated

**Left atrial volume**

**Right ventricle:** size, systolic function

**Right atrial size**

**RA pressure and estimated pulmonary artery pressure** (PH unlikely, possible, likely)

**Aortic valve:** opening area, competence, sub-aortic obstruction

**Mitral valve:** opening area, competence

**Tricuspid valve:** opening area, competence

**Pulmonary valve:** opening area, competence

**Pericardium:** effusion, constriction

**Thoracic aorta:** dimension, atherosclerosis

## CONCLUSION

An echocardiographic study report should end with clear conclusions, emphasizing the main findings of the diagnosis and severity of the heart diseases. Universal grading data are encouraged (e.g. normal-mild dysfunction, moderate dysfunction, severe dysfunction, instead of subjective descriptions (e.g. preserved systolic function).

e.g.: **Dilated LV with severely impaired overall function. A moderate degree mitral regurgitation is also noticed. Shortness of breath of cardiac origin.**

**SIGNATURES**          Sonographer (or trainee physician)          Name of anyone senior who
                        performing exam                            has reviewed the study

# Suggested reading

1. Evangelista A, Flachskampf F, Lancellotti P, et al. on behalf of the European Association of Echocardiography. European Association of Echocardiography recommendations for standardization of performance, digital storage and reporting of echocardiographic studies. *Eur J Echocardiogr* 2008;9:438–48.

2. Lang R, Badano LP, Tsang W, et al. EAE/ASE recommendations for image acquisition and display using three-dimensional echocardiography. *Eur Heart J Cardiovascular Imaging* 2012;13:1–46.

3. Picard M, Adams D, Bierig SM, et al. American Society of Echocardiography recommendations for quality echocardiography laboratory operations. *J Am Soc Echocardiography* 2011;24:1–10.

# CHAPTER 3

# The Standard Transoesophageal Examination

# 3.1 Transoesophageal echocardiography (TOE)

## Clinical indications, procedure, and contraindications

**TOE examination is indicated when TTE is unable or unlikely to answer the clinical question**

### Search for a potential cardiovascular source of embolism

◆ Left ventricular apex or aneurysm (transgastric and low TOE 2CV views)

◆ Aortic and mitral valve (look for vegetations, degenerative changes, or tumours, i.e. fibroelastoma)

◆ Ascending and descending aorta, aortic arch (aneurysm, thrombi, atherosclerotic lesions)

◆ Left atrial appendage (including PW Doppler); note spontaneous contrast

◆ Left atrial body including atrial septum; note spontaneous contrast

◆ Fossa ovalis/foramen ovale/atrial septal defect/atrial septal aneurysm; contrast + Valsalva

### Infective endocarditis

◆ Mitral valve in multiple cross-sections

◆ AV in long- and short-axis views; para-aortic tissue (in particular short-axis views of AV and aortic root) to rule out abscess

- Tricuspid valve in transgastric views, low oesophageal view, and RV inflow–outflow view
- Pacemaker, central intravenous lines, aortic grafts, Eustachian valve, pulmonic valve in high basal short-axis view of the right heart (inflow–outflow view of the RV)

## Aortic dissection, aortic aneurysm

- Ascending aorta in long-axis and short-axis views; note maximal diameter, flap, intramural haematoma, para-aortic fluid
- Descending aorta in long- and short-axis views
- Aortic arch
- Aortic valve (note mechanism of aortic regurgitation)
- Relation of dissection membrane to coronary ostia
- Pericardial effusion, pleural effusion
- Entry/re-entry sites of dissection (colour Doppler)
- Spontaneous contrast or thrombus formation in false lumen (use colour Doppler to characterize flow/absence of flow in false lumen)

## Mitral regurgitation

- Mitral anatomy (transgastric basal short-axis view, multiple lower transoesophageal views). Mechanism and origin of regurgitation (mapping of prolapse/flail to leaflets and scallops, papillary muscle and chordal integrity, vegetations, paraprosthetic leaks)

- Colour Doppler of regurgitant jet (including proximal jet width and proximal convergence zone)
- Left upper and right upper pulmonary venous pulsed Doppler

## Prosthetic valves

- Obstruction (reduced opening/mobility of cusps/discs/leaflets and elevated velocities by CW Doppler)
- Regurgitation, with mapping of the origin of regurgitation to specific sites (transprosthetic, paraprosthetic); dehiscence/rocking of prosthesis
- Pathologic structural changes: calcification, immobilization, rupture, or perforation of bioprosthesis leaflets; absence of occluder in mechanical prostheses
- Presence of paraprosthetic structures (vegetation/thrombus/pannus, suture material, strand, abscess, pseudoaneurysm, fistula)

## Intra-operative or periprocedural (catheterization laboratory)

- Intra-operative monitoring of valvular repair (mainly mitral and aortic)
- Intra-operative monitoring of left ventricular function in high-risk patients
- Monitoring and guidance of valve interventions, e.g. transcatheter aortic valve implantation, transcatheter mitral repair, paravalvular leak closure
- Monitoring and guidance of atrial septal defect closure or left atrial appendage closure

# Competency in TOE

- Part of cardiology and cardiothoracic anaesthesiology training
- Certification in TOE by the European Association of Cardiovascular Imaging and the European Association of Cardiothoracic Anaesthesiologists (requires training under a supervisor, submitting a log book, and passing a multiple-choice question exam testing theoretical knowledge and image interpretation)

## Instrument and procedure

- Miniaturized transducer mounted on an endoscopic shaft. The transducer-containing instrument tip can be mechanically flexed anteriorly, posteriorly, to the right, and to the left
- Transducers are 'multi-plane' (rotatable within their casing, changing the imaging plane orientation around their central axis between 0° and 180°). The knobs for these manoeuvres, together with the control for plane orientation, are located at the handle of the instrument
- 2D or 2D and 3D images, with centre frequencies of 5–7 MHz
- Pulsed-wave, continuous-wave, and colour Doppler
- Probe must be mechanically cleansed and chemically disinfected after each use. Specific prescriptions exist for this, or the probe can be inserted in a dedicated cleaning apparatus. Cleaning procedures take at least 20–30 min
- Instruments should be inspected for damage after use, and periodic leakage current tests are recommended by the manufacturers

# Checklist before TOE

- ◆ Appropriate indication
- ◆ History of difficult earlier TOEs, difficulty in swallowing or serious pharyngeal, laryngeal, or oesophageal disease (i.e. diverticula, tumours, strictures)
- ◆ Patient consent
- ◆ Patient has fasted at least four hours
- ◆ ECG monitoring
- ◆ Intravenous access
- ◆ Conscious sedation, most widely with midazolam 2–4 mg (patient will be unfit for driving thereafter); deep sedation is not advisable
- ◆ Topical pharyngeal anaesthesia (value is unclear)
- ◆ Bite guard
- ◆ Left lateral decubitus position
- ◆ If a lot of sedation is used or the patient is in severely impaired haemodynamic condition, monitor oxygen saturation and blood pressure

## Introduction of TOE probe (Fig. 3.1.1)

- ◆ Probe should be advanced along a posterior and medial line through the pharynx and into the oesophagus

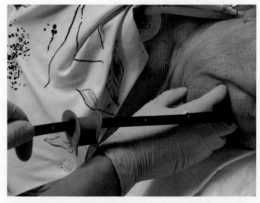

**Fig. 3.1.1** Introduction of TOE probe

- The upper oesophageal sphincter typically offers mild resistance, which waxes and wanes; no more than mild pressure should be applied
- Strong, elastic resistance suggests that the probe tip is caught in one of the recessus piriformes at the sides of the larynx
- No force should ever be applied during intubation. Check that the patient's head is not at a substantial angle with the neck
- Patient should try to swallow
- The tip may be guided with index and middle finger of one hand
- In case of difficulty, try with the patient sitting up
- In ventilated patients, use of a laryngoscope facilitates TOE probe placement

## Safety and contraindications

- Overall very safe
- Complications include laryngospasm, arrhythmias (both fast and slow), oesophageal perforation, and haemorrhage from oesophageal tumours
- Substantial resistance to advancement of probe: postpone TOE and ask for endoscopic exam
- Methaemoglobinaemia due to the topical anaesthetic agents prilocaine and benzocaine
- Electrical current leakage may occur after damage to the probe, such as from the patient's teeth; therefore, the probe has to be inspected after each use for damage
- If sedatives are used, resuscitation equipment and training are mandatory, and a benzodiazepine antagonist, e.g. flumazenil (0.3–0.6 mg), must be available
- Oesophageal or pharyngeal tumours are contraindications

- Anticoagulation, thrombocytopenia, or oesophageal varices increase the risk of bleeding, but are not absolute contraindications
- In aortic dissection, tight and documented blood pressure control during TOE is necessary

## Course of the exam

- The sequence of the examination is not standardized
  - if the procedure is not well tolerated, the main structure of interest should be visualized immediately
  - if the procedure is well tolerated or the patient in anaesthesia, a full systematic examination is advisable
  - a systematic exam has three parts
    1. transoesophageal windows
    2. transgastric windows
    3. aortic windows

## Standard 2D views and Doppler recordings of the TOE examination

**Lower-mid-oesophageal probe position** (Fig. 3.1.2ABC)

The following structures are visualized:

- left and right ventricle. LV often foreshortened, because good contact of the probe tip with the oesophagus often necessitates anteflexion
- atrioventricular valves
- atrial and ventricular septum

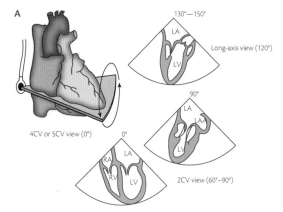

**Fig. 3.1.2A** Lower-mid-oesophageal probe position

After reducing the image depth, the mitral valve is examined by displaying it in the centre of the screen and systematically performing stepwise plane rotation

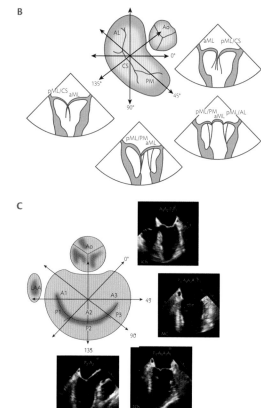

**Fig. 3.1.2BC** Focus on mitral valve

Schematic overview of mitral leaflets and scallops and the main TOE cross-sections used in mitral imaging. A1, A2, A3 are the segments of the anterior mitral leaflet opposite to P1, P2, P3. MC is a 'bicommissural' view of the mitral valve and the LV which bisects both mitral commissures and is found midway between two-chamber and four-chamber view at approximately 45°. 2Ch, two-chamber view, 3Ch, three-chamber view, 4Ch, four-chamber view. Reproduced, with permission, from Hahn RT, et al., *J Am Soc Echocardiogr* 2013;26:921–64

## Upper oesophageal probe position (Figs. 3.1.3–3.1.6)

Main pulmonary artery and cranial atrial view (0°). These views also show the superior vena cava (SVC) in a short axis and the inflow of the upper right pulmonary vein (RUPV) (Fig. 3.1.5).

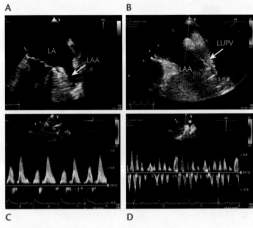

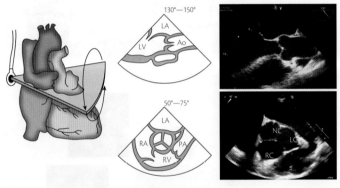

**Fig. 3.1.3**  Upper oesophageal probe position
Aortic valve long- (120°–150°) and short-axis views (30°–60°); the latter also shows the right ventricular inflow and outflow tract with the pulmonary valve. Aortic valve and aortic pathology should be systematically evaluated using long- and short-axis views. Orthogonal simultaneous views as generated by matrix (3D) transducers are helpful; e.g. to ensure that the true maximal anteroposterior diameter of the aortic annulus or the ascending aorta is displayed. In the short-axis view of the aortic valve, the right coronary artery takes off at approximately 6 o'clock and the left at approximately 1 o'clock. The right heart wraps around the aortic valve, with right atrium, tricuspid valve, inflow and outflow of the right ventricle, and pulmonary valve (at best faintly visible).

**Fig. 3.1.4**  Focus on LA appendage
Left atrial appendage and left upper pulmonary vein views (0°–90°; following Figure 3.1.4AB). The configuration of the left atrial appendage is quite variable. If not seen well at 0° slightly cranial from a four-chamber view, the plane should be rotated up to 90° to display the appendage in full length. Note spontaneous contrast, flow velocities (by pulsed Doppler inside the appendage, D) and possible thrombi, not to be confounded with pectinate muscles, which are small wall structures oriented perpendicular to the appendage long axis. Immediately posterior to the appendage, and separated by a tissue ridge, the inflow of the left upper pulmonary vein is located, which should be sampled by pulsed-wave Doppler especially for assessment of mitral regurgitation severity (C).

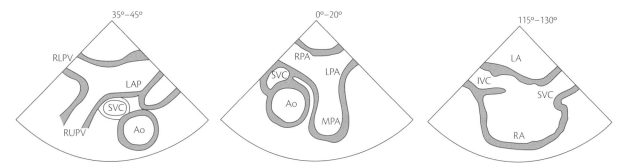

**Fig. 3.1.5** Focus on pulmonary artery (LPA/RPA left/right pulmonary artery; MPA main pulmonary artery

**Fig. 3.1.6** Focus right atrium

Sagittal view of the right and left atrium and superior/inferior caval veins (approximately 90°). This view is important to visualize atrial septal defects of secundum and sinus venosus type, foramen ovale, pacemaker electrodes, and the right atrial appendage (Fig. 3.1.6).

## Transgastric views (Fig. 3.1.7)

◆ Short-axis view of the LV at the papillary muscle level and at the MV level (0°). Inferior wall is on top and anterior wall at the bottom of the screen

◆ 2CV view of the LV (90°). Subvalvular mitral apparatus (chordae, papillary muscles) are very well seen

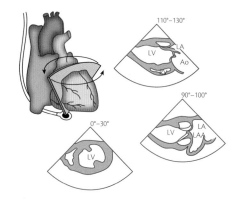

**Fig. 3.1.7** Transgastric views

- A long-axis equivalent at 90–120° shows the aortic valve and LVOT at an angle amenable to spectral-Doppler examination
- Right heart views (long-axis view of the RV inflow and outflow tract)
- Deep transgastric view with maximal anteflexion (transgastric 4CV, 5CV, or long-axis view at 0°–90°). Spectral-Doppler examination of the AV is often possible in these views

## Views of descending aorta and aortic arch (Fig. 3.1.8)

Structures in the aorta should be evaluated changing systematically between short- and long-axis views.

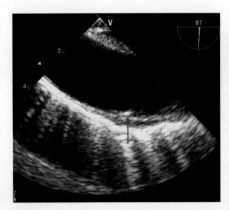 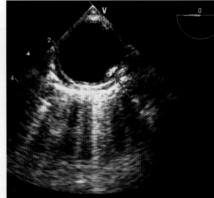

**Fig. 3.1.8** Focus on the aorta. Long- (left) and short- (right) axis view of descending aorta. Note atherosclerotic plaques (arrows)

# Essential imaging for specific clinical indications

## Infective endocarditis

- MV in multiple cross-sections
- AV in long- and short-axis view; aortic wall thickening (possible abscess)?
- TV in transgastric views, low oesophageal view, and right ventricular inflow–outflow view (modified aortic valve short-axis view)
- Pacemaker, central intravenous lines, Eustachian valve in sagittal right atrial view at 90°

## Source of embolism

- LA appendage (including pulsed-wave Doppler of inflow/outflow velocities): spontaneous contrast, sludge, thrombus?
- LA body: spontaneous contrast, thrombus, myxoma?
- Aortic and mitral valve: vegetations, fibroelastoma?
- Ascending and descending aorta and aortic arch: mobile thrombus, dissection flap?
- Interatrial septum: foramen ovale, septal defect, septal aneurysm?

## Aortic dissection and other aortic diseases

- Ascending aorta in long-axis and short-axis views, maximal diameter; note flap or intramural haematoma, para-aortic fluid, pericardial fluid, pleural fluid, entry and re-entry sites, spontaneous contrast or thrombus formation in false lumen

- Descending aorta in long- and short-axis views; note pathology as for ascending aorta
- Aortic arch; note maximal diameter, flap, intramural haematoma, para-aortic fluid
- AV (degree and mechanism of regurgitation, annular diameter, number of cusps). Relation of dissection membrane to coronary ostia

## Mitral regurgitation

- Mitral anatomy (transgastric basal short-axis view, multiple lower transoesophageal views)
- Mechanism and origin of regurgitation (detection and mapping of prolapse/flail to leaflets and scallops, papillary muscle and chordal integrity, vegetations)
- LA colour Doppler mapping with emphasis on jet width and proximal convergence ('PISA') zone (use zoom, modify colour-bar baseline to magnify proximal convergence zone)
- Left and right upper pulmonary venous flow

## Prosthetic valve evaluation

- Morphologic and Doppler evidence of obstruction (reduced opening/mobility of cusps/discs/leaflets, and elevated velocities by continuous-wave Doppler
- Morphologic and Doppler evidence of regurgitation, with mapping of the origin of regurgitation (transprosthetic, paraprosthetic); dehiscence?
- Prosthetic structure: calcification, perforation of bioprostheses, absence of occluder?

◆ Presence of additional paraprosthetic structures (vegetation, thrombus, or pannus; suture material, strand, abscess, pseudoaneurysm, fistula)

# Suggested reading

1. Flachskampf FA, Badano L, Daniel WG, et al. Recommendations for transoesophageal echocardiography—update 2010. *Eur J Echocardiogr* 2010;11:461–76.
2. Hahn RT, Abraham T, Adams MS, et al. Guidelines for performing a comprehensive transesophageal echocardiographic examination: recommendations from the American Society of Echocardiography and the Society of Cardiovascular Anesthesiologists. *J Am Soc Echocardiogr* 2013;26:921-64.
3. Habib G, Badano L, Tribouilloy C, et al; European Association of Echocardiography. Recommendations for the practice of echocardiography in infective endocarditis. *Eur J Echocardiogr* 2010;11:202–19.

# 3.2 The standard transoesophageal 3D echo examination

## General principles (Boxes 3.2.1, 3.2.2)

**Similar to 2D TOE**

## 3D TOE protocol

### Aortic valve (AV)

- 60° mid-oesophageal, short-axis view
- With or without colour (zoomed or full-volume acquisition) (Fig. 3.2.2A)
- 120° mid-oesophageal, long-axis view
- With or without colour (zoomed or full-volume acquisition) (Fig. 3.2.2B)

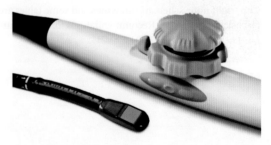

**Fig. 3.2.1** TOE probe

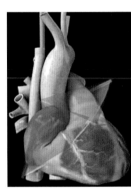

**Fig. 3.2.2AB** Aortic valve

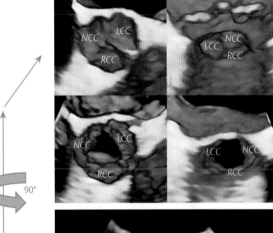

**Fig. 3.2.2A** AV seen from the aorta (left) and from the left ventricle (right) (LCC = left coronary cusp; NCC = non-coronary cusp; RCC = right coronary cusp)

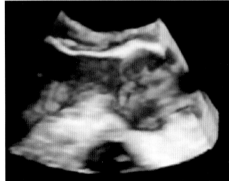

**Fig. 3.2.2B** Longitudinal view of the AV

## Mitral valve (MV)

- 0° to 120° mid-oesophageal views
- With or without colour (zoomed or full-volume acquisition) (Fig. 3.2.3AB)

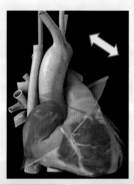

**Figs. 3.2.3AB** Mitral valve

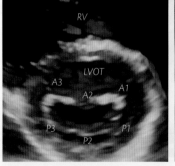

**Fig. 3.2.3A** MV from a ventricular perspective (LVOT = left ventricular outflow tract; RV = right ventricle)

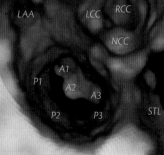

**Fig. 3.2.3B** MV seen from the left atrium (LCC = left coronary cusp; NCC = non-coronary cusp; RCC = right coronary cusp; LAA = left atrial appendage; A = anterior and P = posterior scallops)

## Pulmonary valve (PV)

- 90° high-oesophageal view
- With or without colour (zoomed acquisition) (Fig. 3.2.4AB)

## Tricuspid valve (TV)

- 0° to 30° mid-oesophageal 4CV
- With or without colour (zoomed acquisition)
- 40° transgastric view with anteflexion (Fig. 3.2.5AB)

## Left ventricle (LV)

- 0° to 120° mid-oesophageal views
- Encompassing the entire ventricle (full-volume acquisition) (Fig. 3.2.6)

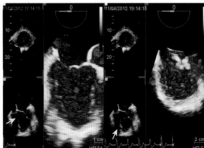

**Fig. 3.2.6** 3D view of the left ventricle

**A**

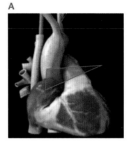

**B**

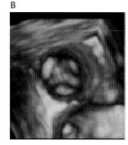

**Fig. 3.2.4** Pulmonic valve

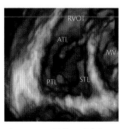

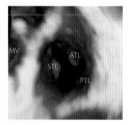

**Fig. 3.2.5A** Right atrial view of the TV (RVOT = right ventricular outflow tract)

**Fig. 3.2.5B** Right ventricular view of the TV (A = anterior; S = septal; P = posterior; TL = tricuspid leaflet)

## Right ventricle (RV)

- 0° to 120° mid-oesophageal views
- Encompassing the right ventricle tilted to be in the centre of the image (full-volume acquisition)

## Interatrial septum

- 0°, the probe is rotated to the interatrial septum (zoomed or full-volume acquisition) (Fig. 3.2.7)

# Specific windows and views

## Before TAVI

- Aortic annulus measure/stepwise approach (Fig. 3.2.8)

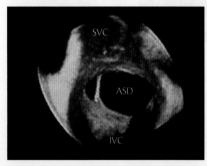

**Fig. 3.2.7** Right atrial view of the interatrial septum with an ASD (ASD = atrial septal defect; SVC = superior vena cava; IVC = inferior vena cava)

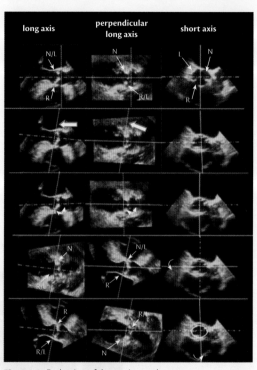

**Fig. 3.2.8** Evaluation of the aortic annulus

- Coronary ostia distance (Fig. 3.2.9)

# Suggested reading

1. Flachskampf FA, Badano L, Daniel WG, et al. Recommendations for transoesophageal echocardiography—update 2010. *Eur J Echocardiogr* 2010;11:461–76.
2. Lang RM, Badano LP, Tsang W, et al. EAE/ASE recommendations for image acquisition and display using three-dimensional echocardiography. *Eur Heart J Cardiovasc Imaging* 2012;13:1–46.
3. Faletra FF, Pedrazzini G, Pasotti E, et al. 3D TEE during catheter-based interventions. *JACC Cardiovasc Imaging* 2014;7:292–308.
4. Faletra FF, Ramamurthi A, Dequarti MC, et al. Artifacts in three-dimensional transesophageal echocardiography. *J Am Soc Echocardiogr* 2014;27:453–62.

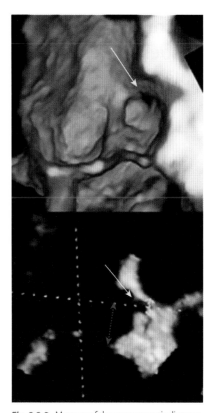

**Fig. 3.2.9** Measure of the coronary ostia distance

# 3.3 The storage and report on transoesophageal echocardiography (Tables 3.3.1, 3.3.2, 3.3.3A, 3.3.3B, 3.3.4)

**Table 3.3.1** Minimal basic dataset to acquire and store

| Projections[a] | 2D[b] | Colour[c] | Spectral[d] PW | Spectral[d] CW |
|---|---|---|---|---|
| **1. Mid-oesophageal views** | | | | |
| A Four-chamber view | e | | | |
| B Left atrial appendage view | | | | |
| C Two-chamber view of LV | | | | |
| D Cross-commissural view of MV | | | | |
| E Long-axis view of LV, MV, AV, and aortic root | | | | |
| F Short-axis view at the level of the AV | | | | |
| G Views of PV, pulmonary artery, and bifurcation | | | | |
| H Bicaval view | e | | | |
| J Views of pulmonary veins | | | | |
| **2. Transgastric view** | | | | |
| A Short-axis view of LV | | | | |

Table 3.3.1 Minimal basic dataset to acquire and store (*continued*)

| Projections[a] | 2D[b] | Colour[c] | Spectral[d] PW | CW |
|---|---|---|---|---|
| B  Two-chamber view of LV | ■ | | | |
| C  Long-axis view of LV (includes LV outflow tract) | ■ | ▨ | | ▨ |
| D  Long-axis view of right heart | ■ | | | |
| E  Short-axis view of right heart | ■ | | | |
| **3. Views of descending thoracic aorta** | | | | |
| A  Short axis | ■ | | | |
| B  Long axis | ■ | c | | |
| **4. Views of aortic arch** | ■ | c | | |
| **5. Views of ascending aorta** | ■ | c | | |

a. Red boxes: mandatory acquisitions; Orange boxes: conditional acquisitions.

b. 2D imaging of these views can be obtained by proper positioning of the transducer along with advancement, pulling out, flexion, retroflexion, sideward flexion, and/or rotation of the probe.

c. Colour-flow Doppler examination may be performed at the end of the grey-scale (B-mode) imaging of all four valves and the atrial septum. Colour Doppler interrogation is essential when the TTE study data are considered suboptimal in quality in comparison with the TOE examination (e.g. dissection of the aorta).

d. PW and CW Doppler are optional when the required assessments (e.g. RV systolic pressure, diastolic LV function, valve gradients, pulmonary venous flow), have already been performed in the previous transthoracic study. A new interrogation is rational when the TTE study data are considered suboptimal in quality in comparison with the TOE examination. Left atrial appendage velocities can only be measured during the TOE study.

e. Occasionally, agitated saline contrast at rest and with release of Valsalva manoeuvre may be required to reveal intracardiac or intrapulmonary shunting.

## Table 3.3.2 3D dataset acquisition and display

| | AV | LV | RV | PV | MV | IAS | TV |
|---|---|---|---|---|---|---|---|
| 60° mid-oesophageal, short-axis view | ■■ FZ | | | | | | |
| 120° mid-oesophageal, long-axis view | ■■ FZ | | | | | | |
| 0° to120° mid-oesophageal views | | | | | ■■ Z | | |
| LV - 0° to120° mid-oesophageal views encompassing the entire ventricle | | ■ F | | | | | |
| RV - mid- 0° to 120° oesophageal views with the RV tilted to be in the centre of the image | | | ■ F | | | | |
| 0° with the probe rotated to the IAS | | | | | | ■ FZ | |
| 90° high-oesophageal view | | | | ■■ Z | | | |
| 120° mid-oesophageal, 3-chamber view | | | | ■■ Z | | | |
| 0° to30° mid-oesophageal, 4-chamber view | | | | | | | ■■ Z |
| 40° transgastric view with anteflexion | | | | | | | ■■ Z |

**F** full-volume acquisition    ■ loops without colour
**Z** zoomed acquisition    ■ loops with colour

## Table 3.3.3A  Recommendations for reporting TOE

Facility i.e. Hospital name, Unit, Department.

| Patient first name | xxxx | Patient last name | xxxx | Date of birth | dd-mm-yyyy |
|---|---|---|---|---|---|
| Gender | F | Patient ID | 12345 | Study quality | Good |
| Referring Physician/Dept. | A.S. (name with initials) | Study ordered | dd-mm-yyyy | Study performed | dd-mm-yyyy |
| Indication for the study | e.g. Shortness of breath | | | | |

| Echo instrument identifier | Brand name of echo machine (e.g. HP) | Location of patient (✓) | ICU | ✓ | Heart rhythm: e.g. atrial fibrillation |
|---|---|---|---|---|---|
| | | | OR | | |
| Intubated (Y/N) | N | | ER | | Heart rate (bpm) : 90 |
| Sedated (Y/N) | Y | | PACU | | |
| Weight (kg) | 70 | | Echo lab | | Blood pressure (mmHg): 120/80 |
| Height (cm) | 167 | | Outpatient | | |
| BSA (m²) | 1, 8 | | | | Probe insertion: easy, difficult, failed |

### B-mode and Doppler measurements

| Aorta | Diameter (mm) | Dissection (Y/N) | Plaque thickness (mm) | | Plaque mobile (Y/N) |
|---|---|---|---|---|---|
| Root (sinus level) | 33 | n | 0-3, | >3 | |
| Sinotubular junction | 32 | n | 0-3, | >3 | |
| Ascending aorta | 33 | n | 0-3, | >3 | |
| Arch | 30 | n | 0-3, | >3 | |
| Descending aorta | 28 | n | 0-3, | >3 | n |

**Table 3.3.3B  Recommendations for reporting TOE**

| Atria | Size (normal, dilated) | Spontaneous contrast (Y/N) | Thrombus (Y/N) | Tumour (Y/N) | Device (Y/N) |
|---|---|---|---|---|---|
| Right atrium | n | n | n | n | n |
| Left atrium | d | n | n | n | n |
| Left atrial appendage | comments, e.g.: thrombus, spontaneous contrast, etc. | | | | |
| Interatrial septum | comments, e.g.: normal, aneurysmal, PFO, ASD (type), shunt (R>L, L>R, bidirectional) | | | | |
| Other comments | | | | | |

| Ventricles | LV | RV | LV regional function (1=normal, 2=hypokinetic, 3=akinetic, 4=dyskinetic) | | | |
|---|---|---|---|---|---|---|
| Size (normal, dilated) | | | **Basal Segments** | **Mid Segments** | **Apical Segments** | |
| | | | 1. Anterior | 7. Anterior | 13. Anterior | |
| Hypertrophy (Y/N) | | | 2. Anteroseptal | 8. Anteroseptal | 14. Septal | |
| | | | 3. Inferoseptal | 9. Inferoseptal | 15. Inferior | |
| Thrombus (Y/N) | | | 4. Inferior | 10. Inferior | 16. Lateral | |
| | | | 5. Posterior | 11. Posterior | 17. Apex | |
| Overall function (normal, ↓, ↓↓, ↓↓↓) | | | 6. Lateral | 12. Lateral | | |
| Comments: | | | | | | |

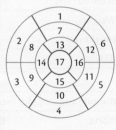

**Table 3.3.3B  Recommendations for reporting TOE** (*continued*)

| Valves | | | | | | | |
|---|---|---|---|---|---|---|---|
| | **Annulus** (normal, dilated, calcified) | **Stenosis** (no, mild, moderate, severe) | **Area** | **Gradient** | **Regurg.** (0–4+) | **Leaflet Morphology** e.g. normal, myxomatous, calcified, vegetation, perforated, bicuspid, thickened | **Leaflet/Disc Motion** e.g. normal, prolapse flail, restricted, SAM |
| **Aortic valve** (NCC/RCC/LCC) | n | no | | | | | |
| **Mitral valve** ($A_1$, $A_2$, $A_3$/$P_1$, $P_2$, $P_3$) | d | no | P2-3 | | ++ | myxomatous | prolapse |
| **Tricuspid** | n | no | | | | | |
| **Prosthetic (1)** | | | | | | | |
| **Prosthetic (2)** | | | | | | | |

**Table 3.3.4  Recommendations for reporting TOE**

**COMMENTS**

As in the transthoracic examination, open-text field or descriptive statements should elucidate the main findings of the study. This part of the report is crucial and answers the clinical queries, highlights the important findings and compares the data of the index study with previous ones. Major limitations or particular conditions (clinical, haemodynamics, etc.) prone to influencing the results should be reported. Additional data that cannot be included in the above tables are also prescribed in this section (e.g. incidental finding of pleural effusion, pericardium description. [etc.]). It is also recommended (especially with computerized report generation) to specify whether certain cardiac structures have or have not been studied. It is mandatory to note all side effects and complications.

**Table 3.3.4 Recommendations for reporting TOE** (*continued*)

**CONCLUSION**

An echocardiographic study report should end with clear conclusions, emphasizing the main findings of the diagnosis and severity of the heart diseases.

**SIGNATURES**

| Sonographer (or trainee physician) performing exam | Name of anyone senior who has reviewed the study |
|---|---|
| | |

# Suggested reading

1. Flachskampf F, Badano L, Daniel WG, et al. Recommendations for transoesophageal echocardiography: update 2010. *Eur J of Echocardiography* 2010;11:557–76.

2. Lang R, Badano LP, Tsang W, et al. EAE/ASE Recommendations for image acquisition and display using three-dimensional echocardiography. *Eur Heart J Cardiovascular Imaging* 2012;13:1–46.

3. Recommendations for a standardized report for adult perioperative echocardiography from the Society of Cardiovascular Anaesthesiologists/American Society of Echocardiography Task Force for standardized perioperative echocardiography report. (<http://www2.scahq.org/sca3/teereport.shtml>).

## List of abbreviations

**2D,** two-dimensional echocardiography; **AV,** aortic valve; **CW,** continuous-wave Doppler; **ER,** emergency room; **IAS,** interatrial septum; **ICU,** Intensive Care Unit; **LV,** left ventricle; **MV,** mitral valve; **OR,** Operating room; **PACU,** postanaesthaesia care unit; **PV,** pulmonic valve; **PW,** pulsed-wave Doppler; **RV,** right ventricle; **TV,** tricuspid valve

# CHAPTER 4

# Assessment of the Left Ventricular Systolic Function

# 4.1 Left chamber quantification

## Left ventricle (LV): Measurement of LV size

### Linear measurements

- **Internal linear dimensions**
  - Use PTLAX view obtained perpendicular to the LV long axis (Fig. 4.1.1A)
  - Measured at the level of the mitral valve leaflet tips
  - Electronic calipers should be positioned on the interface between wall and cavity and the interface between wall and pericardium
- **Techniques**
  - M-mode tracing (Fig. 4.1.1B)
  - 2D-guided linear measurements (Fig. 4.1.1CD)
- **Advantages**
  - Reproducible
  - High temporal resolution
  - Wealth of published data
- **Limitations**
  - Beam orientation frequently off axis
  - Single dimension, i.e. representative only in normally shaped ventricles

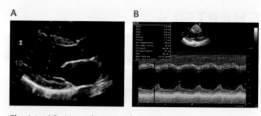

**Fig. 4.1.1AB** M-mode tracing from PTLAX view

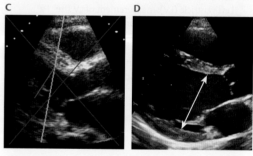

**Fig. 4.1.1CD** M-mode cursor (white) not perpendicular to LV walls (C). Use 2D measurement (arrow) (D)

## Volumetric measurements

- LV volumes are measured using 2DE or 3DE
- Volume calculations derived from linear measurements are not recommended (i.e. Teichholz or Quinones methods)

### End-diastolic (EDV) and end-systolic (ESV) volumes

- Based on tracings of the blood–tissue interface in the AP 4CV and 2CV
- Trace endocardial borders excluding papillary muscles
- Connect MV insertions on the annulus with straight line
- LV length is defined as the distance between the middle of this line and the most distant point of the LV contour
- Acquiring LV views at a reduced depth in order to focus on the LV cavity will reduce the likelihood of foreshortening and minimize errors in endocardial border tracings

### Techniques

- Biplane disc's summation
- Area–length method
- Endocardial border enhancement (contrast echo)
- 3DE imaging

### Tracings

◆ End-diastole = frame preceding MV closure or the frame in the cardiac cycle, in which the LV dimension/volume is the largest

◆ End-systole = frame following AV closure or the frame in which the LV dimension/volume is the smallest

◆ In regular heart rhythm, measurements of the timing of valve openings and closures may be derived from M-mode echo, PW- or CW-Doppler

## Biplane disc's summation (Fig. 4.1.2)

### Indications

◆ The recommended 2DE method

### Advantages

◆ Corrects for shape distortions

◆ Less geometrical assumptions compared to linear dimensions

### Limitations

◆ Apex frequently foreshortened

◆ Endocardial dropout

◆ Blind to shape distortions not visualized in the AP 2CV and 4CV

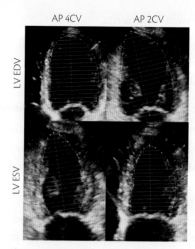

**Fig. 4.1.2** Biplane disc's summation

## Area–length (Fig. 4.1.3)

### Indications

◆ When apical endocardial definition precludes accurate tracing

### Advantages

◆ Partial correction for shape distortion

### Limitations

◆ Apex frequently foreshortened
◆ Heavily based on geometrical assumptions
◆ Limited data on normal population

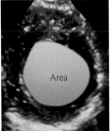
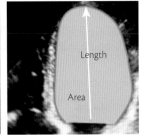

**Fig. 4.1.3** Area–length method. The area is obtained from the PTSAX and the length from AP–4CV

## Endocardial border enhancement (Fig. 4.1.4)

### Indications

◆ Indicated to improve endocardial delineation when ≥ 2 contiguous LV endocardial segments are poorly visualized

### Advantages

◆ Helpful in patients with suboptimal acoustic window
◆ Provides volumes that are closer to those measured with cardiac magnetic resonance

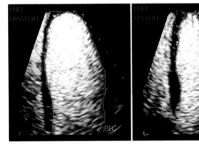

**Fig. 4.1.4** Contrast enhancement echo

## Limitations

- Same limitations as the above non-contrast 2D techniques
- Acoustic shadowing in LV basal segments with excess contrast

### 3D echo imaging (Fig. 4.1.5)

#### Advantages

- No geometrical assumption
- Unaffected by foreshortening
- More accurate and reproducible compared to other imaging modalities

#### Limitations

- Lower temporal resolution
- Fewer published data on normal values
- Image quality dependent

# LV global systolic function

## LV fractional shortening (FS) (Fig. 4.1.6)

- Derived from 2D-guided M-mode or preferably from linear measurements obtained from 2D images (see Table 4.1.1)
- Appropriate only if there are no regional wall motion abnormalities

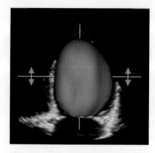

**Fig. 4.1.5** 3D echo imaging (full-volume acquisition centred on the LV)

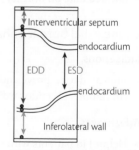

**Fig. 4.1.6** M-mode tracing to assess FS

**Table 4.1.1** Normal ranges and severity partition cut-off values for 2D-derived LV size, function, and mass

| | Male | | | | Female | | | |
|---|---|---|---|---|---|---|---|---|
| | Normal range | Mildly abnormal | Moderately abnormal | Severely abnormal | Normal range | Mildly abnormal | Moderately abnormal | Severely abnormal |
| LV diastolic diameter (cm) | 4.2–5.8 | 5.9–6.3 | 6.4–6.8 | > 6.8 | 3.8–5.2 | 5.3–5.6 | 5.7–6.1 | > 6.1 |
| LV diastolic diameter/BSA (cm/m²) | 2.2–3.0 | 3.1–3.3 | 3.4–3.6 | > 3.6 | 2.3–3.1 | 3.2–3.4 | 3.5–3.7 | > 3.7 |
| LV systolic diameter (cm) | 2.5–4.0 | 4.1–4.3 | 4.4–4.5 | > 4.5 | 2.2–3.5 | 3.6–3.8 | 3.9–4.1 | > 4.1 |
| LV systolic diameter/BSA (cm/m²) | 1.3–2.1 | 2.2–2.3 | 2.4–2.5 | > 2.5 | 1.3–2.1 | 2.2–2.3 | 2.4–2.6 | > 2.6 |
| LV diastolic volume (mL) | 62–150 | 151–174 | 175–200 | > 200 | 46–106 | 107–120 | 121–130 | > 130 |
| LV diastolic volume/BSA (mL/m²) | 34–74 | 75–89 | 90–100 | > 100 | 29–61 | 62–70 | 71–80 | > 80 |
| LV systolic volume (mL) | 21–61 | 62–73 | 74–85 | > 85 | 14–42 | 43–55 | 56–67 | > 67 |
| LV systolic volume/BSA (mL/m²) | 11–31 | 32–38 | 39–45 | > 45 | 8–24 | 25–32 | 33–40 | > 40 |
| LV ejection fraction (%) | 52–72 | 41–51 | 30–40 | < 30 | 54–74 | 41–53 | 30–40 | < 30 |
| Septal wall thickness (cm) | 0.6–1.0 | 1.1–1.3 | 1.4–1.6 | > 1.6 | 0.6–0.9 | 1.0–1.2 | 1.3–1.5 | > 1.5 |
| Posterior wall thickness (cm) | 0.6–1.0 | 1.1–1.3 | 1.4–1.6 | > 1.6 | 0.6–0.9 | 1.0–1.2 | 1.3–1.5 | > 1.5 |
| LV mass (g) | 88–224 | 225–258 | 259–292 | > 292 | 67–162 | 163–186 | 187–210 | > 210 |
| LV mass/BSA (g/m²) | 49–115 | 116–131 | 132–148 | > 148 | 43–95 | 96–108 | 109–121 | > 121 |
| LV mass (g) | 96–200 | 201–227 | 228–254 | > 254 | 66–150 | 151–171 | 172–193 | > 193 |
| LV mass/BSA (g/m²) | 50–102 | 103–116 | 117–130 | > 130 | 44–88 | 89–100 | 101–112 | > 112 |
| Maximum LA volume/BSA (mL/m²) | 16–34 | 35–41 | 42–48 | > 48 | 16–34 | 35–41 | 42–48 | > 48 |

- Proved in uncomplicated hypertension, obesity, or valvular diseases
- FS = ((LVEDD − LVESD)/LVEDD) × 100%
- Reference values = 28–44%

## LV ejection fraction (LVEF)

- 2D (biplane method of discs = modified Simpson's rules) or 3D (to be used if good image quality)
- LVEF = ((LVEDV − LVESV)/LEDV) × 100%
- LVEF is not significantly related to gender, age, and BSA
- Reference upper 2DE limits
  - Men: LVEDV = 74 ml/m$^2$, LVESV = 31 ml/m$^2$
  - Women: LVEDV = 61 ml/m$^2$, LVESV = 24 ml/m$^2$
  - LVEF = 63 ± 5%; range 53–73% above 20 years
- A value of LVEF < 53% is suggestive of abnormal LV systolic function

## Global longitudinal strain (GLS) (Fig. 4.1.7)

- The most commonly used strain-based measure of LV global systolic function
- Obtained often with speckle tracking, less frequently with Doppler tissue imaging (DTI)

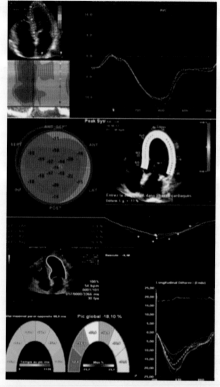

**Fig. 4.1.7** Examples of measurement of GLS using different software

- GLS is the relative length change of the LV myocardium between end-diastole and end-systole
- GLS measurements obtained in the three standard apical views should be averaged
- GLS calculation can be obtained using endocardial, mid-wall, or average deformation
- Most of data come from mid-wall GLS, which is reproducible and robust
- In a healthy person, a peak GLS around −20% can be expected
- GLS decreases with age and is slightly higher in women

## Other parameters

- **Cardiac output:** normal stroke volume > 35 ml/m$^2$ and cardiac output > 4 L/min
- **LV dP/dt:** values < 1000 mmHg are abnormal
- **Myocardial performance index:** values > 0.47 identify systolic dysfunction

# LV regional function

## LV segmental analysis (Figs. 4.1.8, 4.1.9, 4.1.10)

- For the assessment of regional LV function, the LV is divided into a 16, 17, or 18 segments model, which reflect coronary perfusion territories
- The 17-segment model should be used for myocardial perfusion studies or when comparing different imaging modalities, SPECT, PET, or CMR

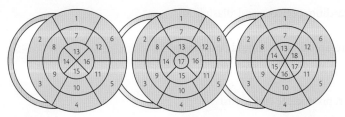

**all models**

1. basal anterior
2. basal anteroseptal
3. basal inferoseptal
4. basal inferior
5. basal inferolateral
6. basal anterolateral
7. mid anterior
8. mid anteroseptal
9. mid inferoseptal
10. mid inferior
11. mid inferolateral
12. mid anterolateral

**16 and 17 segment model**

13. apical anterior
14. apical septal
15. apical inferior
16. apical lateral

**17 segment model only**

17. apex

**18 segment model only**

13. apical anterior
14. apical anteroseptal
15. apical inferoseptal
16. apical inferior
17. apical inferolateral
18. apical anterolateral

**alternatively, walls are commonly labelled as:**

3., 9., 15(18-seg.) : septal;   5., 11., 17(18-seg.) : posterior;   6.,12.,18(18-seg.) : lateral

**Fig. 4.1.8** Schematic diagram of the different LV segmentation models

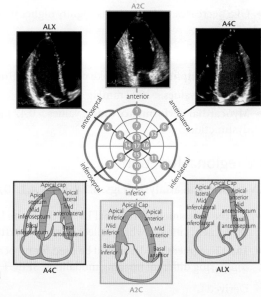

**Fig. 4.1.9** Orientation of apical four-, two-chamber, and long-axis (AP 4CV, AP 2CV, and APLAX) views in relation to the bull's-eye display of the LV segments

- ◆ Scoring to assess wall motion
  - ◆ each segment should be analysed individually in multiple views
  - ◆ 1 = normal or hyperkinetic, 2 = hypokinetic (reduced thickening), 3 = akinetic (absent or negligible thickening), and 4 = dyskinetic (systolic thinning or stretching)

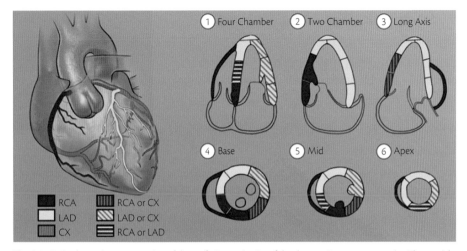

**Fig. 4.1.10** A schematic representation of the perfusion territories of the three major coronary arteries. The arterial distribution varies between patients. Some segments have variable coronary perfusion

- The 16-segment model is recommended for routine studies assessing wall motion, since endocardial excursion and thickening of the tip of the apex is imperceptible

## LV mass

- Most used in epidemiology and treatment studies
- Measurements performed at the end of diastole (frame prior to MV opening)
- Derived from M-mode, 2DE, and 3DE

## Linear measurements (M-mode tracing or 2D-guided)
(Figs. 4.1.1AB and 4.1.11)

- Cube formula = 0.8 (1.04 ([LVIDd + PWTd + IVSTD]$^3$ − [LVIDd]$^3$)) + 0.6 g LVIDd = LV internal diameter in diastole; PWTd = LV posterior wall thickness in diastole
- Advantages
  - Fast and widely used
  - Wealth of published data
  - Demonstrated prognostic value
  - Fairly accurate in normally shaped ventricles (i.e. systemic hypertension, aortic stenosis)
  - Simple for screening large populations
- Limitations
  - Based on the assumption that the LV is a prolate ellipsoid with a 2:1 long-: short-axis ratio and symmetric distribution of hypertrophy
  - Beam orientation frequently off axis
  - Since linear measurements are cubed, even small measurement errors in dimensions or thickness have an impact on accuracy

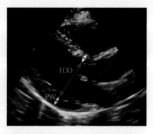

**Fig. 4.1.11** 2D-guided linear measurements

## 2D: Truncated ellipsoid (TE) or area–length (AL) (Fig. 4.1.12)

**LV mass (TE) = 1.05 {(b+t)$^2$ [⅔(a+1) +d − d$^3$/3(a+t)$^2$] − b$^2$ [⅔ a+d − d$^3$/3a$^2$]}**

**LV mass (AL) = 1.05 { [⅚ A$_1$ (a+d+t) ] − [⅚ A$_2$ (a+d)]}**

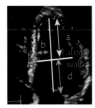 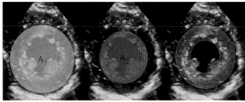

**Fig. 4.1.12** 2D assessment of LV mass

- ◆ Limitations
  - ◆ Good image quality and properly oriented PTSAX views (no oblique planes) are required
  - ◆ Good epicardial definition is required
  - ◆ Higher measurement variability
  - ◆ Few published normative data
  - ◆ Limited prognostic data

## 3D echo LV mass estimation (Fig. 4.1.13)

### Advantages

- ◆ Direct measurement without geometrical assumptions about cavity shape and hypertrophy distribution
- ◆ More accurate than the linear or the 2D measurements
- ◆ Higher inter-measurement and test/retest reproducibility
- ◆ Discriminates small changes within patients better

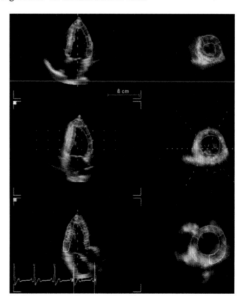

**Fig. 4.1.13** 3D assessment of LV

## Limitations

◆ Normal values less well established
◆ Dependent on image quality
◆ LV myocardial volume = (LV epicardial volume − LV endocardial volume) × 1.05

## Recommendations

◆ In normally shaped LV, both M-mode and 2DE formulas can be used
◆ In abnormally shaped ventricles or in patients with asymmetric or localized hypertrophy, 3D echo is recommended
◆ Reference upper limits
  ◆ Linear measurements: 95 g/m² in women; 115 g/m² in men
  ◆ 2D measurements: 88 g/m² in women; 102 g/m² in men
  ◆ Limited values with 3D echo
  ◆ Relative wall thickness = RWT = (2 × PWT)/LVED internal diameter
  ◆ Concentric LVH (RWT > 0.42) or eccentric LVH (RWT ≤ 0.42) (Fig. 4.1.14)

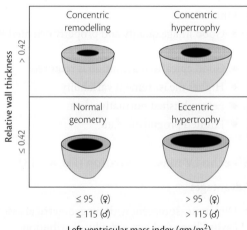

**Fig. 4.1.14** Types of LV hypertrophy

# Left atrial (LA) measurements

**TTE is the recommended approach for assessing LA size (see Table 4.1.2)**
**TOE: the entire LA frequently cannot fit in the image sector**

## Internal linear dimensions → LA anteroposterior diameter—M-mode tracings (Fig. 4.1.15)

◆ PTLAX view perpendicular to the aortic root long axis, and measured at the level of the aortic sinuses by using the leading-edge to leading-edge convention at the end of systole

**Table 4.1.2** Normal values of LA size

|  | Women | Men |
|---|---|---|
| AP dimension (cm) | 2.7–3.8 | 3.0–4.0 |
| AP dimension index (cm/m²) | 1.5–2.3 | 1.5–2.3 |
| AP 4CV area index (cm/m²) | 9.3 ± 1.7 | 8.9 ± 1.5 |
| AP 2CV area index (cm/m²) | 9.6 ± 1.4 | 9.3 ± 1.6 |
| AP 4CV volume index MOD (cm/m²) | 25.1 ± 7.2 | 24.5 ± 6.4 |
| AP 4CV volume index AL (cm/m²) | 27.3 ± 7.9 | 27.0 ± 7.0 |
| AP 2CV volume index MOD (cm/m²) | 26.1 ± 6.7 | 27.1 ± 7.9 |
| AP 2CV volume index AL (cm/m²) | 28.0 ± 7.3 | 28.9 ± 8.5 |

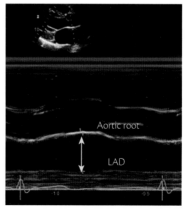

**Fig. 4.1.15** LA measurement: M-mode

## Advantages

- Reproducible, high temporal resolution
- Wealth of published data

## Limitations

- Single dimension not representative of actual LA size (i.e. dilated LA)

## 2D-guided linear measurements (Fig. 4.1.16)

## Advantages

- Facilitates orientation perpendicular to LA posterior wall

## Limitations

- Lower frame rates than in M-mode
- Single dimension only

## 2D echo assessment of LA size

## Area

- Measured in 4CV, at end-systole, on the frame just prior to MV opening by tracing the LA inner border, excluding the area under the MV annulus and the inlet of the pulmonary veins (Fig. 4.1.17A)

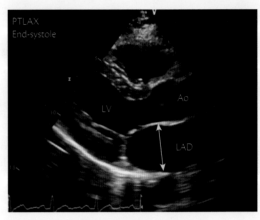

**Fig. 4.1.16** 2D-guided linear LA measurement

### Advantage

♦ More representative of actual LA size than anteroposterior diameter only

### Limitations

♦ Need for a dedicated view to avoid left atrial foreshortening
♦ Assumes a symmetric shape of the atrium

## Volume

### Tracings

♦ 2D volumetric measurements are based on tracings of the blood-tissue interface on AP 4CV and AP 2CV (Fig. 4.1.17AB)
♦ Connect MV insertions on the annulus with straight line
♦ Endocardial tracing should exclude atrial appendage and pulmonary veins
♦ LA length L is defined as the shortest of the two long axes measured in AP 4CV and AP 2CV views (Fig. 4.1.17AB)

### Techniques

♦ Biplane disc's summation (Fig. 4.1.18AB)
♦ Area–length method (Fig. 4.1.17AB)

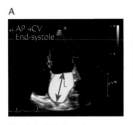
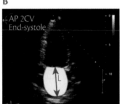

**Fig. 4.1.17** LA tracings

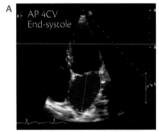
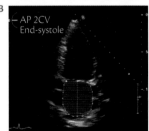

**Fig. 4.1.18** Biplane disc's summation

### Advantages

- ◆ Enables accurate assessment of the asymmetric remodelling of the left atrium
- ◆ More robust predictor of cardiovascular events than linear or area measurements

### Limitations

- ◆ Geometric assumptions about left atrial shape
- ◆ Few accumulated data on normal population
- ◆ Single plane volume calculations are inaccurate since they are based on the assumption that A1 = A2

## 3D echo imaging (Fig. 4.1.19)

- ◆ 3D datasets are usually obtained from the apical approach using a multi-beat full-volume acquisition

### Advantages

- ◆ No geometrical assumption about LA shape
- ◆ More accurate when compared to 2D measurements

### Limitations

- ◆ Dependent on adequate image quality
- ◆ Lower temporal resolution
- ◆ Limited data on normal values

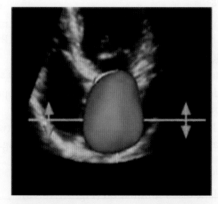

**Fig. 4.1.19** 3D echo imaging
(full-volume acquisition centred on the LA)

## Recommendations for LA measurements

◆ The biplane disc's-summation method is the preferred approach
◆ Indexing to BSA LA parameters is recommended
◆ The upper limit of normality for 2DE LA volume is 34 ml/m$^2$ for both genders

# Aortic annulus and aortic root

◆ The aortic root extends from the basal attachments of the AV leaflets within the LVOT to their distal attachment to the aorta sinotubular junction (see Table 4.1.3)
◆ **The aortic root includes**
  ◆ the aortic valve annulus
  ◆ the inter-leaflet triangles
  ◆ the semilunar aortic leaflets and their attachments
  ◆ the aortic sinuses of Valsalva
  ◆ the sinotubular junction

**Table 4.1.3** Aortic root dimensions in normal adults

| Aortic root | Absolutes Values (cm) | | Indexed Values (cm/m²) | |
|---|---|---|---|---|
| Annulus | 2.6 ± 0.3 | 2.3 ± 0.2 | 1.3 ± 0.1 | 1.3 ± 0.1 |
| Sinuses of Valsalva | 3.4 ± 0.3 | 3.0 ± 0.3 | 1.7 ± 0.2 | 1.8 ± 0.2 |
| Sinotubular junction | 2.9 ± 0.3 | 2.6 ± 0.3 | 1.5 ± 0.2 | 1.5 ± 0.2 |
| Proximal ascending aorta | 3.0 ± 0.4 | 2.7 ± 0.4 | 1.5 ± 0.2 | 1.6 ± 0.3 |

◆ **The aortic annulus** (Fig. 4.1.20)

    ◆ is not a distinct anatomic structure

    ◆ virtual annulus: the basal attachments of the aortic leaflets

    ◆ true anatomic ring: distal attachment to the aorta (shape of a crown)

    ◆ is more often an ellipse than a circle

        ◆ larger diameter in the medial-lateral direction

        ◆ a smaller diameter in the anterior-posterior direction (often measured in 2D TTE PTLAX or TOE long axis)

## Aortic measurements

◆ Annulus (Fig. 4.1.21)

    ◆ PTLAX using 2D echo

    ◆ zoom mode

    ◆ in mid-systole (annulus is slightly larger and rounder than in diastole)

    ◆ measure from inner edge to inner edge

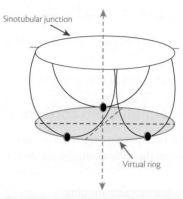

**Fig. 4.1.20** Crown shape of the aortic annulus

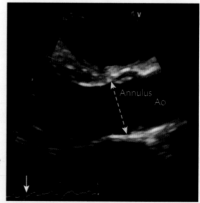

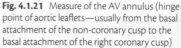

**Fig. 4.1.21** Measure of the AV annulus (hinge point of aortic leaflets—usually from the basal attachment of the non-coronary cusp to the basal attachment of the right coronary cusp)

- ◆ the 2D TTE PTLAX or TOE long axis, usually corresponds to the minor annulus dimension with CT
- ◆ frequently slightly larger with TOE when compared to TTE
- ◆ All other aortic measurements should be made at end-diastole, in a strictly perpendicular plane to that of the long axis of the aorta (Fig. 4.1.22)
  - ◆ PTLAX
  - ◆ focus on the aorta (specific probe angulation)
  - ◆ measure from leading edge to leading edge

# Suggested reading

1. Carerj S, Micari A, Trono A, et al. Anatomical M-mode: an old-new technique. *Echocardiography* 2003;20:357–61.

2. Cheitlin MD, Armstrong WF, Aurigemma GP, et al. ACC/AHA/ASE 2003 guideline update for the clinical application of echocardiography–summary article: A Report of the American College of Cardiology/American Heart Association Task Force on Practice Guidelines (ACC/AHA/ASE Committee to Update the 1997 Guidelines for the Clinical Application of Echocardiography). *J Am Coll Cardiol* 2003 3;42:954–70.

3. Lang RM, Badano LP, Mor-Avi V, et al. Recommendations for chamber quantification. *Eur Heart J Cardiovasc Imag* 2015;16(3):233–70.

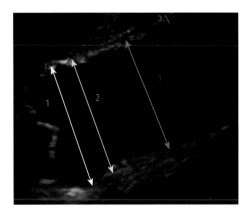

**Fig. 4.1.22** Measure of the (1) sinuses of Valsalva (maximal diameter); (2) sinotubular junction; (3) proximal ascending aorta

4.  Nikitin NP, Constantin C, Loh PH, et al. New generation 3-dimensional echocardiography for left ventricular volumetric and functional measurements: comparison with cardiac magnetic resonance. *Eur J Echocardiogr* 2006;7:365–72.

5.  Kolias TJ, Aaronson KD, Armstrong WF. Doppler-derived dP/dt and -dP/dt predict survival in congestive heart failure. *J Am Coll Cardiol* 2000;36:1594–9.

# CHAPTER 5

# Assessment of Diastolic Function

# 5.1 Left ventricle diastolic function

## Principles and basic physiology

**Diastole is the part of the cardiac cycle starting at aortic valve closure and ending at mitral valve closure (Box 5.1.1)**

**Normal LV diastolic function** allows the swift decrease in LV pressure in early diastole with an adequate filling of the LV at low–normal pressure both at rest and during exercise

The final result of abnormal LV diastolic function is elevation of LV filling pressure

---

**Box 5.1.1  Diastole phases**

Diastole can be divided into four phases (Fig. 5.1.1)
1.  LV pressure fall during isovolumetric relaxation
2.  Early rapid diastolic filling (E)
3.  Diastasis
4.  Late diastolic filling due to atrial contraction (A)

---

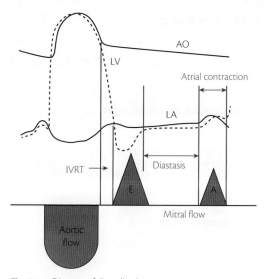

**Fig. 5.1.1** Diagram of diastolic phases

## Factors influencing LV filling (Box 5.1.2)

◆ Active LV myocardial relaxation, such as in sinus rhythm dysfunction, asynchrony

- Intrinsic passive properties of LV compliance, such as myocardial stiffness, tone, chamber geometry, and wall thickness
- Extrinsic passive properties, including pericardial restraint, extrinsic compression, and ventricular interaction
- LA filling pressures, including LA distensibility, LA systolic function, mitral valve orifice, mitral regurgitation

## Echocardiographic assessment of LV diastolic function (Box 5.1.3)

- Assessment of diastolic function includes analysis of LV relaxation and compliance, LA and LV filling pressures

| Box 5.1.2 Diastolic function |
| --- |
| Overall diastolic function is preserved through the perfect match of both active and passive determinants of the LV filling |

| Box 5.1.3 The integrated approach of LV diastolic function |
| --- |
| The integrated approach of LV diastolic function includes: |

- **M-mode and 2D/3D echocardiography**: LV geometry, left atrial size, rate of wall thinning, annular and pericardial displacement
- **PW-Doppler echocardiography**: assessment of mitral inflow and pulmonary venous flow
- **CW-Doppler echocardiography**: assessment of tricuspid regurgitation jet and pulmonary regurgitation jet to derive pulmonary artery pressures
- **PW tissue Doppler echocardiography**: assessment of early and late diastolic mitral annular velocities
- **Colour-flow M-mode Doppler:** measuring flow velocity propagation (Vp)

- ◆ The combination of different techniques and manoeuvres is needed in order to allow for an effective staging of LV diastolic dysfunction

## M-mode and 2D/3D echocardiography

### Structural assessment of LV size and mass and of LA volume (Fig. 5.1.2)

- ◆ In patients with LV diastolic dysfunction, concentric or eccentric hypertrophy can be found (Box 5.1.4)
- ◆ Increased LA volume reflects the cumulative effects of the increased LV filling pressures over time ('chronicity of the disease')—(important to be considered in conjunction with patient's clinical status, other chambers' volumes, and Doppler parameters of LV relaxation and compliance)
- ◆ Abnormal relaxation reduces rate of posterior wall thinning and reduces annular motion in early diastole
- ◆ Severely reduced compliance diminishes LV enlargement in mid and late diastole

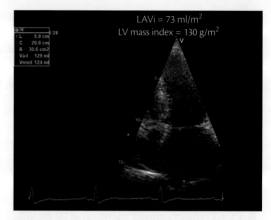

LAVi = 73 ml/m²
LV mass index = 130 g/m²

**Fig. 5.1.2** Measurement of end-systolic (maximum) LA volume in the apical 4CV

---

**Box 5.1.4  LV diastolic dysfunction**

- ◆ LV hypertrophy
  LV mass index > 115 g/m² in men
  LV mass index > 95 g/m² in women
- ◆ LA enlargement
  LA volume index > 34 ml/m²

# PW Doppler echocardiography

## Mitral inflow assessment

(Box 5.1.5, Box 5.1.6, Table 5.1.1, Table 5.1.2)

| **Box 5.1.5** How to assess |
| --- |
| ◆ Apical 4CV |
| ◆ Align the Doppler beam with the inflow direction |
| ◆ Place a 1–3 mm PW Doppler sample volume between the mitral leaflets tips |
| ◆ Reduce/adjust Doppler gain so that modal frequency is seen |
| ◆ Use a sweep speed of 50–100 mm/s |
| ◆ Measure deceleration time (EDT) from the peak of E-wave down to the baseline (Fig. 5.1.3A) |
| ◆ Measure isovolumic relaxation time (IVRT) by placing the PW Doppler sample volume in between LV inflow and outflow to simultaneously display the end of aortic ejection and the onset of mitral E-wave velocity (Fig. 5.1.3BC) |

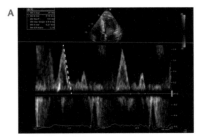
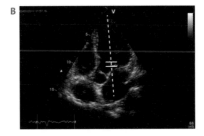
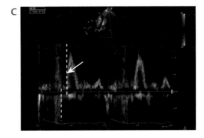

**Fig. 5.1.3** Correct tracing of E deceleration time from the peak of E-wave down to the baseline (A). Measurement of isovolumic relaxation time (IVRT) by placing the PW Doppler sample volume in between LV inflow and outflow (B) to simultaneously display the end of aortic ejection and the onset of mitral E-wave velocity (C)

**Table 5.1.1** Mitral inflow assessment

| Primary measurements | Secondary measurements |
|---|---|
| Peak of early filling (E velocity) | A-wave duration |
| Peak of late atrial filling (A velocity) | Atrial filling fraction (the A-wave velocity time integral/total mitral inflow velocity time integral) |
| The E/A ratio | |
| Deceleration time (DT) of E wave | |
| Isovolumic relaxation time (IVRT) | |

**Table 5.1.2** Normal values of mitral inflow PW Doppler parameters

| Measurement | Age group (y) | | | |
|---|---|---|---|---|
| | 16–20 | 21–40 | 41–60 | >60 |
| IVRT (ms) | 50 ± 9 (32–68) | 67 ± 8 (51–83) | 74 ± 7 (60–88) | 87 ± 7 (73–101) |
| E/A ratio | 1.88 ± 0.45 (0.98–2.78) | 1.53 ± 0.40 (0.73–2.33) | 1.28 ± 0.25 (0.78–1.78) | 0.96 ± 0.18 (0.6–1.32) |
| EDT (ms) | 142 ± 19 (104–180) | 166 ± 14 (138–194) | 181 ± 19 (143–219) | 200 ± 29 (142–258) |
| A duration (ms) | 113 ± 17 (79–147) | 127 ± 13 (101–153) | 133 ± 13 (107–159) | 138 ± 19 (100–176) |

**Box 5.1.6 Tips**

- Do not confound the measurement of EDT with the measurement of PHT (Fig. 5.1.4AB)
- Changes in PW sample volume position towards the mitral annulus or towards the apex can alter significantly the mitral flow velocities (Fig. 5.1.4C)
- Low mid-diastolic velocities can occur in normal subjects, but when increased (>20 cm/s), they often represent delayed LV relaxation and elevated filling pressures (Fig. 5.1.4D)

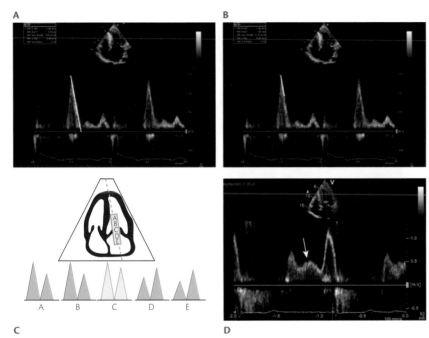

**Fig. 5.1.4** Measurement of EDT (A, B). Mitral flow velocities according to PW sample volume position (C). Mid-diastolic velocity in a patient with delayed LV relaxation (D)

## Mitral inflow pattern

**Classification of diastolic filling patterns based on the E/A ratio and E-wave deceleration time (EDT)** (Figs. 5.1.5ABCD, 5.1.6, Boxes 5.1.7, 5.1.8, 5.1.9, 5.1.10)

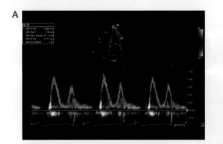
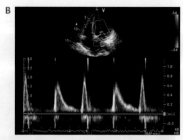
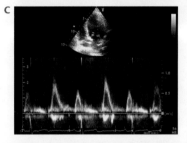
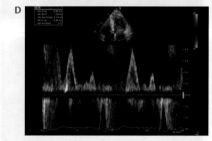

**Fig. 5.1.5** Illustration of diastolic filling patterns: normal (A), delayed relaxation (B), pseudonormal (C), restrictive (D)

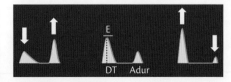

**Fig. 5.1.6** Diagram of diastolic filling patterns

---

**Box 5.1.7  Normal pattern**

E/A ratio = 1–2
DT = 150–200 ms
IVRT = 50–100 ms

---

**Box 5.1.8  Delayed relaxation**

E/A ratio < 0.8
DT > 200 ms
IVRT ≥ 100 ms

---

**Box 5.1.9  Pseudonormal**

E/A ratio = 0.8–1.5

---

**Box 5.1.10  Restrictive**

E/A ratio ≥ 2
DT < 160 ms
IVRT < 80 ms

## Mitral inflow analysis

- The opposing effects of impaired relaxation and increased filling pressure on the mitral inflow pattern (E/A) lead to a parabolic distribution of mitral inflow pattern during progression from normal LV diastolic function to severe diastolic dysfunction, describing a U-shaped curve (Fig. 5.1.7)
- By temporary decreasing of venous return, the Valsalva manoeuvre allows unmasking of an impaired relaxation pattern in patients with pseudonormalization (Fig. 5.1.8ABC)
- Decrease of 50% in the E/A ratio is highly specific for increased LV filling pressures (a smaller magnitude of change does not always indicate normal diastolic function)

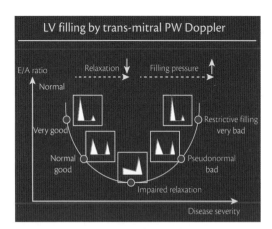

**Fig 5.1.7** Parabolic distribution of mitral inflow pattern during progression from normal LV diastolic function to severe diastolic dysfunction

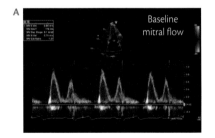
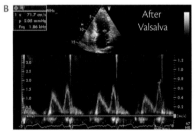
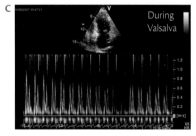

**Fig 5.1.8** Valsalva manoeuvre unmasking an impaired relaxation pattern in a patient with pseudonormalization (A, B, C)

- The Valsalva manoeuvre should be performed in a standardized manner (i.e. by blowing into a sphygmomanometer to raise pressure at 40 mmHg and keep it stable for 10 seconds)

## Mitral inflow influencing factors
(Fig. 5.1.9ABCD, Table 5.1.3)

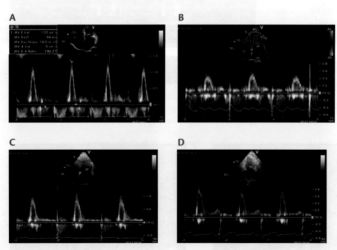

**Fig. 5.1.9** Diastolic filling patterns in: A: Atrial fibrillation, B: Atrial flutter, C: Atrial stunning one day after cardioversion, D: Atrial stunning three days after cardioversion

**Table 5.1.3** Factors influencing velocities of mitral flow

| Factors influencing velocities of mitral inflow | E | A | E/A |
|---|---|---|---|
| Age | ↓ | ↑ | ↓ |
| Tachycardia/atrio ventricular block first degree | | ↑ | ↓ |
| Preload ↓<br>• Hypovolaemia<br>• Diuretics, venodilators<br>• Valsalva manoeuvre | ↓ | N/↑ | ↓ |
| Preload ↑<br>• Hypervolaemia<br>• Left atrial pressure ↑<br>• Mitral regurgitation | ↑ | ↓ | ↑ |
| Left ventricular systolic dysfunction | ↑ | ↓ | ↑ |
| Left atrial dysfunction<br>• Atrial fibrillation/flutter (cardioversion)<br>• Sinus rhythm | | absent ↓ | |

# Pulmonary venous flow

## Pulmonary venous flow assessment
(see Box 5.1.11, Box 5.1.12, Table 5.1.4, Table 5.1.5)

**Table 5.1.4**

| Primary measurements | Secondary measurements |
|---|---|
| Peak systolic (**S**) velocity | The duration of the **Ar wave** |
| Peak anterograde diastolic (**D**) velocity | The time difference between Ar and mitral A-wave duration (**Ar-A**) |
| The **S/D** ratio | D wave velocity deceleration time (DDT) |
| Peak **Ar** velocity in late diastole | End of the PV reversal flow in relation to QRS |
| Systolic filling fraction $(S_{\text{time-velocity integral}}/ [S_{\text{time-velocity integral}}+ D_{\text{time-velocity integral}}]) \times 100$ | |

**Box 5.1.11** How to assess

- Apical 4CV
- 'Open-up' the right upper pulmonary vein (RUPV) by angulating the transducer superiorly (such that the AV is seen)
- Align the Doppler cursor with the PV flow direction (by colour Doppler)
- Place a 2–3 mm PW Doppler sample volume 0.5–1 cm into the RUPV
- Reduce Doppler gain, decrease velocity scale (low pulse repetition frequency)
- Use a sweep speed of 100 mm/sec
- Record tracings during apnoea (Fig. 5.1.10)

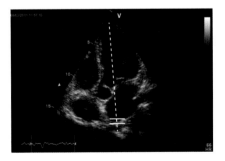

**Fig. 5.1.10** PW Doppler recording of pulmonary vein flow placing the sample volume within the pulmonary vein

### Box 5.1.12 Tips

- With severe mitral regurgitation systolic pulmonary vein flow (S) is decreased or even reversed, limiting the use of S/D ratio in the assessment of LV diastolic function

- MR alters pulmonary venous flow patterns, showing a decreased pulmonary venous systolic flow and prominent diastolic flow (Fig. 5.1.11AB)

- In patients immediately after cardioversion of atrial fibrillation, systolic pulmonary vein flow (S) and atrial reversal (Ar) may be reduced due to 'atrial stunning'

- Pulmonary venous flow velocities can be increased in patients after radiofrequency ablation for supraventricular reentrant tachyarrhythmia, due to PV stenosis

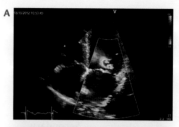

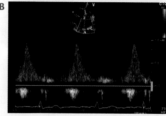

**Fig. 5.1.11** Colour flow imaging in a patient with severe, eccentric mitral regurgitation (A) altering the Doppler recording of PV flow that shows a prominent diastolic component (B)

**Table 5.1.5** Normal values of pulmonary vein flow PW Doppler parameters

| Measurement | Age group (y) | | | |
|---|---|---|---|---|
| | **16–20** | **21–40** | **41–60** | **> 60** |
| PV S/D ratio | 0.82 ± 0.18 (0.46–1.18) | 0.98 ± 0.32 (0.34–1.62) | 1.21 ± 0.2 (0.81–1.61) | 1.39 ± 0.47 (0.45–2.33) |
| PV Ar (cm/s) | 16 ± 10 (1–36) | 21 ± 8 (5–2.37) | 23 ± 3 (17–29) | 25 ± 9 (11–39) |
| PV Ar duration (ms) | 66 ± 39 (1–144) | 96 ± 33 (30–162) | 112 ± 15 (82–142) | 113 ± 30 (53–173) |

## Pulmonary venous flow morphology

- Pulmonary vein flow Doppler recordings normally show four distinct velocity components (Figs. 5.1.12, 5.1.13 Box 5.1.13)
- The biphasic pattern of systolic inflow and atrial reversal may be more difficult to demonstrate on transthoracic compared to transoesophageal echocardiography due to a lower signal-to-noise ratio

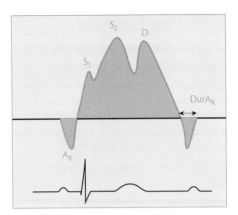

**Fig. 5.1.12** Diagram of pulmonary vein flow Doppler recording in a normal subject

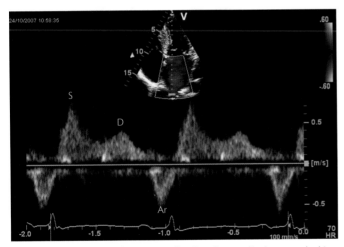

**Fig. 5.1.13** Illustration of pulmonary vein flow Doppler recording in a normal subject

**Box 5.1.13** Velocity components

**S1**—first systolic forward flow: related to left atrial relaxation
**S2**—second systolic forward flow: related to apical systolic displacement of the mitral ring
**D**—diastolic forward flow: corresponds to ventricular relaxation
**AR**—atrial reversal: corresponds to atrial contraction

## Pulmonary venous flow analysis

- There is a parabolic distribution of the S/D ratio with the progression of LV diastolic dysfunction
- When LVEDP increases both the amplitude and duration of Ar wave increase, whereas the duration of mitral inflow A velocity decreases. Thus, the time difference between Ar duration and mitral inflow A duration increases as LVEDP increases (Fig. 5.1.14AB, Table 5.1.6)
- A time difference > 30 ms indicates significantly increased LVEDP

**Table 5.1.6** Pulmonary vein flow Doppler velocities profile corresponding to different mitral inflow patterns

| Mitral inflow pattern | Pulmonary venous flow |
|---|---|
| Normal | S/D > 1 (normal) |
| Delayed relaxation | S/D > 1 (S/D ratio increases whereas E/A ratio decreases) |
| 'Pseudonormal' | S/D < 1, AR↑, DurAR > DurAMitral |
| Restrictive | S/D < 1, AR > 35 cm/s, DurAR − DurAMitral > 30 ms |

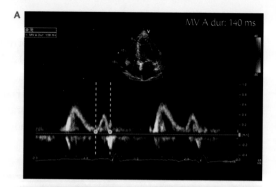

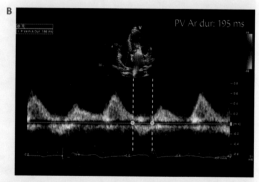

**Fig. 5.1.14** Pulsed-wave Doppler recording of the mitral inflow (A) and pulmonary vein flow velocities (B) in a patient with increased LVEDP

## Pulmonary venous flow influencing factors (Table 5.1.7)

**Table 5.1.7**

| Factors influencing PV flow velocities | S/D |
|---|---|
| Advanced age | > 1 |
| Tachycardia | S-D fusion |
| Atrio ventricular block (first degree) | < 1 |
| Mitral regurgitation | < 1 |
| Preload ↑ | > 1 |
| Left ventricular systolic dysfunction | ↑ |

## PW tissue Doppler echocardiography

### Mitral annulus velocity

**Assessment** (Box 5.1.14, Box 5.1.15, Table 5.1.8, Table 5.1.9)

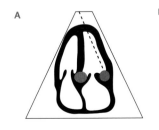
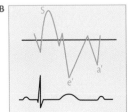

**Box 5.1.14  How to assess**

- Apical 4CV
- Align the Doppler cursor as parallel as possible to the longitudinal annular motion (septal or lateral LV wall)
- Place a 6–8 mm PW DMI sample volume at the septal or lateral insertion sites of the mitral leaflets (Fig. 5.1.15AB). Check that the annulus is moving through the sample volume during the whole cardiac cycle
- Reduce/adjust Doppler gain
- The velocity scale should be set at about +/−20 cm/s to avoid velocity aliasing
- Set the sweep speed at 50–100 mm/s
- Record at end-expiration

**Fig. 5.1.15  Mitral annular velocities measurement by DMI.** Septal (red bullet) and lateral (blue bullet) sites for PW DMI sample volume used to measure annular velocities (A). The DMI tracing pattern shows a rounded wave facing upwards (S) in systole and two sharper waves facing downwards in diastole (e, a') (B)

**Box 5.1.15** Tips

- ◆ Sampling of the septal annulus is less influenced by the translation movement of the heart as it moves parallel to the ultrasound beam but it may be influenced by the right ventricular interaction

- ◆ In patients with normal LVEF, lateral tissue Doppler signals (E/e' and e'/a') have the best correlations with LV filling pressures and invasive indices of LV stiffness

- ◆ e' velocity is usually reduced in patients with significant annular calcification, surgical rings, mitral stenosis, prosthetic mitral valves and with ischaemia or scar in the respective wall (septum/lateral)

- ◆ e' is increased in patients with moderate to severe primary MR and normal LV relaxation due to increased flow across the regurgitant valve. In these patients, abnormal LV relaxation might be indicated by reduced −dP/dt (estimated from MR or AR), while the E/e' ratio should not be used. IVRT/TE-e' ratio can be applied

- ◆ The E/e' ratio is not accurate as an index of filling pressures in normal subjects or in patients with heavy annular calcification, mitral valve disease, and constrictive pericarditis. E/e' ratio may not be accurate in severely dilated LV with severely decreased systolic function

**Table 5.1.8** Mitral annulus velocity assessment

| Primary measurements | Secondary measurements |
|---|---|
| Peak systolic (**S**) velocity | **e'/a'** ratio |
| Peak early diastolic (**e'**) velocity | **E/e'** ratio |
| Peak late diastolic (**a'**) velocity | **TE-e'** (the time interval between QRS complex and the onset of E velocity subtracted from the time interval between the QRS complex and e' onset |

**Table 5.1.9** Normal values of PW Doppler diastolic mitral annular velocities

| Measurement | Age group (y) | | | |
|---|---|---|---|---|
| | 16–20 | 21–40 | 41–60 | >60 |
| Septal e' (cm/s) | 14.9 ± 2.4 (10.1–19.7) | 15.5 ± 2.7 (10.1–20.9) | 12.2 ± 2.3 (7.6–16.8) | 10.4 ± 2.1 (6.2–14.6) |
| Septal e'/a' ratio | 2.4 | 1.6 ± 0.5 (0.6–2.6) | 1.1 ± 0.3 (0.5–1.7) | 0.85 ± 0.2 (0.45–1.25) |
| Lateral e' (cm/s) | 20.6 ± 3.8 (13–28.2) | 19.8 ± 2.9 (14–25.6) | 16.1 ± 2.3 (11.5–20.7) | 12.9 ± 3.5 (5.9–19.9) |
| Lateral e'/a' ratio | 3.1 | 1.9 ± 0.6 (0.7–3.1) | 1.5 ± 0.5 (0.5–2.5) | 0.9 ± 0.4 (0.1–1.7) |

## Morphology (Figs. 5.1.16, 5.1.17, Box 5.1.16, Box 5.1.17)

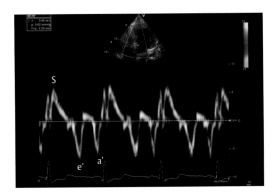

**Fig. 5.1.16** Annular PW DMI recordings using the septal site

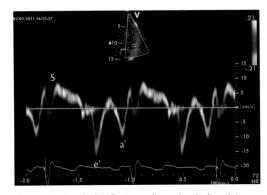

**Fig. 5.1.17** Annular PW DMI recordings using the lateral site

**Box 5.1.16** Annular PW DMI recordings

**Annular PW DMI recordings show three distinct velocity components**

S—systolic wave: related to ventricular contractility

e'—early diastolic velocity: reflects relaxation of the myocardium

a'—late diastolic velocity: corresponds to atrial contraction

**Box 5.1.17** Morphology assessment

- A decrease in e' is one of the earliest markers of LV diastolic dysfunction and this decrease is present in all stages of diastolic dysfunction (Fig. 5.1.18)

- Because e' velocity remains reduced and mitral E velocity increases with higher filling pressure, the ratio between E and e' (the E/e' ratio) correlates with LV filling pressure or pulmonary capillary wedge pressure (Table 5.1.10)

**Table 5.1.10** Factors influencing the annular velocities

| Factors | e' | a' | e'/a' |
|---|---|---|---|
| Ageing (ischaemia, hypertrophy, cardiomyopathy) | ↓ | ↑ | ↓ |
| Preload ↑ (mitral regurgitation) | ↑ | | |
| Afterload ↑ (systemic hypertension) | ↓ | ↑ | |

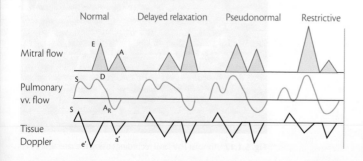

**Fig. 5.1.18** Pulsed-wave Doppler profile of mitral inflow, pulmonary vein flow, and mitral annular velocities with the progressive impairment of LV diastolic function

## Analysis (Box 5.1.18, 5.1.19. 5.1.20, Table 5.1.11)

---

**Box 5.1.18** Measurements and analysis

♦ Because septal e' is usually lower than lateral e´ velocity, the E/e' ratio using septal signals is usually higher than the ratio derived by lateral e', and different cut-off values should be applied

♦ Although single-site measurements are sometimes used in patients with globally normal or abnormal LV systolic function, it is recommended to use the average (septal and lateral) e' velocity in the presence of regional LV dysfunction

---

## Colour-flow M-mode Doppler

**Flow propagation velocity assessment** (Box 5.1.21, 5.1.22, Table 5.1.12)

♦ The ratio of peak E velocity to Vp is directly related to LA pressure and therefore the E/Vp ratio can be used to predict LV filling pressure (see also Box 5.1.23, 5.1.24)

♦ In most patients with depressed LV ejection fraction Vp is reduced. Should other Doppler indices appear inconclusive, an E/Vp ratio > 2.5 predicts a PCWP > 15 mmHg with reasonable accuracy

---

**Box 5.1.19** Correlation between septal E/e' ratio and LV filling pressure

♦ In the case of **lateral site, E/e' ratio > 12** is associated with high LVFP

♦ When **averaging septal and lateral values, E/e' ratio > 13** should be used to define an undoubtedly LVFP increase

---

**Box 5.1.20** Explanation of TE-e'

**TE-e'** is particularly useful in subjects with normal cardiac function or those with mitral valve disease and when the E/e´ ratio is 8:15. The average of four annular sites is more accurate than a single-site measurement **IVRT/TE-e' ratio < 2** has reasonable accuracy in identifying patients with increased LVFP

---

**Table 5.1.11** Correlation between septal E/e ratio and LV filling pressure

| E/e' < 8 | LV filling pressure—normal |
|---|---|
| E/e' > 15 | LV filling pressure—increased |
| E/e' between 8 and 15 | Other echocardiographic indices should be used |

## Box 5.1.21  How to assess

- Apical 4CV, magnified to encompass the LV
- Colour Doppler flow from M annulus into the LV
- M-mode cursor aligned with colour inflow
- Colour M-mode, at a sweep speed of 100 mm/s
- Shift the colour-flow baseline to lower the Nyquist limit so that the central highest velocity jet is blue (Fig. 5.1.19)
- Slope the first aliasing velocity during early filling, measured from the mitral valve plane to approx. 4 cm distally into the LV cavity, or the transition from no colour to colour

## Box 5.1.22  Tips

- Patients with normal LV volume and LVEF but abnormal filling pressures can have a misleadingly normal Vp
- Vp can be falsely high in small ventricles

**Table 5.1.12**  Factors influencing flow Vp

|  | **Vp** |
|---|---|
| Age | ↓ |
| LV delayed relaxation | ↓ |

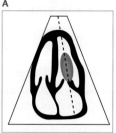 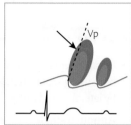

**A**      **B**

**Fig. 5.1.19** Diagram showing the M-mode cursor aligned with colour inflow in apical 4CV (A) and the slope of the first aliasing velocity during early filling measured from the mitral valve plane (B)

## Box 5.1.23  LV filling pressure

**Vp > 55 cm/s is considered normal**

## Box 5.1.24  Prediction of LV filling pressure

- The reduction of mitral-to-apex flow propagation measured by colour M-mode Doppler represents a semiquantitative marker of LV diastolic dysfunction (Figs. 5.1.20, 5.1.21AB)
- Vp in conjunction with mitral E predicts LV filling pressures

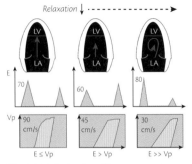

**Fig. 5.1.20** Reduction of flow propagation velocity with the progressive impairment of LV diastolic function

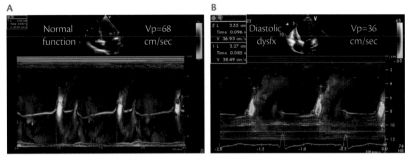

**Fig. 5.1.21** Flow propagation velocity in a normal subject (A). Reduced flow propagation velocity in a patient with diastolic dysfunction (B)

# Echocardiographic assessment of LV diastolic function

Although both LV relaxation and compliance can be impaired, it is useful to know which is the main factor contributing to LV diastolic dysfunction by separately assessing indicators of abnormal relaxation and of decreased compliance (Fig. 5.1.22)

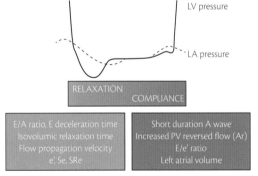

**Fig. 5.1.22** Diagram emphasizing the interplay between left ventricular diastolic components (relaxation and compliance) and their main echocardiographic parameters

# Presence and severity of diastolic dysfunction
(Table 5.1.13, Table 5.1.14, Figs. 5.1.23-25)

**Table 5.1.13** Presence and severity of diastolic dysfunction (STEP 1)

| Pathophysiology | Normal | relaxation ↓ | relaxation ↓<br>LVFP ↑ | relaxation↓<br>compliance↓<br>LVFP↑ | relaxation ↓<br>compliance ↓↓<br>LVFP↑↑ |
|---|---|---|---|---|---|
| | **Normal** | **Mild** | **Mild–Moderate** | **Moderate** | **Severe** |
| E/A | 1–2 | < 1 | < 1 | 1–2 | > 2 |
| e'/a' | 1–2 | < 1 | < 1 | < 1 | > 1 |
| IVRT (ms) | 50–100 | > 100 | Normal | ↓ | ↓ |
| DT (ms) | 150–200 | > 200 | > 200 | 150–200 | < 150 |
| S/D | ≥ 1 | S > D | S > D | S < D | S << D |
| Ar (m/s) | < 0.35 | < 0.35 | ≥ 0.35 | ≥ 0.35 | ≥ 0.35 |
| Ar dur–A dur (ms) | < 20 | < 20 | > 20 | > 20 | > 20 |

**Table 5.1.14** Estimation of LV filling pressure (STEP 2)

| LA | E/A | EDT | Ar | Ar dur – A dur | S/D | DDT | E/e' | E/Vp |
|---|---|---|---|---|---|---|---|---|
| ↑ | > 2 | < 150 ms | > 0.35 m/s | > 30 ms | S < D | < 175 ms | > 15 | > 2 |

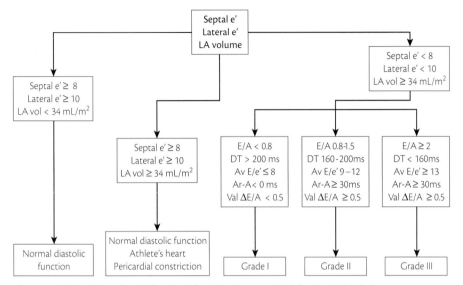

**Fig. 5.1.23** Scheme for grading LV diastolic dysfunction. Av: average; LA: left atrium; Val: Valsalva

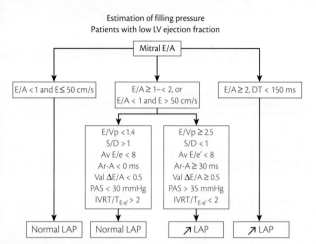

**Estimation of filling pressure**
**Patients with low LV ejection fraction**

Mitral E/A

- E/A < 1 and E ≤ 50 cm/s
- E/A ≥ 1–< 2, or E/A < 1 and E > 50 cm/s
- E/A ≥ 2, DT < 150 ms

E/Vp < 1.4
S/D > 1
Av E/e < 8
Ar-A < 0 ms
Val ΔE/A < 0.5
PAS < 30 mmHg
IVRT/T$_{E-e'}$ > 2

E/Vp ≥ 2.5
S/D < 1
Av E/e' < 8
Ar-A ≥ 30 ms
Val ΔE/A ≥ 0.5
PAS > 35 mmHg
IVRT/T$_{E-e'}$ < 2

Normal LAP | Normal LAP | ↗ LAP | ↗ LAP

**Fig. 5.1.24** Scheme for grading LV filling pressure. Av: average; LA: left atrium; Val: Valsalva

**Patients with normal LV ejection fraction**

E/e'

- Av E/e' < 8
- Av E/e' 9–14
- Sep E/e' ≥ 15 or Lat E/e' ≥ 12 or Av E/e' ≥ 13

LA volume < 34 mL/m$^2$
Ar-A < 0 ms
Val ΔE/A < 0.5
PAS < 30 mmHg
IVRT/T$_{E-e'}$ > 2

LA volume ≥ 34 mL/m$^2$
Ar-A ≥ 30 ms
Val ΔE/A ≥ 0.5
PAS > 35 mmHg
IVRT/T$_{E-e'}$ < 2

Normal LAP | Normal LAP | ↗ LAP | ↗ LAP

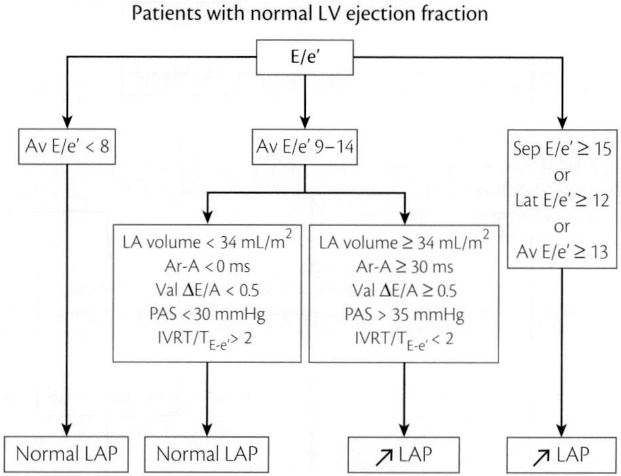

**Fig. 5.1.25** Scheme for grading LV filling pressure. Av: average; LA: left atrium; Val: Valsalva

# Suggested reading

1. Nagueh SF, Appleton CP, Gillbert TC, et al. EAE/ASE recommendations for the evaluation of left ventricular diastolic function by echocardiography. *Eur J Echocardiogr* 2009;10:165–93.

2. Galderisi M, Mondillo S, et al. Assessment of diastolic function. In: Galiuto L, Badano L, Fox K, et al. (eds). *The EAE Textbook of Echocardiography*. Oxford: Oxford University Press, 2011:135–49.

3. Beladan CC, Calin A, et al. Functia diastolica. In: Popescu BA, Ginghina C (eds). *Ecocardiografia Doppler*. Bucharest: Editura Medicala, 2011:81–102.

# CHAPTER 6

# Ischaemic Cardiac Disease (ICD)

# Introduction

## Role of echo in ICD

### Diagnostic value of echo

- **Segmental wall motion abnormalities**
  - hypokinesis: < 40% in systolic wall thickening
  - akinesis: < 10% in systolic wall thickening
  - dyskinesis: wall moves outward during systole with wall thinning
  - evaluation of the wall thickening, systolic wall motion and diastolic wall thickness: conservation of the diastolic thickness in recent myocardial infarction (MI)
  - location and extent
    - 16-segment model or 17-segment model
    - Determine a wall motion score index (WMSI: extension)

### Ruling out acute MI in prolonged or suspect chest pain

- **Estimation of extension and risk stratification**
- **Detection of complications**

# 6.1 Assessment of acute myocardial infarction (AMI)

## Role of echo: the risk stratification

◆ **Ejection fraction**: a global ejection fraction less than 40% indicates a higher mortality and morbidity. A bi-dimensional Simpson method should be used (and better 3D method if available). Additional prognostic information can be derived from other estimates of the global function (systolic strain, dP/dt, etc.) (Fig. 6.1.1ABC)

◆ **Wall motion abnormalities**: a WMSI ≥ 1.7 indicates a poor prognosis

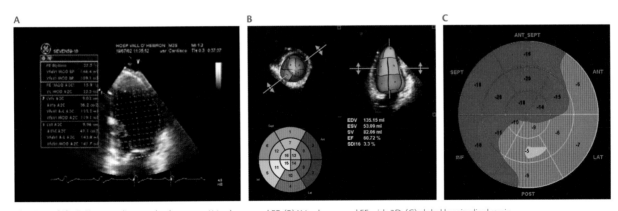

**Fig. 6.1.1** (A) 2D Simpson discs method to assess LV volumes and EF; (B) LV volumes and EF with 3D; (C) global longitudinal strain

- ◆ **Left cavities diameter and volume**
  - ◆ An LV enlargement (LEDD ≥ 60 mm or 40 mm/m$^2$) within the first hours to days after the acute event corresponds to expansion. A global remodelling can occur within days to months after MI and also indicates a poor prognosis. A concomitant dilatation of the right ventricle or an RV dysfunction is also associated with a poorer prognosis. Sphericity index > 0.25 is a predictor of remodelling
  - ◆ An increase in left atrial volume index ≥ 31 mL/m$^2$ is associated with a bad prognosis
- ◆ **Diastolic filling pattern:** a restrictive Doppler filling pattern (especially non reversible) indicates a poor prognosis (see diastolic function section for assessing)
- ◆ **Complications are also** responsible for a dismal prognosis

# 6.2 Complications of AMI

## LV aneurysm

- Incidence 10–22% with first anterior MI
- Most often in transmural infarction
- May be detected as early as five days post MI
- Higher mortality rate (60% in three years)
- Increased risk of thrombus formation/systemic embolization (Fig. 6.2.1)
- Association with ventricular arrhythmias
- Aneurysm causes a deformity of the LV during ventricular systole and diastole (dyskinesis deforms LV only during ventricular systole)

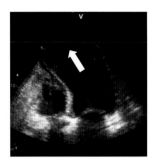

**Fig. 6.2.1** TTE 4CV showing an apical aneurysm with a thrombus (arrow)

## LV pseudoaneurysm (PSA)

- Free wall rupture of the LV and haemopericardium is confined by the pericardium (3% of all AMI), also due to cardiac surgery, blunt trauma, or endocarditis
- Significantly increased risk of sudden death, common cause of death within the first two weeks of AMI (5–10%)
- Increased risk of thromboembolism, associated with congestive heart failure
- PSA often associated with left circumflex artery occlusion
- **Echo findings**
  - narrow perforation with sharp edges of the left ventricular free wall with a globular contour of the false chamber (Fig. 6.2.2)

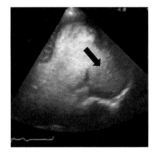

**Fig. 6.2.2** TTE modified 4CV with contrast showing a PSA of the lateral wall (arrow)

- ◆ systolic expansion of the pseudoaneurysm
- ◆ extension of the aneurysmal space behind the left ventricular wall ( ≠ true aneurysm)
- ◆ displacement of surrounding cardiac chambers
- ◆ 'neck' diameter/true diameter ratio (< 0.5 indicates pseudoaneurysm)
- ◆ Doppler: PW at the mouth of PSA → two peaks: atrial and ventricular systolic colour-flow Doppler: turbulent flow at the orifice, abnormal flow within the PSA (decrease colour velocity scale/wall filter)

## LV thrombus

- ◆ May be visualized as early as two days (50%) and almost 95% present within the first two weeks after AMI (early > worse prognosis)
- ◆ Common complications after MI (up to 40%) (Fig. 6.2.3)
- ◆ Often associated with anterior MI
- ◆ Timing of the echo evaluation of an LV thrombus: 24–48 h post MI, 10–15 days and 1–3 months
- ◆ May be as small as 2 mm (thin < 0.6 cm may not be detected)
- ◆ Pedunculated or irregular thrombi represent an increased risk for embolization
- ◆ **Echo findings**
  - ◆ density generally greater than adjacent endocardium (contrast helpful)
  - ◆ associated with segmental wall motion abnormalities
  - ◆ describe location, type (mural, non-protruding, sessile, protruding, pedunculated, mobile), echodensity, and dimensions

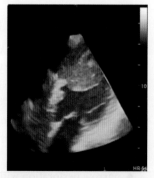

**Fig. 6.2.3** 3D TTE 4CV showing an apical thrombus

- pedunculated generally < early stages; mural generally < older
- new thrombi, generally hypoechogenic; older clots generally brighter
- colour Doppler may be useful to demonstrate a 'filling defect' in the area of the thrombus (low velocity scale and wall filter)

# Mitral regurgitation (MR) (Fig. 6.2.4)

- Determine the presence and the severity of MR (quantification), severity of the MR may be underestimated by colour Doppler due to Coanda effect as well as a reduced LV–LA gradient
- Determine the direction of the jet
- Assess the mechanism of the MR (papillary muscle dysfunction and its most severe form, papillary muscle rupture)
- TOE may be helpful

# Wall rupture (septal or free) (Fig. 6.2.5ABCD)

- Must be suspected when new, loud systolic murmur, associated with a thrill
- 1–5% of deaths in AMI
- Associated with a 65% mortality within two weeks
- Over one-half occur in the setting of anterior MI

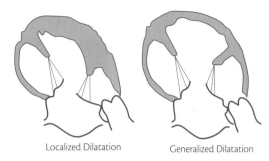

Localized Dilatation          Generalized Dilatation

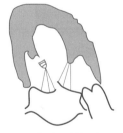

Ruptured Muscle

**Fig. 6.2.4** Schematic drawing of the mechanisms of MR in MI

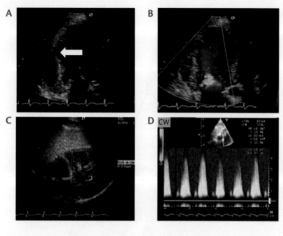

**Fig. 6.2.5** TTE A: Apical 3CV of a free wall rupture (arrow); B: Doppler colour flow showing the flow; C: subcostal view of septal defect; D: CW Doppler of the left to right flow at the level of the septal defect

- Usually seen within two to seven days after MI
- Requires urgent surgical closure in patients with unstable haemodynamics (delayed > three weeks in stable patients)

## RV infarction

- Associated most often with inferior infarction (up to one-third of patients with inferior wall infarction)
- Isolated RV infarction is rare (3–5%)
- RV dilatation (Fig. 6.2.6)

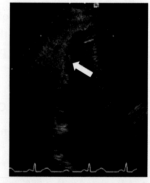

**Fig. 6.2.6** TTE 4CV showing a thin wall and akinetic RV (arrow)

- Paradoxical septal motion
- Inferior vena cava dilatation
- Bulging of the IAS in the LA
- Tricuspid regurgitation with low pulmonary pressures (Fig. 6.2.7)
- Pulmonary regurgitation with steep PHT (Fig. 6.2.8)

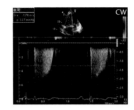 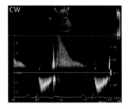

**Fig. 6.2.7** Tricuspid regurgitation with low pulmonary pressures

**Fig. 6.2.8** Pulmonary regurgitation with steep PHT

## Pericardial effusion

- Common in AMI (two to four days): about 30% (Fig. 6.2.9)
- Higher incidence in transmural AMI
- Associated with larger infarction and anterior MI
- May predict a more complex course (CHF, atrial/ventricular arrhythmias, one-year mortality)
- Symptomatic or not
- Cardiac tamponade is rare
- Implications
  - relative CI for anticoagulation
  - absolute CI for thrombolysis
- Dressler's syndrome (1–12 weeks after AMI), fever, polyserositis, pain

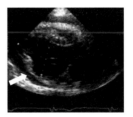

**Fig. 6.2.9** TTE PTLAX view showing a pericardial effusion (arrow) complicating a pseudoaneurysm

# 6.3 Determinants of prognosis in chronic ICD

## Role of echo: poor prognosis risk factors

- LV ejection fraction: when < 25%, it indicates a higher mortality and morbidity. A bi-dimensional Simpson method should be used (and better 3D method if available)
- PW TDI systolic septal annular velocity < 3 cm/s
- Left cavities diameter
  - A LV enlargement (LEDD ≥ 65 mm)
  - LA volume ≥ 31 mL/m²
- Diastolic filling pattern: a restrictive Doppler filling pattern (especially non-reversible) indicates a poor prognosis (see diastolic function section for assessing), E/e' > 15, indicating high LV filling pressures
- PW DMI of the mitral septal annulus early diastolic velocity (e') < 3 cm/s
- RV fractional area change < 32%, TAPSE < 14 mm, PW DMI peak systolic velocity RV free wall < 11 cm/s
- Pulmonary hypertension: tricuspid regurgitation velocity > 2.5 m/s
- Complications: secondary mitral regurgitation (ERO ≥ 0.20 cm²)
- Absence of viability (dobutamine echo, thin wall < 5 mm and/or residual ischaemia (stress echo))

# Suggested reading

1. Wu J, You J, Jiang G, et al. Noninvasive estimation of infarct size in a mouse model of myocardial infarction by echocardiographic coronary perfusion. *J Ultrasound Med* 2012;31:1111–21.
2. Verma A, Pfeffer MA, Skali H, et al. Incremental value of echocardiographic assessment beyond clinical evaluation for prediction of death and development of heart failure after high-risk myocardial infarction. *Am Heart J* 2011;161:1156–62.
3. Ruiz-Bailén M, Romero-Bermejo FJ, Ramos-Cuadra JÁ, et al. Evaluation of the performance of echocardiography in acute coronary syndrome patients during their stay in coronary units. *Acute Card Care* 2011;13:21–9.

# CHAPTER 7

# Heart Valve Disease

# 7.1 Aortic valve stenosis

## Role of echo

### Imaging of AS patients should evaluate the aetiology

- Severity of stenosis
- Repercussions

## Aetiologies (Fig. 7.1.1ABC)

- Calcific stenosis of a trileaflet valve
  - calcifications located in the central part of each cusp (no commissural fusion) resulting in a stellate-shaped systolic orifice
- Bicuspid aortic valve with superimposed calcific changes
  - often results from fusion of the right and left coronary cusps
  - diagnosis is most reliable when the two cusps are seen in systole
- Rheumatic valve disease
  - commissural fusion resulting in a triangular systolic orifice
  - thickening/calcifications most prominent along the edges of the cusps
- Congenital AS are rare in adults

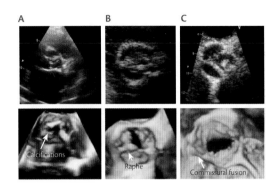

**Fig. 7.1.1** Aortic stenosis aetiology (top: 2D imaging; bottom: 3D imaging)
A: Degenerative tricuspid valve, B: Bicuspid valve, C: Rheumatic AS
Imaging AV: PTLAX and PTSAX views
Features to report: number of cusps, raphe, mobility, calcifications, commissural fusion

# Assessment of AS severity

## Haemodynamic measurements

- Haemodynamic assessment of AS severity relies mainly on three parameters which should be concordant
  - Peak velocity of the anterograde flow across the narrowed aortic orifice measured using CW Doppler
  - Mean transaortic pressure gradient obtained from the same recording as peak velocity
  - Aortic valve area (AVA) calculated according to the continuity equation (Fig. 7.1.2)

  $AVA = Stroke\ volume\ (SV)/TVI_{AV} = \pi \times (D^2/4) \times (TVI_{LVOT} / TVI_{AV})$

  - D: diameter of the left ventricular outflow tract (LVOT)
  - $TVI_{LVOT}$: time–velocity integral recorded with PW Doppler from the apical 5CV just proximal to the valve
  - $TVI_{AV}$: time–velocity integral of the jet crossing the aortic orifice recorded with CW Doppler
  - the dimensionless index (DI) can be used when measurement of the LVOT diameter is considered not reliable. DI = $(TVI_{LVOT} / TVI_{AV})$

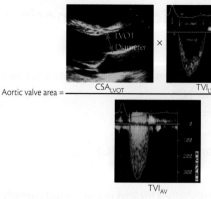

Aortic valve area = $\dfrac{CSA_{LVOT} \times TVI_{LVOT}}{TVI_{AV}}$

**Fig. 7.1.2** The continuity equation

# Measurement of LVOT diameter

## Recordings

♦ PTLAX view, zoom mode
♦ Measurement between insertion of leaflets or 0.5–1.0 cm of the AV orifice (Fig. 7.1.3)
♦ From inner edge to inner edge (white–black interface of the septal endocardium to the anterior mitral leaflet)
♦ Perpendicular to the aortic wall
♦ During mid-systole
♦ Averaging three to five beats

## Limitations

♦ Off-axis measurement: underestimation of LVOT diameter (Fig. 7.1.4)
♦ Careful angulation of the transducer to find maximal LVOT diameter
♦ Error in diameter is squared for calculation of cross-sectional area
♦ Error of 1mm in diameter error of 0.1 cm$^2$ in valve area
♦ Diameter is used to calculate a circular cross-sectional area ($CSA_{LVOT} = \pi \times (D^2/4)$) that is assumed to be circular (Fig. 7.1.5)
♦ Below aortic cusps, LVOT often becomes progressively more elliptical (Fig. 7.1.6)

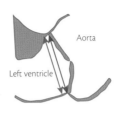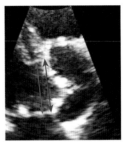

**Fig. 7.1.3** LVOT diameter measurement. Blue arrow: 0.5–1.0 cm of the AV orifice. Red arrow: insertion of aortic cusps

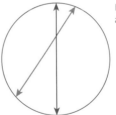

**Fig. 7.1.4** LVOT diameter. Green arrow: off-axis measurement

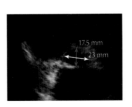

**Fig. 7.1.5** Non-circular LVOT

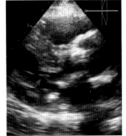

**Fig. 7.1.6** Elliptical LVOT due to upper septal hypertrophy

## What to do if LVOT diameter cannot be measured?

- ◆ Never use apical view
- ◆ Use other echo methods
  - ◆ Measurement of LVOT diameter with TOE
  - ◆ Aortic valve area planimetry
  - ◆ Velocity ratio or DI
  - ◆ Use modified continuity equation (2D/3D echo)
- ◆ Use non-echo methods (CT, MRI, catheterization)

## LVOT velocity

### Recordings

- ◆ Apical long-axis or 5CV
- ◆ PW Doppler as close as possible to Ao valve, in the centre of the $CSA_{LVOT}$
- ◆ Sample volume positioned just on LV side of valve and moved carefully into the LVOT if required to obtain laminar flow curve (Fig. 7.1.7AB)
- ◆ Velocity baseline and scale adjusted to maximize size of velocity curve
- ◆ Time axis (sweep speed) 100 mm/s
- ◆ Low wall filter setting

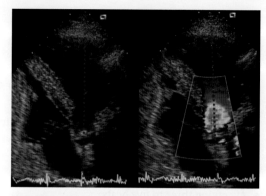

**Fig. 7.1.7A** AP 5CV. LVOT velocity recording

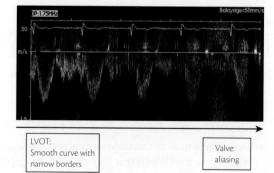

LVOT:
Smooth curve with narrow borders

Valve:
aliasing

**Fig. 7.1.7B** LVOT velocity recording

## Measurement

♦ Smooth velocity curve with a well-defined peak and a narrow velocity range at peak velocity
♦ Maximum velocity from peak of dense velocity curve
♦ Do not stop tracing unless you hit baseline
♦ Measure at least three times

## LVOT velocity: pitfalls

♦ Underestimation of LVOT velocity (Fig. 7.1.8)
  ♦ non-parallel alignment of ultrasound beam
  ♦ sample volume too far from aortic orifice
♦ Overestimation of LVOT velocity (Fig. 7.1.9)
  ♦ sample volume too close from aortic orifice
♦ Dynamic subaortic obstruction: non laminar LVOT flow (Fig. 7.1.10)
  ♦ continuity equation cannot be used (planimetry)
  ♦ pressure gradients cannot be calculated
♦ High LVOT velocity (> 1.5 m/s) (AR, High CO) (Fig. 7.1.11)
  ♦ simplified Bernoulli equation cannot be used

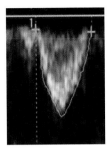

**Fig. 7.1.8** Underestimation of LVOT velocity

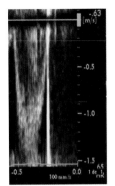

**Fig. 7.1.9** Overestimation of LVOT velocity

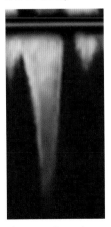

**Fig. 7.1.10** Dynamic subaortic obstruction

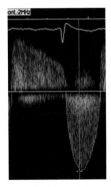

**Fig. 7.1.11** High LVOT velocity

## High LVOT velocity

- Clinical situations: high cardiac output, aortic regurgitation
- Simplified Bernoulli equation : $\Delta P = 4 V_2^2$ (V2 = AS velocity)
- V1 cannot be ignored if > 1.5 m/s and modified Bernoulli equation should be used: $\Delta P = 4 (V2^2 - V1^2)$ (V1 = LVOT velocity)
- Example
  V2 = AS velocity = 4 m/s
  V1 = LVOT velocity = 2 m/s
  $4 (V2^2 - V1^2) = 48$ mmHg
  $4 V2^2 = 64$ mmHg (overestimation by 33%)
- Modified Bernoulli equation allows calculation of maximum gradients but is more problematic for calculation of mean gradients

# AS jet velocity

## Recordings

- CW Doppler (dedicated transducer)
- Multiple acoustic windows (e.g. apical, suprasternal, right parasternal) (Fig. 7.1.12AB)
- Decrease gains, increase wall filter, adjust baseline, and scale to optimize signal

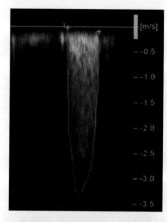

**Fig. 7.1.12A** AP 5CV. AS jet velocity tracing (the outer edge of the dark 'envelope' of the velocity curve is traced)

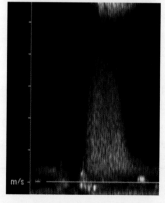

**Fig. 7.1.12B** Right parasternal view with Pedof probe (feasibility: 85%)

- Identify jet direction in the ascending Ao using colour-flow imaging (CFM)

## Measurement

- Maximum velocity at peak of dense velocity curve
- Avoid noise and fine linear signals
- Mean gradient calculated from traced velocity curve
- Report window where maximum velocity obtained (for further examinations)
- The curve is more rounded in shape with more severe obstruction. Mild obstruction, the peak is in early systole

## AS jet velocity: underestimation

- Non-parallel alignment between CW Doppler beam and AS jet results in underestimation of AS velocity and gradients

## AS jet velocity: overestimation

- Confusion between MR and AS (Fig. 7.1.13)
- Measurement of velocity on a post-extrasystolic beat (or measurement of higher velocity in AF without averaging peak velocities)

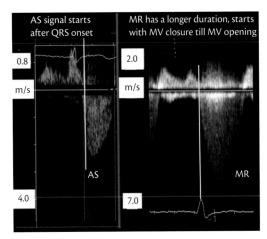

**Fig. 7.1.13** CW Doppler MR jet signal

- Inclusion in measurement of fine linear signals at the peak of the curve (due to transit time effect and not to be included) (Fig. 7.1.14)
- Pressure recovery (if ascending aorta diameter at STJ < 30 mm use the 'energy loss coefficient' = ELCo = (EOA × Aa/(Aa – EOA))/BSA, where Aa is the aorta diameter

## Should aortic valve area be indexed?

- The role of indexing for BSA is controversial
- Indexing valve area is important in children, adolescents, and small adults
  - BSA < 1.5 m$^2$
  - BMI < 22 kg/m$^2$
  - height < 135 cm
- In obese patients, valve area does not increase with excess body weight, and indexing for BSA is not recommended

## What to do in the presence of arrhythmia?

- Do not use TVI of a premature beat or of the beat after it
- Atrial fibrillation: average the velocities from three to five consecutive beats (Fig. 7.1.15)

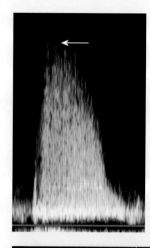

**Fig. 7.1.14** CW Doppler AS jet. Fine linear signals (arrow)

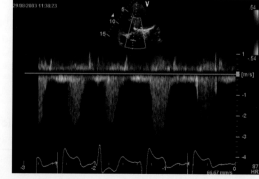

**Fig. 7.1.15** CW Doppler AS jet in a patient with atrial fibrillation

# Discrepancy between echo and cath lab (Fig. 7.1.16)

- Cath lab: peak-to-peak (ΔP net) gradient
  - not simultaneous
  - non-physiologic
- Doppler:
  - max instantaneous gradient (ΔP max) > to ΔP net gradient
  - Doppler mean gradient correlates well with Cath
  - AVA cath > AVA Doppler

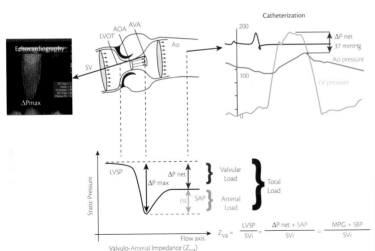

**Fig. 7.1.16** Top: AS CW Doppler signal vs catheterization data. Bottom: evaluation of global LV load

MPG = mean aortic pressure gradient using CW Doppler; PR = pressure recovery; SAP = systolic arterial pressure; SBP = systolic blood pressure; $Z_{va}$ = valvulo-arterial impedance

# Aortic valve area planimetry

## Recordings

- TTE PTSAX (Fig. 7.1.17)
- TOE 45–60° (Fig. 7.1.18)
- TOE often more reliable
- Zoom mode

## Measurement

- Minimal orifice must be identified

## Limitations

- Appropriate view
- Calcium (opening not well defined)

## Interpretation

- Nl = 2.5 – 4.5 cm$^2$
- AVA planimetry > AVA Doppler due flow contraction in the orifice

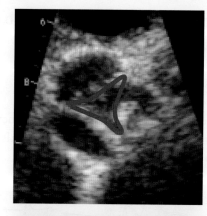

**Fig. 7.1.17** AS AVA planimetry (TTE)

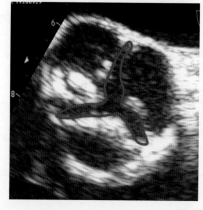

**Fig. 7.1.18** AS AVA planimetry (TOE)

# Velocity ratio (dimensionless index: DI) (Box 7.1.1)

- Velocity ratio ≤ 25% = severe AS
- High sensitivity
- Lower specificity

# Modified continuity equation (CE)

## 3D echo assessment of SV (Figs. 7.1.20, 7.1.21, Box 7.1.2)

- 3D is more accurate than Doppler CE and than 2D volumetric methods to calculate AVA
- Limitations: arrhythmias, significant mitral regurgitation

| Box 7.1.1 Formula to calculate DI (Fig. 7.1.19) |
| --- |
| Velocity ratio = $TVI_{LVOT}$ / $TVI_{AV}$ |

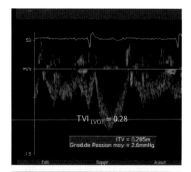

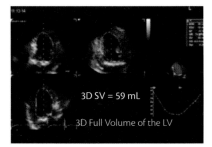

**Fig. 7.1.20** 3D volume assessment

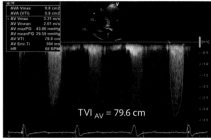

**Fig. 7.1.21** CW AS jet velocity

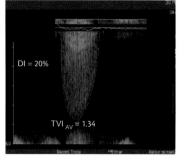

**Fig. 7.1.19** Calculation of DI

# Grades of AS severity (Table 7.1.1)

- ◆ Discrepancy between criteria:
  - ◆ Inappropriate cut-off values or errors in measurements or small body size
  - ◆ Severe AS with low ejection fraction
  - ◆ Paradoxical low-flow, low-gradient AS with preserved LV ejection fraction

# Consequences of AS

## LV geometry/function

- ◆ Evaluate LV function
  - ◆ LVEF often underestimates myocardial dysfunction
  - ◆ global longitudinal function is more sensitive to identify intrinsic myocardial dysfunction (i.e. GLS < 16%, Fig. 7.1.22)

**Table 7.1.1** AS classification (report also blood pressure at the time of examination)

|  | Sclerosis | Mild AS | Moderate AS | Severe AS |
|---|---|---|---|---|
| **Peak aortic velocity, m/sec** | < 2.5 | 2.5–3 | 3–4 | > 4 |
| **Mean gradient (MPG), mmHg** | Normal | < 25 | 25–40 (or 50) | 40 (US) 50 (Europe) |
| **Aortic valve area (AVA), cm²** | Normal | ≥ 1.5 ≥ 0.8 cm²/m² | 1–1.5 0.6–0.8 cm²/m² | < 1 < 0.6 cm²/m² |
| **Dimensionless index** | – | – | – | 0.25 |
| **Energy Loss Index (ELI), cm²/m²** | – | – | – | ≤ 0.5–0.6 |

- Evaluate LV mass (normalized to BSA)
  - identify inadequate/inappropriate LV hypertrophy (Fig. 7.1.23)
    - no hypertrophy despite severe AS
    - severe hypertrophy despite mild AS (coexistent hypertension)
  - evaluate relative wall thickness (RWT)
    - RWT = (2 × PW thickness)/LV end-diastolic diameter
    - identify concentric/eccentric remodelling

## Left atrial (LA) size

- LA area or LA volume

## Pulmonary hypertension

- PSAP > 50 mmHg at rest
- PSAP > 60 mmHg at exercise

# Associated features

## Aortic regurgitation (AR)

- Associated trace or mild AR is common and does not affect the evaluation of AS severity

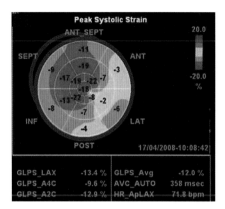

**Fig. 7.1.22** Decrease in GLS in a patient with severe AS

**Fig. 7.1.23** LV remodelling/mass evaluation

◆ Moderate or severe AR is responsible for higher gradient and peak velocity for a given valve area but the continuity equation remains valid
  ◆ it is worth noting that moderate AS and moderate AR may be consistent with a severe combined aortic valve disease

### Mitral regurgitation (MR)

◆ Often MR severity does not affect evaluation of AS severity
◆ It affects AS evaluation when MR leads to a low cardiac output and low gradient
◆ Mitral stenosis (MS) may result in low cardiac output and, therefore, low-flow, low-gradient AS
◆ High cardiac output (haemodialysis, with anaemia, AV fistula, etc.)
  ◆ high cardiac output may cause relatively high gradients in the presence of mild or moderate AS

## Exercise echocardiography

◆ Should not be performed in symptomatic patients
◆ Can be useful in asymptomatic patients
  ◆ criteria for positive exercise ECG (less accurate in elderly subjects > 70 y)
    ◆ symptom development +++ (recommendation for surgery class IC)
    ◆ abnormal blood pressure response: lack of rise (≤ 20 mmHg) or fall in blood pressure ++ (recommendation for surgery class IIaC)
    ◆ ST changes or complex ventricular arrhythmias (minor criteria)

- quantify exercise-induced changes
  - in mean pressure gradient
  - in contractile reserve (changes in LV ejection fraction/strain)
  - in pulmonary arterial systolic pressure (PASP)
- criteria of poor outcome with exercise echo
  - an increase in mean aortic gradient > 18–20 mmHg (recommendation for surgery class IIbC)
  - a weak change in LV ejection fraction
  - a pulmonary hypertension (PASP > 60 mmHg)

## Monitoring

### When?

- mild AS and no significant calcification → evaluation every two to three years
- mild to moderate AS + significant calcification → evaluation every year
- severe AS → clinical examination + echo every six months

### What for?

- occurrence of symptoms—change in exercise tolerance
- progression of AS
  - mean AVA decrease (0.1 cm²/y)
  - mean MPG increase (7 mmHg/y)

- rapid progression = peak aortic velocity > 0.3 m/s/y
- evelution of haemodynamic progression, LV function and hypertrophy, and the ascending aorta

**Surgical class I indications for aortic valve replacement for severe AS**

- symptoms (rest or exercise)
- LVEF < 50%

## Discordant AS grading

**Low ejection fraction (EF) and low-gradient AS**

- **Definition**
  AVA < 1 cm$^2$ (< 0.6 cm$^2$/m$^2$)
  + LV dysfunction (EF ≤ 40%)
  + Mean Ao pressure gradient ≤ 30 (AHA/ACC) − 40 (ESC) mmHg
- Rest TTE cannot differentiate true severe from pseudo-severe AS
- The transaortic velocity is flow-dependent and the aortic valve area (AVA) is not/ less flow-dependent
- In true severe AS, LV dysfunction is secondary to AS and the low cardiac output is responsible for the low gradient
- In pseudo-severe AS,
  - the AS is mild to moderate

- the associated LV dysfunction is due to a ventricular disease
- the low cardiac output due to LV dysfunction limits the AV opening (weak opening forces)

## Dobutamine stress echocardiography (DSE)

- Dosage
  - Rate: start at 2.5 µg/kg/min or 5 µg/kg/min and increase by 2.5 every 5 min
  - Maximum: 10–20 µg/kg/min
  - Performed under supervision and discontinuation of beta-blockers ≥ 24 hours before is usually recommended
- Target
  - Increase heart rate ≥ 10–20 bpm (not exceeding 100 bpm)
  - Avoid ischaemic response that could limit flow recruitment
  - Measure LVOT TVI, AV TVI, MPG, and calculate the AVA at each stage
- Interpretation
  - Flow reserve: increase in stroke volume (SV) ≥ 20% (Figs. 7.1.24, 7.1.25)
- Changes in mean aortic pressure gradient (MPG) and AVA

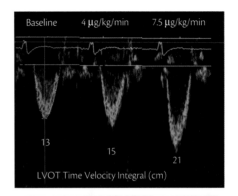

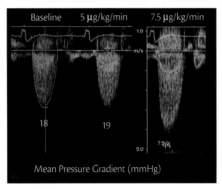

**Fig. 7.1.24** Changes in LVOT TVI and AV TVI under dobutamine infusion in a patient with flow reserve and fixed severe AS. Note the increase in SV and MPG

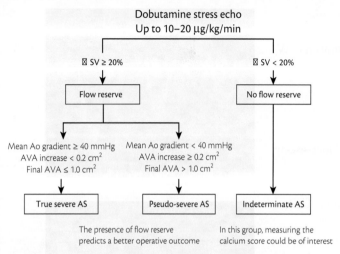

Dobutamine stress echo
Up to 10–20 µg/kg/min

☒ SV ≥ 20%          ☒ SV < 20%

Flow reserve          No flow reserve

Mean Ao gradient ≥ 40 mmHg      Mean Ao gradient < 40 mmHg
AVA increase < 0.2 cm²          AVA increase ≥ 0.2 cm²
Final AVA ≤ 1.0 cm²            Final AVA > 1.0 cm²

True severe AS          Pseudo-severe AS          Indeterminate AS

The presence of flow reserve          In this group, measuring the
predicts a better operative outcome    calcium score could be of interest

**Fig. 7.1.25** Types of dobutamine responses in low-flow, low-gradient AS and LV dysfunction

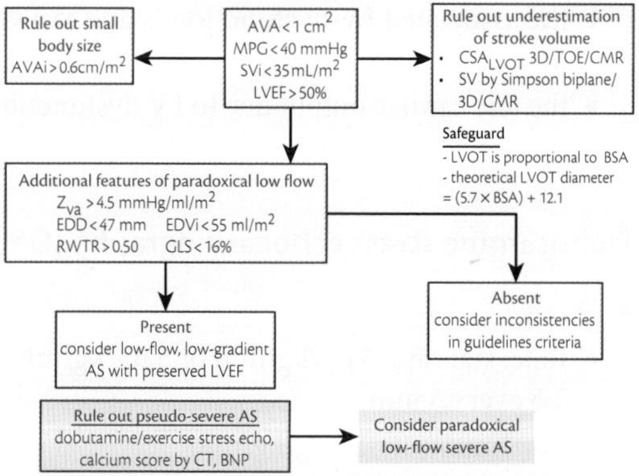

Rule out small
body size
AVAi > 0.6cm/m²

AVA < 1 cm²
MPG < 40 mmHg
SVi < 35 mL/m²
LVEF > 50%

Rule out underestimation
of stroke volume
• CSA$_{LVOT}$ 3D/TOE/CMR
• SV by Simpson biplane/
  3D/CMR

Safeguard
- LVOT is proportional to BSA
- theoretical LVOT diameter
  = (5.7 × BSA) + 12.1

Additional features of paradoxical low flow
Z$_{va}$ > 4.5 mmHg/ml/m²
EDD < 47 mm    EDVi < 55 ml/m²
RWTR > 0.50    GLS < 16%

Present
consider low-flow, low-gradient
AS with preserved LVEF

Absent
consider inconsistencies
in guidelines criteria

Rule out pseudo-severe AS
dobutamine/exercise stress echo,
calcium score by CT, BNP

Consider paradoxical
low-flow severe AS

**Fig. 7.1.26** Stepwise approach to the differential diagnosis of paradoxical low-flow, low-gradient severe AS and LVEF > 50%. CMR: cardiac magnetic resonance; CT: computed tomography; BNP: brain natriuretic peptide

## Preserved LVEF and low-gradient AS
## Paradoxical low-flow, low-gradient AS

♦ **Definition** (Fig. 7.1.26)
AVA < 1 cm² (< 0.6 cm²/m²)
+ LV ejection fraction (EF > 50%)

+ Mean Ao pressure gradient < 40 mm Hg
+ SV index < 35 mL/m²
+ Severely thickened/calcified

- ◆ **Additional echo features in favour of paradoxical AS**
  - ◆ End-diastolic diameter < 47 mm
  - ◆ End-diastolic volume index < 55 mL/m$^2$
  - ◆ Relative wall thickness (RWT) ratio > 0.50
  - ◆ Valvulo-arterial impedance ($Z_{va}$) > 4.5 mmHg/ml/m$^2$ (Fig.7.1.16)
  - ◆ Impaired LV filling
  - ◆ Global longitudinal strain (GLS) < 16%

# 7.2 Pulmonary stenosis (PS)

## Role of echo

**Assessment of the presence, severity, and consequence of PS**

**Aetiology** (cause of the valve disease)

- **congenital** (most frequently)
  - isolated: dysplastic, unileaflet, bileaflet
  - associated with complex congenital malformation: tetralogy of Fallot, double outlet RV, complete atrioventricular, univentricular heart
- **acquired**: rheumatic (rare), carcinoid disease, compression by tumour (internal RVOT or external), deterioration of a bioprosthesis/homograft (Ross surgery)
- **subvalvular stenosis**
  - congenital: RVOT obstruction in case of VSD
  - acquired: infiltrative disease, severe RV hypertrophy
  - iatrogenic (i.e. residual post-surgery for congenital defect)
- **supravalvular stenosis**: rare (congenital)

## Assessment of PS severity

**Valve anatomy** (Fig. 7.2.1)

- Thickening and mobility of the leaflets

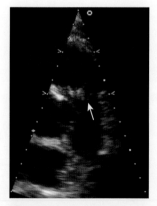

**Fig. 7.2.1** TTE evaluation of PS (arrow)

- Presence of calcification (rare)
- Dome-shaped valve → suspect bicuspid valve
- Inspection of the sub and supravalvular area

## Planimetry

Not possible, except with 3D but not validated

## Pressure gradient (Fig. 7.2.2)

- Most reliable method to ascertain the severity of valve stenosis
- Bernoulli equation: $\Delta P = 4V^2$
- CW Doppler aligned with flow (use colour for help)
- Optimize gain setting
- Use multiple window (PT-SAX, modified 5CV, subcostal)
- Highest velocity obtained must be used for severity assessment

## Functional valve area

- Continuity equation: PW Doppler for RVOT velocity (be aware of subvalvular stenosis)
- RVOT measurement: difficult! (may be easier using TOE)
- CW Doppler for transvalvular gradient
- PVA: $TVI_{PV} / ((RVOT/2)^2 \times 3.14) \times TVI_{RVOT}$

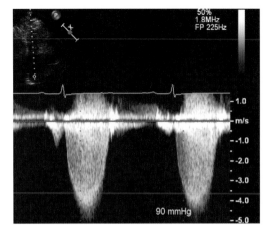

**Fig. 7.2.2** CW Doppler of PV flow

- Not frequently used due to difficulties in RVOT measurement

## Colour Doppler aliasing level

- To localize sub (Fig. 7.2.3) or supra (Fig. 7.2.4) valvular stenosis
- HPRF helps localize stenosis level if the velocity is not too high

## Indices of PS severity

- RV systolic pressure could be measured from TR velocity plus RAP (estimated)
- PASP = RV systolic pressure – PV pressure gradient
- Limitations: in presence of multiple stenoses in the RVOT or pulmonary branch, PV gradient may be different from RV systolic pressure

## Consequence of PS severity

- RV remodelling, RV hypertrophy (Fig. 7.2.5AB), RV function
- Severe PS may be associated with RV hypertrophy, enlargement, and RA enlargement
- RV hypertrophy (PTLAX and PTSAX, apical 4CV, subcostal 4CV)

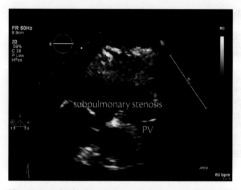

**Fig. 7.2.3** Subvalvular stenosis

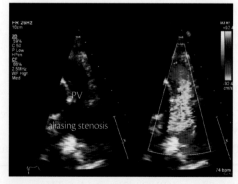

**Fig. 7.2.4** Supravalvular stenosis

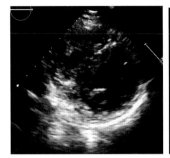

**Fig. 7.2.5A** RV hypertrophy (SAX)

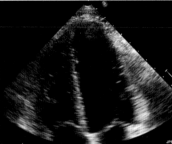

**Fig. 7.2.5B** RV hypertrophy (AP 4CV)

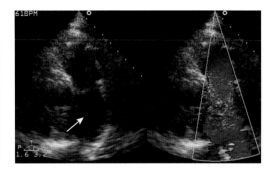

**Fig. 7.2.6** Dilated pulmonary artery (arrow)

- ◆ > 5 mm thickness is considered as hypertrophy
- ◆ RV enlargement: apical 4CV, subcostal 4CV
- ◆ Dilated pulmonary artery (Fig. 7.2.6)

## Grades of PS severity (Table 7.2.1)

**Table 7.2.1** Grades of PS severity

|  | mild | moderate | severe |
|---|---|---|---|
| Peak velocity (m/sec) | < 3 | 3–4 | > 4 |
| Peak gradient (mmHg) | < 36 | 36–64 | > 64 |

# 7.3 Mitral stenosis (MS)

## Role of echo

**Imaging of MS patients should evaluate the aetiology**

- Mechanism
- Dysfunction
- Severity of regurgitation
- Upstream consequences
- Disease progression
- Decision regarding therapy

## Definition

- MS generates obstruction of left atrial (LA) to left ventricle (LV) blood flow
- The presence of a turbulent diastolic jet through the MV orifice, as revealed by colour Doppler interrogation of the LV inflow, should raise the suspicion of mitral stenosis (MS)

## Aetiology (cause of the valve disease)

- **Primary MS (morphological changes of the MV):** rheumatic disease (predominant cause of MS, commissural fusion, multivalve involvement), degenerative (calcifications), congenital (very rare in adults), malignant carcinoid disease, mucopolysaccharidoses, systemic lupus erythematosus, rheumatoid arthritis, methysergide therapy, post-radiation therapy

- **Secondary/functional MS (mitral valve is morphologically intact):** 1) LV inflow obstruction related to extrinsic compression of the MV (usually in the presence of a non-diseased valve), 2) intermittent flow obstruction created by a voluminous LA mass (myxoma/LA thrombus)

## Morphology assessment in rheumatic MS (Box 7.3.1, Tables 7.3.1 and 7.3.2)

- **Thickening of leaflets edges**—first change in RMS, significant if ≥ 5 mm (Fig. 7.3.1)
- **Fusion of commissures**—pathognomonic (Fig. 7.3.2. PMC: posteromedial commissure, ALC: anterolateral commissure; AML: anterior mitral leaflet; PML: posterior mitral leaflet)
- **Chordae shortening and fusion**—contributes less to MS, more to associated MR (Fig. 7.3.3. Systolic apical displacement (red arrow) of the leaflet closure line in relation to the mitral annular plane (green dotted line) due to systolic restriction of the leaflets. Carpentier IIIa MR can be suspected)
- **Calcific deposits**
  - more frequent and in larger quantities in men

---

> **Box 7.3.1** Morphology assessment
>
> Morphology assessment is crucial for therapeutic decision making, best assessed by TOE, can be completed by a 3D echocardiographic study. Several morphological scores (Wilkins and Cormier) can be used to predict the feasibility of PMC

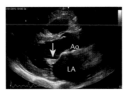

**Fig. 7.3.1** TTE PTLAX: Free edge thickening of AML (arrow) transthoracic

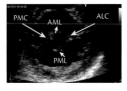

**Fig. 7.3.2** TTE PTSAX zoom mode at the MV opening: Commissural fusion (arrows)

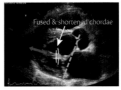

**Fig. 7.3.3** TTE modified PTLAX showing the subvalvular apparatus with chordae thickening

- results in acoustic shadowing
- if doubt regarding the presence of calcific deposits by echo, it can be confirmed by fluoroscopy

## Reduced leaflet mobility

- **diastolic doming** of anterior mitral leaflet (AML) in PSLA view, most specific echo sign for RMS (Fig. 7.3.4)
- '**fish-mouth**' appearance of the MV in diastole in the PSSA view (Fig. 7.3.5)
- '**hockey-stick**' appearance of the AML created by the leaflet edges thickening + the diastolic doming of the AML (Fig. 7.3.6)
- '**funnel shape**', complete loss of mobility, in the late stages of RMS, frequently associated with Carpentier IIIa MR

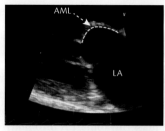

**Fig. 7.3.4** TTE PTLAX: Diastolic doming of the AML (dotted line)

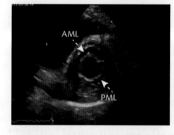

**Fig. 7.3.5** TTE PTSAX: 'Fish-mouth'-like opening of the mitral valve in a patient with RMS

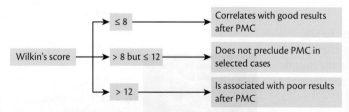

| Wilkin's score | ≤ 8 | Correlates with good results after PMC |
| | > 8 but ≤ 12 | Does not preclude PMC in selected cases |
| | > 12 | Is associated with poor results after PMC |

**Fig. 7.3.7** Wilkin's score: Interpretation

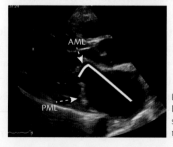

**Fig. 7.3.6** TTE PTLAX: 'Hockey stick' appearance of the AML in diastole

**Table 7.3.1** Wilkin's score

| Grade | Mobility | Thickening | Calcification | Subvalvular thickening |
|---|---|---|---|---|
| 1 | Highly mobile valve. Only leaflet tips have restricted motion | Leaflet thickness normal or thickening in the range of 4–5 mm | A single area of increased echo brightness | Minimal thickening just below the leaflets |
| 2 | Leaflet mid and basal segments have normal mobility | Mid segments of the leaflet are normal but there is considerable thickening of the edges (5–8 mm) | Scattered areas of brightness confined to leaflet's edges | Thickening of chordae extending to one of the chordae length |
| 3 | Valve continues to move forward in diastole mainly from the basal segments | Thickening of the leaflets on all segments (edges, mid and basal segments) between 5–8 mm | Calcifications extending to the mid segment of the leaflets | Thickening extending to distal third of the chordae |
| 4 | No or minimal forward movement of the leaflets in diastole | Considerable thickening of all leaflets (> 8–10 mm) | Extensive calcification extended to all segments of the leaflets | Extensive thickening and shortening of all chordae structures extending down to the papillary muscles |

**Table 7.3.2** Cormier score

| Echocardiographic group | Mitral valve anatomy |
|---|---|
| Group 1 | Pliable non-calcified anterior mitral leaflet and mild subvalvular disease (thin chordae ≥ 10 mm long) |
| Group 2 | Pliable non-calcified anterior mitral leaflet and severe subvalvular disease (thickened chordae < 10 mm long) |
| Group 3 | Calcification of mitral valve of any extent, whatever the state of subvalvular apparatus |

# Assessment of MS severity

## MV anatomic area by planimetry

- **2D planimetry** is the **reference method**
    - offers best correlations to anatomic MV area
    - less dependent on flow, heart rate, chamber compliance
    - not influenced by concomitant MR
    - the most **reliable** tool to estimate MS severity **after PMC**
- **Image acquisition: PTSAX**
    - careful scanning, starting from the mid papillary muscle level, going up towards the base of the mitral annulus, in a parallel plane to the MV opening plane (Fig. 7.3.8A)
    - scanning stops at the level of the MV leaflet tip's plane (will allow definition of the smallest opening orifice)
    - the two fused commissures should be visible in this plane, giving a 'fish-mouth' appearance of the MV orifice in diastole
- **Measurement** (Fig. 7.3.8B)
    - zoom mode
    - lower gain to avoid underestimation
    - measurement in mid-diastole
    - tracing is made at the black–white interface
    - measure at least three cardiac cycles in sinus rhythm
    - measure at least five cardiac cycles in atrial fibrillation

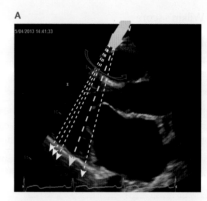

**Fig. 7.3.8** Image acquisition and measurement of the MVA by planimetry with 2D TTE

# 3D TTE planimetry

## Biplane/x-plane modality

◆ allows optimization of the position of the sagittal plane in relation to MV orifice, increasing accuracy of measurement

◆ image acquisition is done from the PTLAX view and the lateral plane is adjusted to transect the edges of the MV leaflets in diastole (Fig. 7.3.9)

◆ zoom mode can be applied to perform the measurement

## 3D zoom mode or full volume acquisition focused on the MV

◆ A pyramidal volume on one cardiac cycle focused on the MV is taken from the apical view by 3D TTE (Fig. 7.3.10AB)

◆ Planimetry of the MV orifice can be made using multi-planar reformat of the 3D data (Fig. 7.3.10C)

◆ With some vendors, planimetry can be directly made from the 3D image (yellow dotted tracing, Fig. 7.3.10D)

## Limitations of the planimetry

◆ Tomographic plane does not coincide with the smallest MV orifice

  ◆ too close to the mitral annulus plane or transecting the mid portion of the MV leaflets → **overestimates MVA** (Fig. 7.3.8A)

  ◆ oblique in relation to the real MV orifice → excludes one of the commissures from the image plane → overestimates MVA

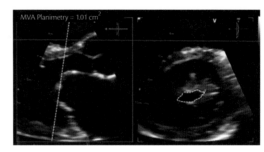

**Fig. 7.3.9** 3D TTE—biplane modality

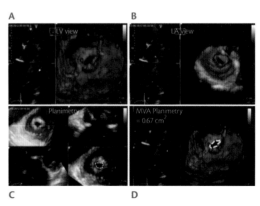

**Fig. 7.3.10** 3D TTE MVA planimetry

- 2D gain settings
- Poor acoustic access
- Deformed valve anatomy (i.e. post-valvuloplasty). It could be overcome by 3D echo (Figs. 7.3.9, 7.3.10ABCD)
- MV orifice anatomy is complex and non-planar

### Trans-mitral diastolic pressure gradient (Fig. 7.3.11, Box 7.3.2)

- **Maximum pressure gradient (PPG)** across the valve is related to the high velocity jet in the stenosis through the simplified Bernoulli equation: $PPG = 4 \times V^2$
- **Mean pressure gradient (MPG)** is calculated by averaging the instantaneous gradients over the flow period
- Pressure gradient depends on
  - MVA
  - LV–LA compliance
  - heart rate
  - transvalvular flow
- **Re-evaluation** is mandatory **after adequate heart rate control** (adjustment of betablocker treatment, optimal HR < 80 bpm)
- **Always report the HR** at which gradient was measured (important for follow-up studies and disease's progression)

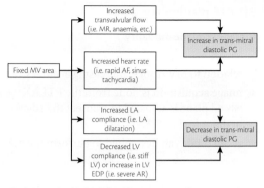

**Fig. 7.3.11** Trans-mitral diastolic pressure gradient

---

**Box 7.3.2** Trans-mitral diastolic pressure gradient

Not reliable in the first 24–72 h after percutaneous mitral commissurotomy (PMC). However, it yields prognostic value in follow-up studies after PMC and should always be reported

## Trans-mitral diastolic PG image acquisition (Box 7.3.3)

**Box 7.3.3** Trans-mitral diastolic PG image acquisition

- Apical 4CV (2CV and 3CV are also useful: the goal is to allow optimal alignment with the flow)
- Colour Doppler-guided detection of diastolic jet direction, optimal alignment of the CW Doppler is needed. Angle (θ) between the direction of the flow and CW Doppler line < 20° to avoid underestimation of PG (Fig. 7.3.12A)
- CW (preferably) or PW Doppler (PW, including HPRF to prevent signal aliasing) can be used by taking care of an adequate position the sample volume at the level of the minimal valve opening plane (into the stenotic orifice)
- Baseline is shifted and velocity scale adjusted so that velocities fill but fit the vertical axis of the tracing
- To avid beat-to-beat variation of the signal, patients should suspend respiration during image acquisition

**Box 7.3.4** Measurement

Optimal sweep speed 100–150 mm/s
Measurement is done at the black–white interface (Fig. 7.3.12B)

- Careful tracing of the outer edge of the signal is done, avoiding the fine linear echoes at the peak of the curve—due to the transit time effect
- Repeated measurements (three in SR or five if AF)

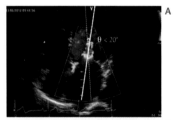

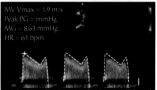

**Fig. 7.3.12** Colour Doppler-guided detection. To avoid underestimation of PG (A) and measurement (B)

## Pressure half-time (PHT)

- Is the time interval (in milliseconds) between the maximal trans-mitral PG and the time point at which this gradient attains the half of its maximal value
- The rate of pressure decline across the stenotic MV
  - is **independent of HR and flow rate**
    - associated MR, or LV diastolic dysfunction or increased LVEDP lowers PHT → underestimate MVA
  - is **inversely correlated to MVA**
    - the more severe the MS → the longer the PHT
- The formula linking MVA to PHT
  - MVA (cm$^2$) = 220/PHT (ms)
  - gives the functional MV area ≠ MVA by planimetry
  - is validated for native MV stenosis only
- MVA estimation through PHT is **not valid in the first 24–72 h after PMC**
- Not feasible if:
  - concave diastolic flow tracings
  - short diastolic filling time (i.e. first degree AV block)

### Pressure half-time (PHT) measurement (Fig. 7.3.13)

- Optimal sweep speed 100–150 mm/s

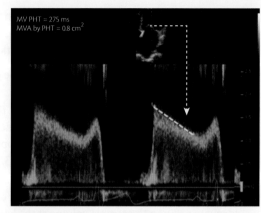

MV PHT = 275 ms
MVA by PHT = 0.8 cm$^2$

**Fig. 7.3.13** MVA assessment by PHT
Notice that sample volume is position at the level of the minimal valve opening

- Measurement is done at the black–white interface where the edge of the diastolic slope is clearly defined
- A clearly defined peak velocity is needed for an accurate measurement
- The deceleration slope of the early trans-mitral flow is used
- In cases with two distinct slopes, the measurement is done on the slowest of the slopes (Fig. 7.3.14)
- Repeated measurements (three in SR or five if AF)

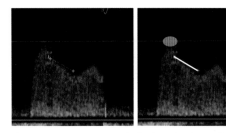

**Fig. 7.3.14** MVA assessment by PHT. Use the slowest slope to evaluate the PHT

## Continuity equation, the Doppler volumetric method

- Time-consuming, more prone to error measurements
- Recommended if discordance between other methods
- Estimates functional MV area ($\neq$ anatomic valve area)
- Doppler volumetric method cannot be applied if more than mild AR or MR is present, but PISA method is applicable
- Relies on the law of volume conservation: in any steady-state process, the rate at which volume enters a system is equal to the rate at which volume leaves the system (Fig. 7.3.15, Box 7.3.5)

## The Proximal Isovelocity Surface Area (PISA) method

- It is technically more difficult to assess
- It can be affected by error measurements

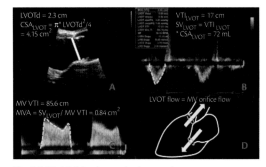

LVOTd = 2.3 cm
$CSA_{LVOT} = \pi^* LVOTd^2/4$
= 4.15 cm$^2$

$VTI_{LVOT}$ = 17 cm
$SV_{LVOT} = VTI_{LVOT}$
$^* CSA_{LVOT}$ = 72 mL

MV VTI = 85.6 cm
$MVA = SV_{LVOT}/ MV VTI = 0.84$ cm$^2$

LVOT flow = MV orifice flow

A    B    C    D

**Fig. 7.3.15** MVA by the continuity equation

### Acquisition (Fig. 7.3.16, Box 7.3.6)

◆ Colour Doppler of the mitral orifice, shifting baseline in the direction of flow in order to detect a correct PISA radius ($V_a$ usually between 25–30 cm/s)

◆ A correct measurement should be done in mid-diastole in a frame where the flow convergence, the jet expansion into the LV, and the proximal isovelocity surface area are best seen

◆ CW Doppler of the trans-mitral flow in diastole in order to detect the highest velocity, flow alignment is guided by colour Doppler

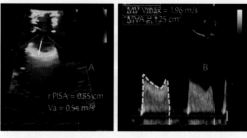

**Fig. 7.3.16** MVA estimation using the PISA method

---

**Box 7.3.5** Equations for the Doppler volumetric method

$$\frac{\text{Blood volume at LV}}{\text{inflow in diastole}} = \frac{\text{Blood volume at LV}}{\text{outflow in systole}}$$

$$CSA_{LVOT} \times TVI_{LVOT} = MVA \times TVI_{MV}$$

$CSA_{LVOT}$ = cross-sectional area of the LVOT

$TVI_{LVOT}$ = time velocity integral of the LVOT

MVA = mitral valve area

$TVI_{MV}$ = time velocity integral of the trans-mitral flow

$CSA_{LVOT} = \pi \times D^2/4$, where D is the LVOT diameter

---

**Box 7.3.6** Equations for the PISA method

$$2\pi r^2 \times V_a = MVA \times V_{max}$$
$$MVA = 2\pi r^2 \times V_a/V_{max}$$
$$MVA = 2\pi r^2 \times V_a/V_{max} \times (\alpha/180)$$

◆ r is the PISA radius

◆ $2\pi r^2$ is the surface of the hemisphere corresponding to the velocity of aliasing

◆ $V_a$ is the aliasing velocity

◆ $V_{max}$ is the maximal trans-stenotic velocity measured by CW Doppler

◆ $\alpha$ = MV leaflets opening angle (red lines)

# Grades of MS severity

**MV stenosis is considered haemodynamically significant if MVA < 1.5 cm²**
**An MVA < 1.0 cm² designates a severe MV stenosis** (Table 7.3.3)

- It is strongly recommended to assess MS severity with at least two methods available

# Consequences of MS

## LA dilatation

- LA surface and volume assessment is recommended as LA dilation may be asymmetric
- LA area > 20 cm² and/or a LA indexed volume > 22 ± 6 mL/m² are considered abnormal

**Table 7.3.3** Recommendations for classification of MS according to current guidelines (report heart rate at the time of examination)

|  | Mild | Moderate | Severe |
|---|---|---|---|
| **Direct findings** |  |  |  |
| Valve area | > 1.5 cm² | 1.5–1.0 cm² | < 1.0 cm² |
| **Supportive findings** |  |  |  |
| Mean pressure gradient* | < 5 mmHg | 5–10 mmHg | > 10 mmHg |
| Pulmonary artery pressure | < 30 mmHg | 30–50 mmHg | > 50 mmHg |

* in patients in sinus rhythm and heart rate < 80 bpm

- LA M-mode diameter > 50 mm or/and LA indexed volume > 60 mL/m$^2$ should prompt the initiation of anticoagulation in MS patients (recommendation class IIa, level of evidence C)

## Pulmonary hypertension

- PSAP > 50 mmHg at rest
- PSAP > 60 mmHg at exercise

## Right ventricle remodelling and function

- Increased chronic PASP leads to RV hypertrophy and dilatation and ultimately, to RV dysfunction and failure
- The presence of RV systolic dysfunction does not preclude PMC or surgery in a patient with MS, but it reflects a higher mortality rate

# Stress echocardiography

- Exercise testing is indicated in
  - asymptomatic patients with significant MS (MVA < 1.5 cm$^2$)
  - patients with equivocal symptoms or discordant symptoms with the severity of MS (i.e. mild to moderate MS in a patient describing exertional dyspnoea)
- Exercise stress echocardiography provides additional information by assessing changes in trans-mitral pressure gradient and pulmonary artery pressures during exercise

- In patients unable to perform an exercise test, dobutamine stress echocardiography can be used
- Changes in trans-mitral pressure gradient and pulmonary pressure during exercise help in selecting patients with significant MS at higher risk for future cardiovascular events

## Echo criteria for PMC

TOE evaluation is mandatory in patients considered for PMC

- Allows accurate evaluation of the MV morphology
- Excludes LA appendage thrombosis
- Reevaluates MS severity and the severity of concomitant MR
- Evaluates interatrial septal morphology (may predict some of the technical difficulties related to transseptal puncture)

Unfavourable echo characteristics

- Severe pulmonary hypertension
- Wilkin's score > 8 or Cormier score = 3
- Very small mitral valve area
- Severe tricuspid regurgitation

Contraindication to PMC

- MV area > 1.5 cm$^2$
- LA thrombus
- More than mild MR
- Severe or bicommissural calcification

Evaluation of successful PMC/stop the procedure

- MV area by planimetry > 1.0 cm/m$^2$
- Complete opening of at least one commissure
- Appearance or increment of MR greater than one grade
  → **is indicative of procedure abortion**

# Evaluation after PMC (before hospital discharge)

The following features are evaluated (usually by TTE)

- MV morphology, extent of commissural opening (Fig. 7.3.17)

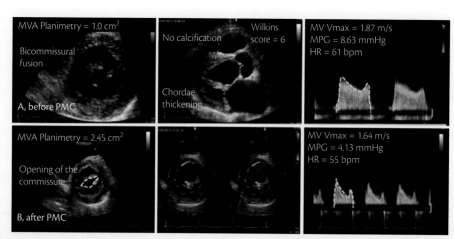

**Fig. 7.3.17** 2D TTE evaluation before and after PMC

- MVA by planimetry (3D is useful when MV orifice might be non-planar)
- MVA by PISA or continuity equation is useful if MVA by planimetry is not feasible
- Mean pressure gradient is assessed and reported, not to quantify the residual MS, but for its prognostic value
- Quantification of the associated MR
- Evaluation of interatrial septum, direction of shunt, Qp/Qs quantification in significant shunts
- Estimation of pulmonary arterial systolic pressure and RV function

# 7.4 Tricuspid stenosis (TS)

## Role of echo

**Assessment of the presence, severity, and consequences of TS**

### Aetiology

- TS is certainly the least common valvular lesion in countries where incidence of rheumatic disease is low
- TS is frequently associated with tricuspid regurgitation, high flow through the valve. Increase the gradient across the valve and increase the pressure in RA
- Cause of the valve disease
  - Rheumatic
  - Rarely isolated and frequently associated with other rheumatic valve disease (mainly mitral rheumatic lesions)
  - Congenital malformation
  - Carcinoid disease
  - Lupus valvulitis
  - Masses obstructing flow (i.e. myxoma, metastatic tumours, thrombus)
  - Device lead impairing valve function (i.e. pacemaker)

# Assessment of TS severity

## Valve anatomy (Fig. 7.4.1)

- Thickening and mobility of the leaflets
- Presence of calcification (rare)

## Pressure gradient (Fig. 7.4.2)

- Most reliable method to ascertain the severity of TS
- Bernoulli equation: $\Delta P = 4V^2$
- CW Doppler aligned with flow (use colour Doppler)
  - optimize gain setting
  - use multiple windows (PS–RV inflow, apical 4CV)
  - highest velocity obtained must be used
  - respiratory variation of RV inflow, measurement in end expiratory apnoea, or average through respiratory cycle
  - repeated measures: average three cycles in SR, five cycles in AF
- Interpretation
  - MPG > 5 mmHg indicates severe TS

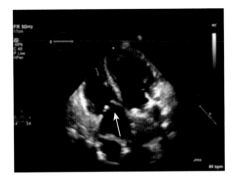

**Fig. 7.4.1** TTE evaluation of TS (arrow)

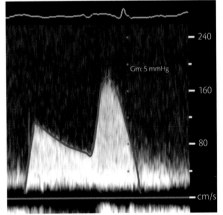

**Fig. 7.4.2** CW Doppler of TV inflow

## Pressure half-time (PHT) (Fig. 7.4.3)

- Proposed for assessment of TS severity
- A constant of 190 was proposed rather than 220 for MS
- TVA with PHT = 190/T1/2
- PHT ≥ 190 ms is indicative of significant TS

## Continuity equation (Fig. 7.4.4)

- PW Doppler for RVOT velocity
  - be aware of subvalvular stenosis
- CW Doppler for transvalvular gradient
- Area → $TVI_{TV}/ ((RVOT/2)^2 \times 3.14) \times TVI_{RVOT}$
- Not frequently used due to difficulties in RVOT measurement and multiple errors possible (use TOE)

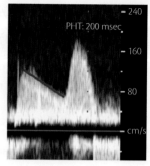

**Fig. 7.4.3** Measure of PHT

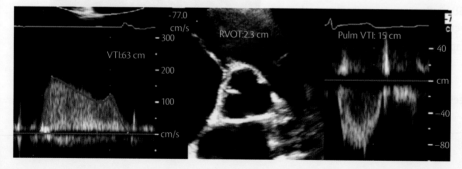

**Fig. 7.4.4** Assessment of TS severity by continuity equation

- Presence of TR = main limitation (if severe, TVA is underestimated)
- TVA < 1 cm$^2$ indicates severe TS regardless of TR

## 3D planimetry (3D) (Fig. 7.4.5)

- 3D echo is the only method allowing direct planimetry of the tricuspid orifice
- Few data and no external validation → not recommended alone

## Consequences of TS

- right atrial dilatation (Fig. 7.4.6A)
- inferior vena cava dilatation (Fig. 7.4.6B)

## Grades of TS severity (Table 7.4.1)

**Table 7.4.1** Findings indicative of haemodynamically significant TS

|  | Severe |
| --- | --- |
| **Specific findings** |  |
| **Mean pressure gradient** | ≥ 5 mmHg |
| TV inflow TVI | > 60 cm |
| $T_{\frac{1}{2}}$ (PHT) | ≥ 190 ms |
| TVA with continuity equation* | ≤ 1 cm$_2$ |
| **Supportive findings** |  |
| **RA dilatation** | ≥ moderate |
| **IVC dilatation** | +++ |

*In the presence of mild TR, the TVA might be underestimated (however, a TVA < 1cm$^2$ indicates severe TS)

A 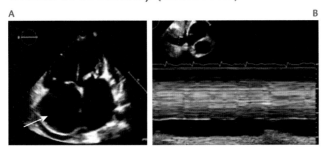 B

**Fig. 7.4.6** Consequences of TS

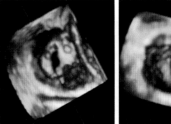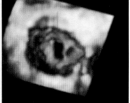

**Fig. 7.4.5** 3D visualization of TV with significant stenosis

# 7.5  Aortic regurgitation (AR)

## Role of echo

Imaging of AR patients should evaluate the aetiology—mechanism—dysfunction—severity of regurgitation—consequences—possibility of repair

### Aetiology

#### Primary AR (organic/structural): Primary pathology of the valve

◆ Congenital (most frequently bicuspid aortic disease, Fig. 7.5.1A)
◆ Rheumatic disease (Fig. 7.5.1B)
◆ Infective endocarditis
◆ Degenerative disease (frequently combined with aortic stenosis, Fig. 7.5.1C)

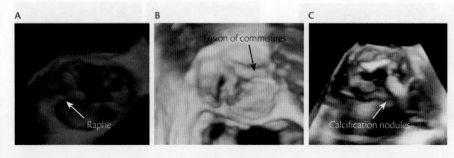

**Fig. 7.5.1** Pathology of the valve. Congenital (A), rheumatic (B), degenerative (C)

## Secondary AR (functional/non-structural)

- Aortic aneurysm with sinotubular junction dilatation (congenital: bicuspid, Marfan, inflammatory or infectious, atherosclerosis, and hypertension) (Fig. 7.5.2B)
- Aortic dissection (Fig. 7.5.2A)
  - aortic dissection extending into the aortic root and disrupting the normal leaflet attachment
  - redundant dissection flap prolapsing through intrinsically normal leaflets

**A**  Aortic dissection with disruption of normal leaflet attachment

**B**  Aortic aneurysm with dilatation of the sinotubular junction

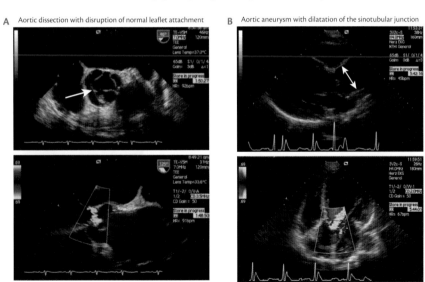

**Fig. 7.5.2** Examples of secondary AR

# Aortic valve anatomy/imaging

- ◆ Three cusps of semi-lunar shape
  - ◆ which are attached to
    - ◆ the aorta media
    - ◆ the myocardium of the LVOT
    - ◆ the anterior mitral leaflet
  - ◆ meet at three commissures that are equally spaced
  - ◆ called left coronary (LCC), right coronary (RCC) and non-coronary cusps (NCC) based on the location of the coronary ostia (Fig. 7.5.3AB)
- ◆ The PTLAX view is classically used to measure the LVOT, the aortic annulus, the sinotubular junction and the aortic sinuses (Fig. 7.5.3C)
- ◆ Leaflet thickening and morphology can be visualized from PTLAX, PTSAX, and apical 5CV
- ◆ If 2D TTE does not allow to correctly identify the anatomy and causes of AR, 3D echo, and especially TOE can better evaluate AR aetiology and mechanisms

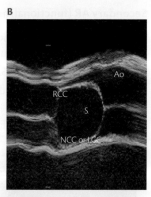

**Fig. 7.5.3B** Aortic cusps (M-mode PTLAX)

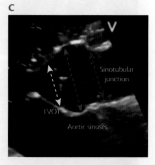

**Fig. 7.5.3C** Normal morphology of the aorta (PTLAX)

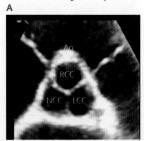

**Fig. 7.5.3A** Aortic cusps (PTSAX)

# Mechanism of dysfunction (Carpentier's classification) (Table 7.5.1)

**Table 7.5.1**  Carpentier's classification and echo findings

| Dysfunction | Echo findings |
| --- | --- |
| **I:** Enlargement of the aortic root with normal cusps (**Fig. 7.5.4**) | ◆ Dilatation of any components of the aortic root (aortic annulus, sinuses of Valsalva, sinotubular junction) |
| **IIa:** Cusp prolapse with eccentric AR jet (**Fig. 7.5.5**) <br> ◆ cusp flail <br> ◆ partial cusp prolapse <br> ◆ whole cusp prolapse | ◆ Complete eversion of a cusp into the LVOT in long-axis views <br> ◆ Distal part of a cusp prolapsing into the LVOT (clear bending of the cusp body on long-axis views and presence of a small circular structure near the cusp free edge on short-axis views) <br> ◆ Free edge of a cusp overriding the plane of aortic annulus with billowing of the entire cusp body into the LVOT (presence of a large circular or oval structure immediately beneath the valve on short-axis views) |
| **IIb:** Free edge fenestration with eccentric AR jet | ◆ Presence of an eccentric AR jet without definite evidence of cusp prolapse |
| **III:** Poor cusp quality or quantity (**Fig. 5.7.6**) | ◆ Thickened and rigid valves with reduced motion <br> ◆ Tissue destruction (endocarditis) <br> ◆ Large calcification spots/extensive calcifications of all cusps interfering with cusp motion |

**Fig. 7.5.4** Type I: Enlargement of the aortic root (Ao) with normal cusps (AV) (dilatation of the aortic root (aortic annulus))

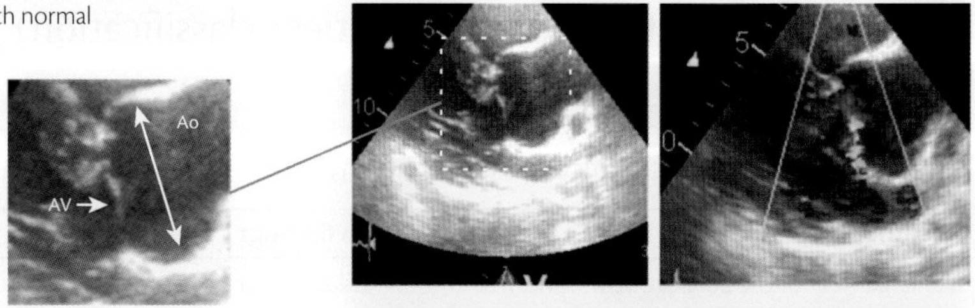

**Fig. 7.5.5** Type IIa: Cusp prolapse with eccentric AR jet due to enormous vegetation (complete eversion of a cusp into the LVOT in long-axis views)

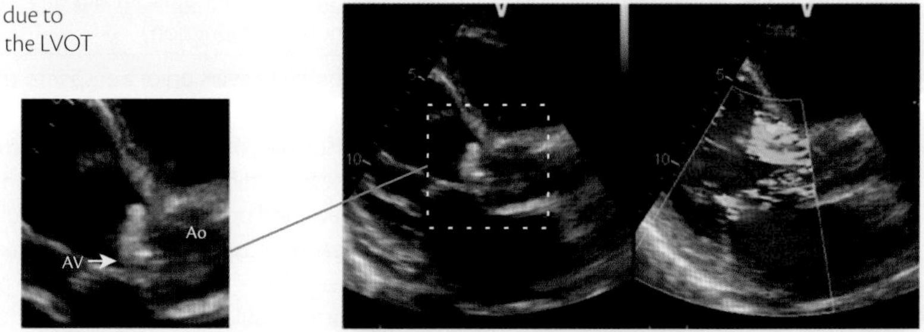

**Fig. 7.5.6** Type III: Poor cusps quality or quantity (thickened and rigid valves with reduced motion)

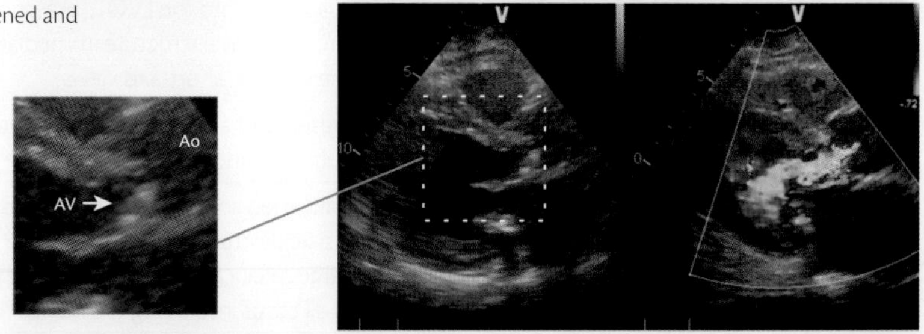

# Assessment of AR severity

## Aortic valve morphology

- Visual assessment
- Multiple views

**Usefulness/Advantages**

- Flail valve (Figs. 7.5.5 and 7.5.7) is specific for significant AR

**Limitations**

- Other abnormalities are non-specific of significant AR

## Colour-flow imaging in AR

- Optimize colour gain/scale
- Parasternal long- and short-axis views

**Usefulness/Advantages**

- Ease of use
- Evaluates the spatial orientation of AR jet
- Quick screen for AR

**Limitations**

- Influenced by technical and haemodynamic factors
- Inaccurate for eccentric jet
- Expands unpredictably below the orifice (Fig. 7.5.8)

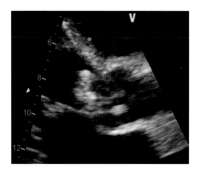

**Fig. 7.5.7** AV morphology PTLAX view of an AV prolapse on endocarditis

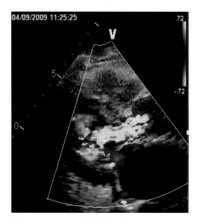

**Fig. 7.5.8** Example of colour-flow image in AR

## Proximal jet width or the cross-sectional jet area to LVOT diameter ratio (Fig. 7.5.9)

♦ Although this measurement suffers from a high inter-observer variability, a jet width ratio > 65% is a strong argument for severe AR

♦ A limitation of this measure is the potential underestimation of eccentric jets and the overestimation of central jets, which expand fully

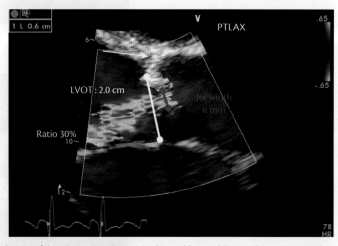

**Fig. 7.5.9** Evaluation of the AR severity using proximal jet width to LVOT ratio. The maximum colour jet diameter (width) is measured in diastole immediately below the aortic valve (at the junction of the LVOT and aortic annulus) in the PTLAX view

## Vena contracta width in AR

- PTLAX is preferred (AP 4CV if not available) (Fig. 7.5.10ABC)
- Optimize colour gain/scale
- Identify the three components of the regurgitant jet (VC, PISA, jet into LV)
- Reduce the colour sector size and imaging depth to maximize frame rate
- Expand the selected zone (zoom)
- Use the cine loop to find the best frame for measurement
- Measure the smallest VC (immediately distal to the regurgitant orifice, perpendicular to the direction of the jet)

### Usefulness/Advantages

- Relatively quick and easy
- Relatively independent of haemodynamic and instrumentation factors
- Not affected by other valve leak
- Good for extremes AR: mild vs severe
- Can be used in eccentric jet

### Limitations

- Not valid for multiple jets
- Small values; small measurement errors leads to large % error
- Intermediate values need confirmation
- Affected by systolic changes in regurgitant flow

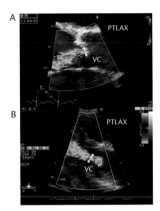

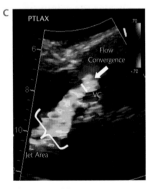

**Fig. 7.5.10** PTLAX vena contracta

### Interpretation

- Mild AR VC < 3 mm
- Severe AR VC > 6 mm

## PISA method in AR: recordings

- Apical 4CV (Fig. 7.5.11ABCDEF)
- Optimize colour-flow imaging of MR
- Zoom the image of the regurgitant mitral valve
- Decrease the Nyquist limit (colour-flow zero baseline)
- With the cine mode select the best PISA
- Display the colour off and on to visualize the MR orifice
- Measure the PISA radius at mid-systole using the first aliasing and along the direction of the ultrasound beam
- Measure MR peak velocity and TVI (CW)
- Calculate flow rate, EROA, R Vol (Box 7.5.1)

### Usefulness/advantages

- Can be used in eccentric jet
- Small influence of haemodynamics
- Quantitative: estimate lesion severity (EROA) and volume overload (R Vol)

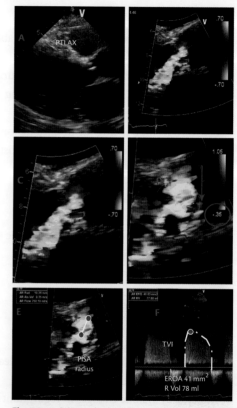

**Fig. 7.5.11** PISA method in AR

## Limitations

- PISA shape affected
  - by the aliasing velocity
  - in case of non-circular orifice (Fig. 7.5.12)
  - by systolic changes in regurgitant flow
  - by adjacent structures (flow constrainment)
- PISA radius is more a hemi-ellipse
- Errors in PISA measurement are squared
- Inter-observer variability
- Not valid for multiple jets (Fig. 7.5.13)
- Feasibility limited by aortic valve calcifications

## Interpretation

- Mild AR EROA < 10 mm$^2$
- Severe AR EROA ≥ 30 mm$^2$

**Box 7.5.1** Formulas to calculate PISA

$$EROA = flow/peak\ velocity$$
$$EROA = (2\pi r^2 \times Va)/peak\ velocity$$
$$EROA = (2 \times 3.14 \times 1.03 \times 35)/578$$
$$EROA = 233/578 = 0.41\ cm^2$$
$$R\ Vol = EROA \times TVI$$
$$R\ Vol = 0.41\ cm^2 \times 190\ cm = 78\ mL$$

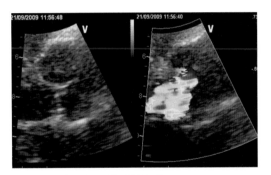

**Fig. 7.5.12** Distortion of the PISA in AR

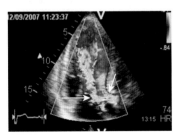

**Fig. 7.5.13** Presence of two AR jets (arrows)

## 3D vena contracta (VC)—PISA in AR

- ◆ VC area calculation assumes a circular or elliptical orifice
- ◆ The orifice geometry is often variable depending on the shape of the orifice and aortic cusps surrounding the orifice
- ◆ Careful consideration of the 3D geometry of VC/PISA may be of interest in evaluating the severity of AR
- ◆ The best 3D echo method to quantitate AR severity is still not defined
  - ◆ VC area < 30 mm$^2$ suggests mild AR
  - ◆ VC area > 50 mm$^2$ suggests severe AR (Fig. 7.5.14AB)

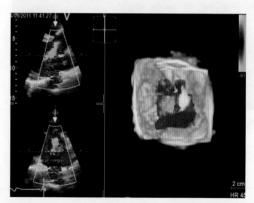

**Fig. 7.5.14A** 3D evaluation of AR

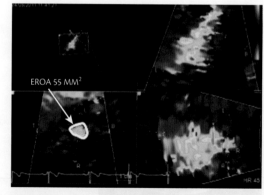

EROA 55 MM$^2$

**Fig. 7.5.14B** 3D evaluation of AR

## Diastolic aortic flow reversal

- Suprasternal approach (Fig. 7.5.15)
- PW Doppler
- Proximal descending aorta/abdominal aorta

### Usefulness/Advantages

- Simple

### Limitations

- Affected by sample volume location
- Affected by the acuity of AR
  - fast equalization of Ao-LV diastolic pressure with no end-diastolic flow reversal
- Affected by aortic compliance
  - flow reversal may be extended with stiffer aorta (i.e. elderly)
- Brief velocity reversal is normal
- Cut-off validated for distal aortic arch

### Interpretation

- Mild AR: early diastolic flow reversal (Fig. 7.5.16AB)
- Suggestive of severe AR (Fig. 7.5.17AB)
  - holodiastolic flow reversal
  - end-diastolic flow reversal velocity > 20 cm/sec (arrow)

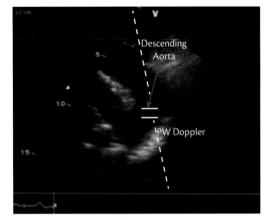

**Fig. 7.5.15** PW Doppler sample positioning

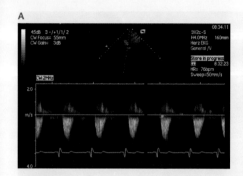

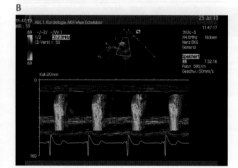

**Fig. 7.5.16** Mild AR (early diastolic flow reversal)
(A: PW Doppler, B: Colour M-mode)

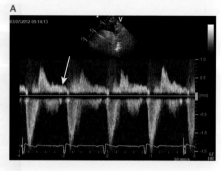

**Fig. 7.5.17** Severe AR (holodiastolic flow reversal)
(A: PW Doppler, B: Colour M-mode)

## Pressure half-time (PHT)

- Apical 3CV or 5CV
- CW AR jet

### Usefulness/Advantages

- Simple

### Limitations

- Qualitative
- Complementary finding
- Requires adequate spectrum definition (alignment)
- Complete signal difficult to obtain in eccentric jet
- Lengthening (↑) of PHT with
  - chronic LV adaptation (↑ LV compliance) to AR
- Shortening (↓) of PHT with
  - ↑ LV end-diastolic pressure
  - ↑ systemic vascular resistance
  - ↑ aortic compliance (i.e. dilated aorta)
  - ↓ LV relaxation

### Interpretation (Fig. 7.5.20)

- Mild AR > 500 ms (Fig. 7.5.18)
- Severe AR < 200 ms (Fig. 7.5.19)

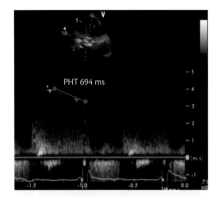

**Fig. 7.5.18** Mild AR

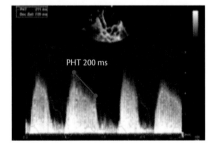

**Fig. 7.5.19** Severe AR. While faint spectral display is compatible with trace or mild AR, significant overlap between moderate and severe AR exists in more dense jet tracings

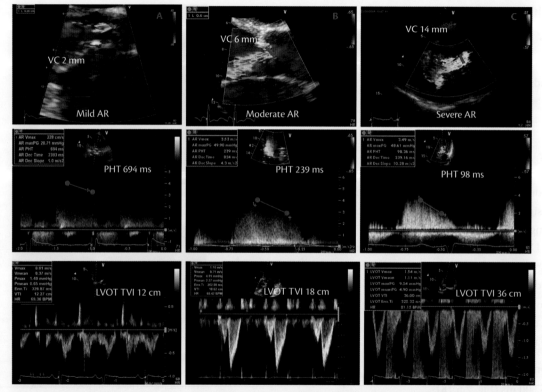

**Fig. 7.5.20** Examples of various degrees of AR (A: mild; B: moderate; C: severe). The LVOT flow (CO > 8 L/min in favour of severe AR) and VC increase with the AR severity while the PHT shortens

## Doppler quantitation from two valves flow (Box 7.5.2)

◆ Not applicable in case of significant mitral regurgitation

---

**Box 7.5.2** Doppler volumetric method (Fig. 7.5.21)

Calculate LVOT stroke volume
$SV_{LVOT} = LVOT\ diameter^2 \times 0.785 \times TVI_{LVOT}$
Calculate mitral inflow stroke volume
$SV_{MI} = mitral\ annulus\ diameter^2 \times 0.785 \times TVI_{MI}$
Subtract MI SV from LVOT SV
Measure AR TVI by continuous-wave Doppler
$EROA = R\ Vol_{AV}/TVI_{AR}$
AR fraction $(RF) = R\ Vol_{AV}/SV_{LVOT}$

---

◆ This approach is time-consuming and is associated with several drawbacks

### Interpretation

◆ Severe AR: RF $\geq$ 50%

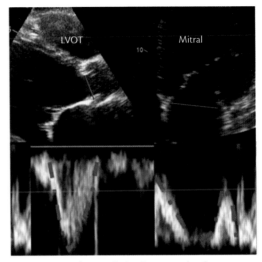

**Fig. 7.5.21** Doppler quantitation from two valves flow

## LV adaptation to AR (Fig. 7.5.22)

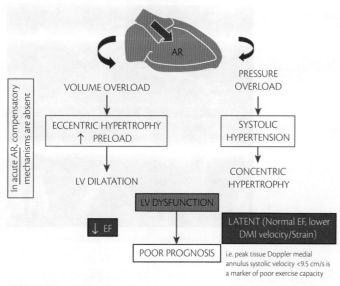

VOLUME OVERLOAD

PRESSURE OVERLOAD

In acute AR, compensatory mechanisms are absent

ECCENTRIC HYPERTROPHY
↑ PRELOAD

SYSTOLIC HYPERTENSION

LV DILATATION

CONCENTRIC HYPERTROPHY

LV DYSFUNCTION

↓ EF

LATENT (Normal EF, lower DMI velocity/Strain)

POOR PROGNOSIS

i.e. peak tissue Doppler medial annulus systolic velocity <9.5 cm/s is a marker of poor exercise capacity

**Fig. 7.5.22** LV adaptation to AR

# Integrating indices of AR severity (Table 7.5.2)

**Table 7.5.2** Integrating indices of AR severity

| | Mild | Moderate | Severe |
|---|---|---|---|
| **Qualitative structural and Doppler parameters** | | | |
| Valve morphology (2D/3D) | Normal or abnormal | Normal or abnormal | Abnormal/flail or large coaptation defect |
| Jet width (colour flow) | Small in central jets | Intermediate | Large (central jets), variable (eccentric jets) |
| Jet density (CW) | Incomplete/Faint | Dense | Dense |
| Diastolic flow reversal in descending aorta (PW) | Early diastolic | Intermediate | Holodiastolic (end-diastolic velocity > 20 cm/s) |
| Diastolic flow reversal in abdominal aorta (PW) | Absent | Absent | Present |
| **Semi-quantitative parameters** | | | |
| Pressure half-time, ms (CW) | > 500 | Intermediate | < 200 |
| Vena contracta width, mm (colour flow) | < 3 | Intermediate | > 6 |
| **Quantitative parameters** | | | |
| EROA, cm$^2$ | < 10 | 10–19 and 20–29 | ≥ 30 |
| Regurgitant volume, ml | < 30 | 30–44 and 45–59 | ≥ 60 |
| Regurgitant fraction, % | < 30 | Intermediate | ≥ 50 |
| | **+ LV size** | | |

# Monitoring of asymptomatic patients with AR

## When?

◆ Mild to moderate AR → clinical examination every year + echo every two years

◆ Severe AR and normal LV function → echo six months after initial examination
  ◆ if stable, yearly follow-up
  ◆ if significant changes of LV diameters/LV EF or close to the thresholds for intervention → follow-up every six months

◆ Aortic root dilatation → echo six months after initial examination
  ◆ yearly follow-up
  ◆ shorter intervals if close to the threshold for intervention or increase in aortic diameter

## What for?

◆ Progression of AR: marked individual differences

◆ Progression of the lesion: new flail leaflet, increase of annulus size

◆ Evolution of LV end-systolic dimension or volume and EF

## Surgical class I indications for AV surgery in AR

◆ Severe AR +
  ◆ symptoms
  ◆ no symptoms but LV ejection fraction ≤ 50% and/or ESD > 50 mm or ESD > 25 mm/m$^2$ or LVEDD > 70mm

# Chronic/acute AR: differential diagnosis (Box 7.5.3)

**Box 7.5.3** Chronic and acute AR. A differential diagnosis

|  | Acute | Chronic |
|---|---|---|
| Cardiac output | ↓ | N |
| Pulse pressure | N↓ | ↓ |
| Syst. pressure | ↓ | ↑ |
| LV ED pressure | ↑↑ | N |
| LV size N | N | ↑ |

# 7.6  Mitral regurgitation (MR)

## Role of echo

### Imaging of MR patients should evaluate the aetiology

◆ mechanism
◆ dysfunction
◆ severity of regurgitation
◆ consequences
◆ possibility of repair

## Definition

◆ Backflow of blood from left ventricle (LV) to left atrium (LA)
◆ Typically MR occurs during systole, but in rare conditions (i.e. AV block) it may occur also during diastole

## Aetiology: cause of the valve disease

### Primary MR (organic/structural): Primary pathology of the valve

◆ **Non-ischaemic:** degenerative disease (Barlow, fibroelastic degeneration, Marfan, Ehler–Danlos, annular calcification), rheumatic disease, toxic valvulopathy, infective endocarditis
◆ **Ischaemic:** ruptured (complete/partial) papillary, scarred/retracted papillary muscle

**Secondary MR (functional/non-structural): malcoaptation related to LV (LA) remodelling with no structural abnormalities of the valve → non-ischaemic and ischaemic**

# Mechanism: lesion/deformation resulting in valve dysfunction

## Degenerative disease (primary MR)

◆ The most common surgical MR cause
◆ Covers a large spectrum of lesions
  ◆ isolated scallop to multi-segment (or generalized) prolapse
  ◆ thin/non-redundant leaflets to thick (> 5 mm)/excess-tissue

## Phenotypes

◆ Barlow (diffuse leaflet thickening)
◆ fibroelastic degeneration (thickening of the prolapsed area)

## Morphotypes (Fig. 7.6.1)

◆ isolated billowing: leaflets tips remaining intraventricular
◆ prolapse: leaflet tip below the mitral annulus plane and directed towards the LV
◆ flail leaflet: leaflet eversion (leaflet tip is directed towards the LA)

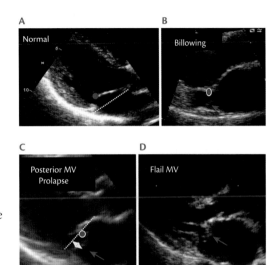

**Fig. 7.6.1** Morphotypes, different stages: (A) normal; (B) billowing; (C) posterior MV prolapse; (D) flail MV

## Factors affecting the possibility of repair: prolapse location, valvular/annular calcifications and severity of annulus dilatation

### Secondary (functional) MR

- ◆ Structurally normal mitral valve
- ◆ Mitral tethering secondary to:
  - ◆ ventricular deformation/remodelling
  - ◆ annular dilatation/dysfunction
  - ◆ insufficient LV-generated closing forces
- ◆ **Echo-morphological parameters**
  - ◆ global LV remodelling: LV sizes, volumes, function, sphericity index (SI) (Fig 7.6.2A)
  - ◆ local LV remodelling: papillary muscles displacement, regional wall motion abnormality
  - ◆ mitral valve (MV) deformation: tenting area (TA), coaptation distance (CD), posterolateral angle (PLA) (Fig 7.6.2B, Box 7.6.1)

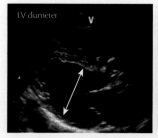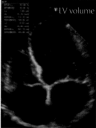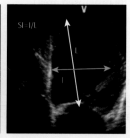

**Fig. 7.6.2A** Echo-morphological parameters: global LV remodelling

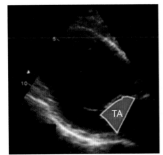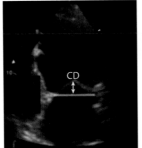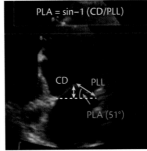

$$PLA = sin{-1} (CD/PLL)$$

**Fig. 7.6.2B** Mitral deformation

**Box 7.6.1** Unfavourable characteristics for **mitral valve repair** in secondary MR

ED diameter > 65 mm, ES diameter > 51 mm, SI > 0.7

TA > 2.5–3 cm²; CD ≥ 1 cm; PLA > 45°

Severe apical and lateral displacement of papillary muscles

# Dysfunction (Carpentier's classification): leaflet motion abnormality

## Type I : Normal leaflet motion

- Annular dilatation (rarely isolated)
- Leaflet perforation (infective endocarditis)

- Cleft MV (Fig. 7.6.3A)

## Type II : Excessive leaflet mobility

- Prolapse
- Flail leaflet (Fig. 7.6.3B)

## Type III : Reduced leaflet mobility or motion

- **IIIa:** systolic+diastolic restriction due to chordae shortening, leaflet thickening (rheumatic disease, toxic valvulopathy, radiation-induced mitral valve disease) (Fig. 7.6.3C)
- **IIIb:** systolic restriction: secondary MR (Fig. 7.6.3D)

## Combination

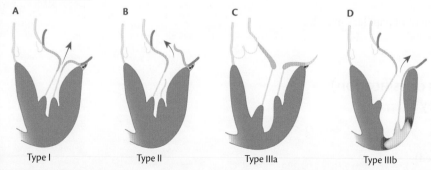

**Fig. 7.6.3** Carpentier's classification

# Mitral valve anatomy/imaging (Figs. 7.6.4AB)

- Two leaflets (each with a thickness about 1 mm)
- Posterior leaflet
  - quadrangular shape
  - two well-defined indentations
  - three individual scallops (P1–P2–P3)
  - two-thirds of the annular circumference
- Anterior leaflet
  - semi-circular shape
  - in continuity with the non-coronary cusp of the aortic valve (intervalvular fibrosa)
  - artificially divided into three portions (A1–A2–A3)

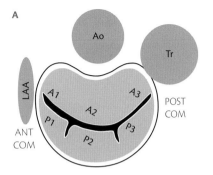

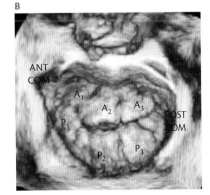

**Fig. 7.6.4** (A) Diagram of the mitral valve.
(B) 3D TOE volume rendering of the mitral valve.
ANT COM: anterior commissure POST COM:
posterior commissure

# Mitral valve analysis: transthoracic echo (TTE) (Figs. 7.6.5, 7.6.6)

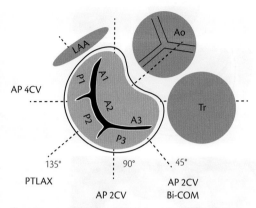

**Fig. 7.6.5** Transthoracic diagram of the mitral valve (Box 7.6.2)

**Box 7.6.2** Definitions

AP 4CV = apical 4-chamber
AP 2CV = apical 2-chamber
PTLAX = parasternal long-axis
PTSAX = parasternal short-axis
Bi–COM = bi-commissure

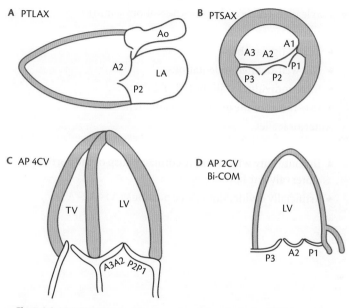

**Fig. 7.6.6** MVI: TTE Diagrams of each section of the mitral valve: (A) PTLAX; (B) PTSAX; (C) AP 4CV; (D) AP 2CV

# Mitral valve imaging (TTE) (Fig. 7.6.7ABCD)

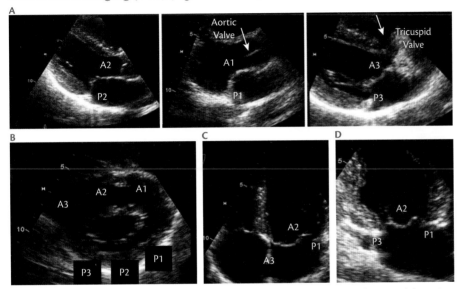

**Fig. 7.6.7** MVI: TTE echograms of each section of the mitral valve: (A) PTLAX; (B) PTSAX; (C) AP 4CV; (D) AP 2CV

# Mitral valve analysis: transoesophageal echo (TOE) (Figs. 7.6.8, 7.6.9ABCD)

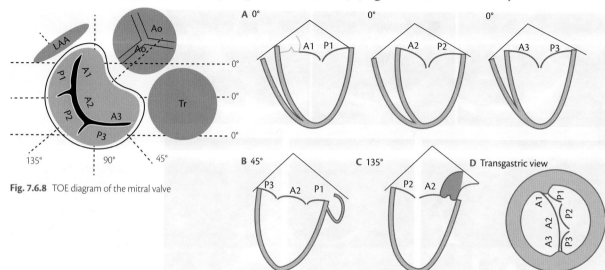

**Fig. 7.6.8** TOE diagram of the mitral valve

**Fig. 7.6.9** TOE diagrams of each section of the mitral valve: (A) 4-chamber-view at 0°; (B) bicommissural view at 45°; (C) long-axis view at 135°; (D) transgastric view

# Mitral valve imaging (TOE) (Figs. 7.6.10ABCD, 7.6.11AB)

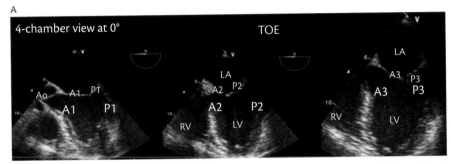

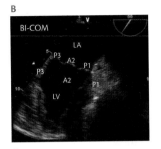

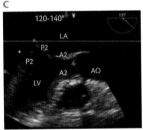

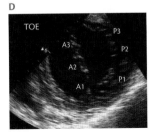

**Fig. 7.6.10** TOE echocardiograms of each section of the mitral valve: (A) 4-chamber view at 0°; (B) bicommissural view at 30–70°; (C) long-axis view at 120–135°; (D) transgastric view

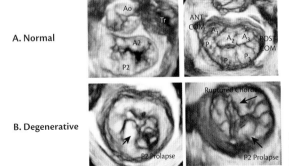

**A. Normal**

**B. Degenerative**

**Fig. 7.6.11** 3D TOE volume rendering of the mitral valve: LA perspective. (A) normal; (B) degenerative

# Probability of successful mitral valve repair in MR (Table 7.6.1)

**Table 7.6.1** Probability of successful mitral valve repair in MR

| Aetiology | Dysfunction | Calcification | Mitral annulus dilatation | Probability of repair |
|---|---|---|---|---|
| Degenerative | II: Localized prolapse (P2 and/or A2) | No/Localized | Mild/Moderate | Feasible |
| Secondary | I or IIIb | No | Moderate | |
| Barlow | II: Extensive prolapse (≥ three scallops, posterior commissure) | Localized (annulus) | Moderate | Difficult |
| Rheumatic | IIIa but pliable anterior leaflet | Localized | Moderate | |
| Severe Barlow | II: Extensive prolapse (≥ three scallops, anterior commissure) | Extensive (annulus + leaflets) | Severe | Unlikely |
| Endocarditis | II: Prolapse but destructive lesions | No | No/Mild | |
| Rheumatic | IIIa but stiff anterior leaflet | Extensive (annulus + leaflets) | Moderate/Severe | |
| Secondary | IIIb but severe valvular deformation | No | No or Severe | |

# Assessment of MR severity

## Mitral valve morphology

- ◆ Visual assessment
- ◆ Multiple views

### Usefulness/Advantages

- ◆ Flail valve (Fig. 7.6.12) or ruptured PMs are specific for significant MR

### Limitations

- ◆ Other abnormalities are non-specific of significant MR

## Colour-flow imaging in MR

- ◆ Optimize colour gain/scale
- ◆ Evaluate in two views
- ◆ Need blood pressure evaluation

### Usefulness/Advantages

- ◆ Ease of use
- ◆ Evaluates the spatial orientation of MR jet
- ◆ Good screening test for mild vs severe MR

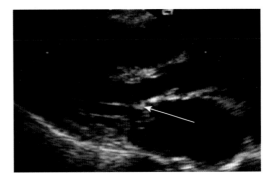

**Fig. 7.6.12** MV morphology (flail)

**Limitations**

- Can be inaccurate for estimation of MR severity
- Influenced by technical and haemodynamic factors
- Underestimates eccentric jet adhering the LA wall (Coanda effect) (Fig. 7.6.13)

## Vena contracta width in MR

- Two orthogonal planes: PTLAX (Fig. 7.6.14) and AP-4CV (Fig. 7.6.15)
- Optimize colour gain/scale (40–70 cm/s)
- Identify the three components of the regurgitant jet (VC, PISA, jet into LA)

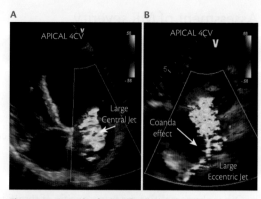

**Fig. 7.6.13** Example of colour-flow image in MR

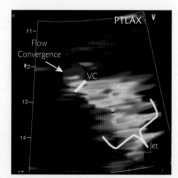

**Fig. 7.6.14** PTLAX vena contracta

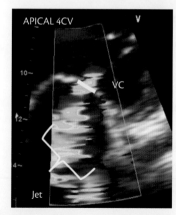

**Fig. 7.6.15** AP-4CV vena contracta

- Reduce the colour sector size and imaging depth to maximize frame rate
- Expand the selected zone (zoom)
- Use the cine-loop to find the best frame for measurement
- Measure the smallest VC (immediately distal to the regurgitant orifice, perpendicular to the direction of the jet)
- The VC is the area of the jet as it leaves the regurgitant orifice; it reflects thus the regurgitant orifice area

## Usefulness/Advantages

- Relatively quick and easy
- Relatively independent of haemodynamic and instrumentation factors
- Not affected by other valve leak
- Good for extreme MR: mild vs severe
- Can be used in eccentric jet

## Limitations

- Not valid for multiple jets
- Small values; small measurement errors leads to large % error
- Intermediate values need confirmation
- Affected by systolic changes in regurgitant flow

## Interpretation

- Mild MR VC < 3 mm
- Severe MR VC > 7 mm

## Proximal isovelocity surface area (PISA)

### Definition

◆ Flow converges toward a restrictive orifice remaining laminar and forming isovelocity surfaces that approximate hemispheres (Fig. 7.6.16)

### Conservation of mass principle

◆ Flow across any isovelocity surface = flow through orifice

### PISA method in MR: recordings

◆ Apical 4CV (Fig. 7.6.17ABCDEF)
◆ Optimize colour-flow imaging of MR
◆ Zoom the image of the regurgitant mitral valve
◆ Decrease the Nyquist limit (colour-flow zero baseline)
◆ With the cine mode select the best PISA

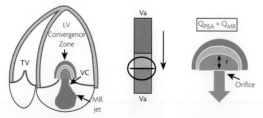

**Fig. 7.6.16** PISA. Va = flow velocity at radius r (cm/s). r = radius of the isovelocity shell (cm)

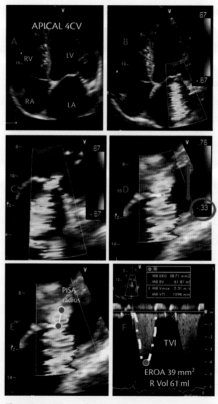

**Fig. 7.6.17** PISA method in MR

- Display the colour off and on to visualize the MR orifice
- Measure the PISA radius at mid-systole using the first aliasing and along the direction of the ultrasound beam
- Measure MR peak velocity and TVI (CW)
- Calculate flow rate, EROA, R Vol (Box 7.6.3)

## Usefulness/Advantages

- Can be used in eccentric jet
- Not affected by the aetiology of MR or other valve leak
- Quantitative: estimate lesion severity (EROA) and volume overload (R Vol)
- Flow convergence at 50 cm/s alerts to significant MR

## Limitations

- PISA shape affected
  - by the aliasing velocity
  - in case of non-circular orifice
  - by systolic changes in regurgitant flow (Fig. 7.6.18EF)
  - by adjacent structures (flow constrainment) (Fig. 7.6.18AD)
- PISA is more a hemi-ellipse (Fig. 7.6.18B)
- Errors in PISA radius measurement are squared
- Inter-observer variability
- Not valid for multiple jets (Fig. 7.6.18C)

---

**Box 7.6.3** Formulas to calculate PISA

$EROA = Flow/Peak\ velocity$

$EROA = (2\pi r^2 \times Va)/Peak\ velocity$

$EROA = (2 \times 3.14 \times 1 \times 3[IT9]3)/531$

$EROA = 207/531 = 0.39\ cm^2$

$R\ Vol = EROA \times TVI$

$R\ Vol = 0.39\ cm^2 \times 158\ cm = 61\ mL$

## Interpretation

- Mild MR EROA < 20 mm$^2$
- Severe MR EROA ≥ 40 mm$^2$

## Haemodynamics of MR (Fig. 7.6.19)

Under basal conditions, regurgitant volume (RV) is determined by the MR orifice area, the systolic pressure gradient across the orifice, and the duration of the systole (Box 7.6.4)

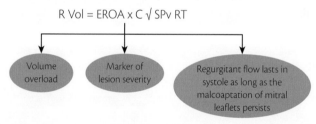

$$R\ Vol = EROA \times C \sqrt{SPv}\ RT$$

Volume overload

Marker of lesion severity

Regurgitant flow lasts in systole as long as the malcoaptation of mitral leaflets persists

**Fig. 7.6.19** Haemodynamics of MR. SPG: systolic pressure gradient; RT: regurgitant time.

---

**Box 7.6.4  EROA and R Vol are dynamic (systole/anaesthesia/exercise)**

Prolapse: EROA may appear or increase in mid-to-late systole
Secondary MR: EROA decreases in mid-systole
In significant MR, the EROA is usually holosystolic
It is advocated to evaluate MR out of the operating room and under routine loading conditions
The EROA is typically lower in secondary than in primary MR

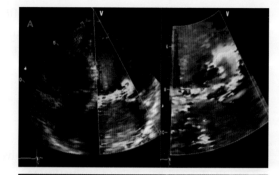

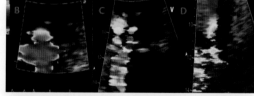

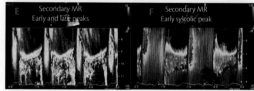

**Fig. 7.6.18** PISA method limitation and M-mode changes in regurgitant flow during systole

## 3D vena contracta (VC)—PISA in MR

- Calculations of VC area and flow convergence zone from 2DE are based on the geometric assumption that the VC area is either circular or elliptical
- So the geometry can be variable depending on the shape of the orifice and mitral valve leaflets surrounding the orifice
  - Secondary MR looks like an **ellipsoidal** shape and two separate MR jets originating from the medial and lateral sides of the coaptation line can be observed on 2D echo (Fig. 7.6.20)
    - In primary MR, the shape of the PISA is **often rounder**, which minimizes the risk of EROA underestimation (Fig. 7.6.21)
- Careful consideration of the 3D geometry of VC/PISA may be of interest in evaluating the severity of MR. The best 3D echo method to quantitate MR severity is still not defined

## Doppler quantitation from two valves flow (Box 7.6.5)

- Not applicable in case of significant aortic regurgitation
- **This approach is time-consuming and is associated with several drawbacks**

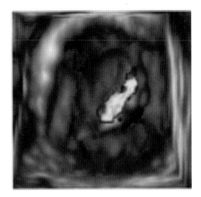

**Fig. 7.6.20** Secondary MR

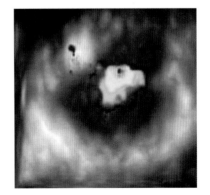

**Fig. 7.6.21** Primary MR

**Box 7.6.5** Doppler volumetric method (Fig. 7.6.22)

Calculate LVOT stroke volume (SV)

$SV_{LVOT} = LVOT\ diameter^2 \times 0.785 \times TVI_{LVOT}$

Calculate mitral inflow (MI) stroke volume

$SV_{MI} = mitral\ annulus\ diameter^2 \times 0.785 \times TVI_{MI}$

Subtract LVOT SV from MI SV

Measure MR TVI by continuous-wave Doppler

$EROA = R\ Vol_{MV}\ /\ TVI_{MR}$

$MR\ fraction\ (RF) = R\ Vol_{MV}\ /\ SV_{MI}$

### Interpretation

- Severe AR: RF > 50%

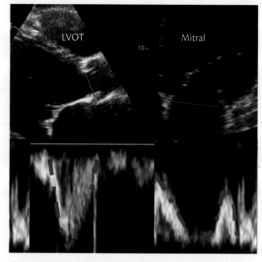

**Fig. 7.6.22** Doppler quantitation from two valves flow

## Complementary findings

### PW mitral inflow (Fig. 7.6.23a) Recordings

- Apical 4CV
- Sample volume of PW-Doppler places at mitral leaflet tips

**Usefulness/Advantages**
- Simple, easily available
- Dominant A-wave almost excludes severe MR

**Limitations**
- Affected by LA pressure, atrial fibrillation

- More applicable in patients older than 50 years old or in conditions of impaired myocardial relaxation.

### CW RJ profile (Fig. 7.6.23b) Recordings

- Apical 4CV

**Usefulness/Advantages**
- Simple, easily available

**Limitations**
- Qualitative
- Complete signal difficult to obtain in eccentric jet

- Peak velocity: four and six m/s
- Cutoff sign: ↗ LA pressure/severe MR

### Pulmonary vein (PV) flow (Fig. 7.6.23d) Recordings

- Apical 4CV
- Sample volume of PW places into (1 cm) the PV (often right upper PV)
- Identify the PV orifice on the back flow of the LA
- Interrogate the different PVs when possible

**Usefulness/Advantages**
- Simple
- Systolic flow reversal is specific for severe MR

**Limitations**
- Affected by LA pressure, atrial fibrillation
- Not accurate if MR jet directed into sampled vein

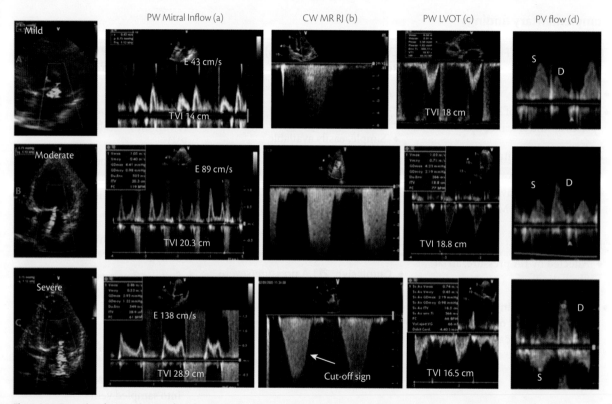

**Fig. 7.6.23** Examples of various degrees of MR (A: mild; B: moderate; C: severe; **(a)** PW mitral inflow **(b)** CW MR RJ **(c)** PW LVOT **(d)** PV flow (CW: continuous wave; PW: pulse wave, PV: pulmonary vein)

# Consequences of MR

## LV size and function (Fig. 7.6.24ABC)

- ◆ LV enlargement is measured by LV diameters (2D diameters) and/or volumes (2D method of discs or 3D echo when imaging is of high quality)
  - ◆ dilatation sensitive for chronic significant MR
  - ◆ normal size almost excludes significant chronic MR unless it is acute
- ◆ LV dysfunction is evaluated by either ejection fraction or end-systolic LV size
- ◆ LV ejection fraction is load-dependent, often overestimates LV systolic performance
- ◆ Other parameters of LV dysfunction
  - ◆ global longitudinal strain < 18.1% or strain rate value < 1.07/s
  - ◆ peak tissue Doppler lateral annulus systolic velocity < 10.5 cm/s

## LA size (Figs. 7.6.24D)

- ◆ LA volume can be reliably measured by 2D method of discs
  - ◆ a normal sized LA is inconsistent with severe MR unless it is acute
  - ◆ significant enlargement: LA volume index > 40 mL/m²

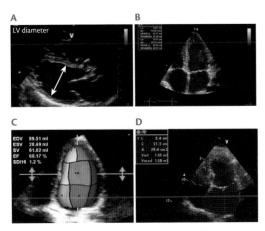

**Fig. 7.6.24** Consequence of MR: ABC LV size and function; D LA size

**Pulmonary systolic arterial pressure** (significant increase: PSAP > 50 mmHg at rest)

**Tricuspid annular dilatation** (significant: ≥ 40 mm or > 21 mm/m²)

## Specificities in secondary MR

◆ LV and LA dilatation are in excess to the degree of MR
◆ LA pressure is often elevated despite lower R Vol than in primary MR

# Integrating indices of MR severity (Table 7.6.2)

**Table 7.6.2** Integrating indices of MR severity

| | Mild | Moderate | Severe |
|---|---|---|---|
| **Qualitative structural and Doppler parameters** | | | |
| Valve morphology (2D/3D) | Normal or abnormal | Normal or abnormal | Flail/Ruptured papillary muscle |
| Colour-flow MR jet | Small, central jets | Intermediate | Very large central jet or eccentric jet adhering, swirling and reaching the posterior LA wall |
| Jet density (CW) | Faint/Parabolic | Dense/Parabolic | Dense/Triangular |
| Flow convergence zone | No or small | Intermediate | Large |
| **Semi-quantitative parameters** | | | |
| Vena contracta width, mm (colour flow) | < 3 | Intermediate | ≥ 7 (≥ 8 for biplane) |
| Pulmonary vein flow | Systolic dominance | Systolic blunting | Systolic flow reversal |
| Mitral inflow | A wave dominant | Variable | E wave dominant (> 1.5 m/s) |
| TVI mit/TVI Ao | < 1 | Intermediate | ≥ 1.4 |

| | Mild | Moderate | Severe |
|---|---|---|---|
| **Quantitative parameters** | | | |
| EROA, cm$^2$ | < 20 | 20–29 and 30–39 | ≥ 40 |
| Regurgitant volume, ml | < 30 | 30–44 and 45–59 | ≥ 60 |
| Regurgitant fraction, % | < 30 | Intermediate | ≥ 50 |
| **+ LV and LA sizes + sPAP** | | | |

## Chronic/acute MR: differential diagnosis (Box 7.6.6)

**Box 7.6.6** Chronic and acute MR. A differential diagnosis

| | Acute | Chronic |
|---|---|---|
| Cardiac output | ↓ | N |
| LV ejection fraction | N↓ | N↑ |
| Hyperdynamic heart | + | +/− |
| Tachycardia | + | +/− |
| LV size | N | ↑ |
| LA compliance | N | ↑ |
| LV ED pressure | ↑↑ | N |
| Low-velocity MR jets | + | − |
| Triangular-shaped MR jet | + | if severe |

# Monitoring of asymptomatic patients with primary MR

## When?

- Moderate MR → clinical examination every year + echo every two years
- Severe MR → clinical examination every six months + echo every year
- Severe MR → clinical examination every six months + echo every six months if LV ejection fraction 60–65% or end-systolic diameter close to 40 mm (22 mm/m²)

## What for?

- Progression of MR: marked individual differences
- Progression of the lesion: new flail leaflet, increase of annulus size
- Evolution of LV end-systolic dimension or volume
  - LV ejection fraction
  - LA size and area
  - pulmonary systolic pressure
  - exercise capacity
  - occurrence of atrial arrhythmias

## Surgical class I indications for mitral valve surgery (repair preferred) in primary MR

- Severe MR +
  - symptoms and LV ejection > 30% and ESD < 55 mm
  - no symptoms but LV ejection fraction ≤ 60% and/or ESD ≥ 45 mm

# Exercise echocardiography in MR

## Asymptomatic patients with moderate to severe primary MR

- Symptom onset
- Contractile reserve
  - LVEF increases by > 4%
  - global longitudinal strain increases > 1.9%
- Worsening of MR severity
- Pulmonary arterial systolic pressure (PSAP) > 60 mmHg

## Heart failure patients with moderate secondary MR

- Exercise-induced dyspnoea
- Viability/ischaemia
- Global/regional contractile reserve
- Increase in MR (EROA $\geq$ 13 mm$^2$)
- Significant increase in PSAP

# 7.7 Tricuspid regurgitation (TR)

## Role of echo

**Imaging of TR patients should evaluate the aetiology—mechanism—dysfunction—severity of regurgitation—consequences—possibility of repair**

## Definition

- Backflow of blood from right ventricle (RV) to right atrium (RA)
- Typically TR occurs during systole, but in rare conditions (i.e. AV block) it may occur also during diastole

## Aetiology

**Primary TR (organic, structural):** evident structural abnormalities of TV leaflets

- **acquired** (i.e. rheumatic disease, degenerative or Barlow disease, infective endocarditis, carcinoid, traumatic, pacemaker-related, connective tissue disease, radiotherapy)
- **congenital** (i.e. Ebstein anomaly, atrioventricular septal defect, etc.)

**Secondary TR (functional, non-structural):** TV malcoaptation due to enlargement and/or dysfunction of TV annulus/RV/RA, with no significant structural abnormalities of TV leaflets (i.e. pulmonary hypertension, RV dilation, RV dysfunction, atrial fibrillation)

# Tricuspid valve anatomy/imaging

Normally, TV is located slightly more apical than mitral valve

- TV complex includes:
  - three leaflets of unequal size (anterior usually the largest, posterior, and septal) (Fig. 7.7.1)
  - annulus
  - subvalvular apparatus (chordae and papillary muscles)
  - RV and RA
- TV annulus has an oval, non-planar structure with a saddle-shaped pattern, having two high points (oriented superiorly towards the RA) and two low points (oriented inferiorly toward the RV)

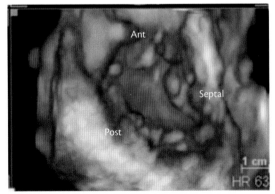

**Fig. 7.7.1** Normal tricuspid valve morphology (3D imaging)

# Tricuspid valve imaging (Fig. 7.7.2ABCD 2D imaging; EF 3D imaging)

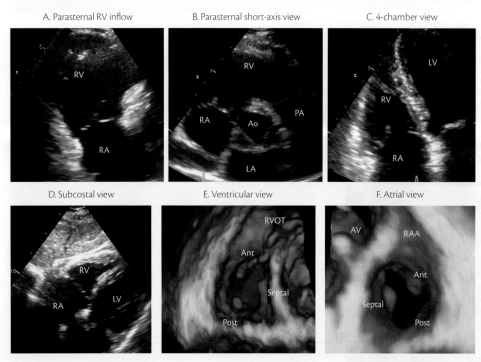

A. Parasternal RV inflow

B. Parasternal short-axis view

C. 4-chamber view

D. Subcostal view

E. Ventricular view

F. Atrial view

**Fig. 7.7.2 2D** imaging; EF 3D imaging
AV, aortic valve; RAA, right atrial appendage; RVOT, RV outflow tract

# Mechanism: lesion/deformation resulting in valve dysfunction

## Mechanism of TR

- **Primary TR:** prolapse/flail (Fig. 7.7.3AB), thickened leaflets with commissural fusion (Fig. 7.7.3CD), restricted mobility (Fig. 7.7.3EF), vegetations (Fig. 7.7.3GH), interference by catheters, etc.

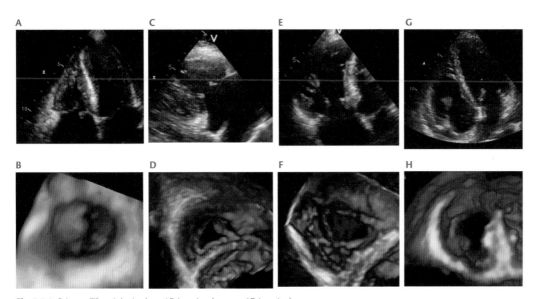

**Fig. 7.7.3** Primary TR aetiologies (top: 2D imaging; bottom: 3D imaging)

- **Secondary TR**
  - no structural abnormalities of leaflets
  - annular dilation/planar annulus
  - tethering of leaflets
  - papillary muscle displacement
  - ventricular deformation/remodelling
  - **echo-morphological parameters**
    - RV remodelling: RV sizes, volumes, function
    - Tricuspid valve (TV) deformation (Fig. 7.7.4)
      - tenting area (TA)
      - coaptation distance (CD)

## Mechanism of dysfunction (Carpentier's classification)

### Type I: Normal Leaflet Motion

- Annular dilatation (rarely isolated) (Fig. 7.7.5)
- Leaflet perforation (infective endocarditis)

### Type II: Excessive Leaflet Mobility

- Prolapse
- Flail leaflet (Fig. 7.7.3AB)

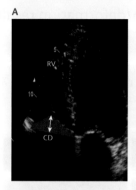
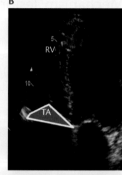

**Fig. 7.7.4** Tricuspid valve deformation (AB: 2D imaging; C: 3D imaging)

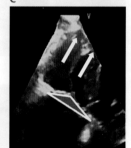

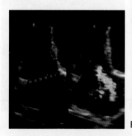

**Fig. 7.7.5** Carpentier type I

### Type III: Reduced Leaflet Mobility or Motion

- **IIIa:** systolic + diastolic restriction due to chordae shortening, leaflet thickening (rheumatic disease, toxic valvulopathy, radiation-induced TV disease) (Fig. 7.7.6)
- **IIIb:** systolic restriction: secondary TR (Fig. 7.7.3C)

### Combination

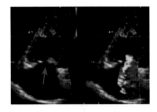

**Fig. 7.7.6** Carpentier type IIIa

## Assessment of TR severity

### Tricuspid valve

#### Morphology

- ◆ Visual assessment
- ◆ Multiple views

#### Usefulness/Advantages

- ◆ Flail valve is specific for significant TR (Fig. 7.7.7)

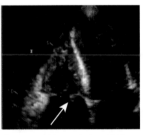

**Fig. 7.7.7** TV morphology (flail)

#### Limitations

- ◆ Other abnormalities are non-specific of significant TR

### Colour-flow imaging in TR

- ◆ Optimize colour gain/scale
- ◆ Need blood pressure evaluation

## Usefulness/Advantages

- ◆ Ease of use
- ◆ Evaluates the spatial orientation of TR jet
- ◆ Good screening test for mild vs severe TR

## Limitations

- ◆ Can be inaccurate for estimation of TR severity
- ◆ Influenced by technical and haemodynamic factors (Fig. 7.7.8)
- ◆ Underestimates eccentric jet adhering the RA wall (Coanda effect) (Fig. 7.7.9)

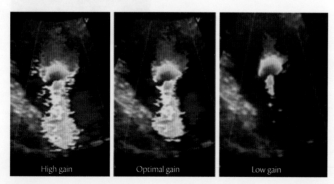

**Fig. 7.7.8** Impact of gain setting

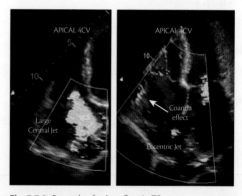

**Fig. 7.7.9** Example of colour flow in TR

## Vena contracta width in TR

- Apical 4CV (Fig. 7.7.10ABC)
- Optimize colour gain/scale (40–70 cm/s Nyquist limit)
- Identify the three components of the regurgitant jet (VC, PISA, jet into RA)
- Reduce the colour sector size and imaging depth to maximize frame rate
- Expand the selected zone (zoom)
- Use the cine loop to find the best frame for measurement
- Measure the smallest VC (immediately distal to the regurgitant orifice, perpendicular to the direction of the jet)
- The VC is the area of the jet as it leaves the regurgitant orifice; it reflects thus the regurgitant orifice area

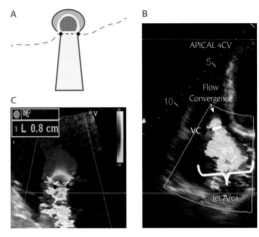

**Fig. 7.7.10** AP-4CV vena contracta imaging

### Usefulness/Advantages

- Relatively quick and easy
- Relatively independent of haemodynamic and instrumentation factors
- Not affected by other valve leak
- Good for extreme TR: mild vs severe
- Can be used in eccentric jet

## Limitations

- Not valid for multiple jets
- Small values; small measurement errors leads to large % error
- Intermediate values need confirmation
- Affected by systolic changes in regurgitant flow

## Interpretation

- Severe TR VC > 7 mm

## PISA method in TR: recordings (Box 7.7.1)

- Apical 4CV (Figs. 7.7.11 and 7.7.12ABCDEF)
- Optimize colour-flow imaging of TR
- Zoom the image of the regurgitant TV
- Decrease the Nyquist limit (colour-flow zero baseline)
- With the cine mode select the best PISA
- Display the colour off and on to visualize the TR orifice
- Measure the PISA radius at mid-systole using the first aliasing and along the direction of the ultrasound beam
- Measure TR peak velocity and TVI (CW)
- Calculate flow rate, EROA, R Vol

**Box 7.7.1** Formulas to calculate PISA

$$EROA = Flow/Peak\ velocity$$
$$EROA = (2\pi r^2 \times Va)/Peak\ velocity$$

$$EROA = (2 \times 3.14 \times 0.71 \times 33)/362$$
$$EROA = 147/368 = 0.40\ cm^2$$

$$R\ Vol = EROA \times TVI$$
$$R\ Vol = 0.40\ cm^2 \times 98\ cm = 49\ mL$$

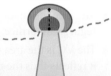

PISA radius

**Fig. 7.7.11** PISA illustration showing the convergent hemispheres

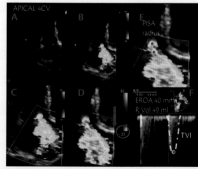

**Fig. 7.7.12** PISA method in TR

## Usefulness/Advantages

- Can be used in eccentric jet (Fig. 7.7.13)
- Not affected by the aetiology of TR or other valve leak
- Quantitative: estimate lesion severity (EROA) and volume overload (R Vol)

## Limitations

- PISA shape affected
  - by the aliasing velocity
  - in case of non-circular orifice (Fig. 7.7.14)
  - by systolic changes in regurgitant flow
  - by adjacent structures (flow constrainment)
- Errors in PISA radius measurement are squared
- Inter-observer variability
- Validated in only few studies

## Interpretation

- A TR PISA radius > 9 mm at a Nyquist limit of 28 cm/s indicates severe TR
- Severe TR EROA $\geq 40$ mm$^2$

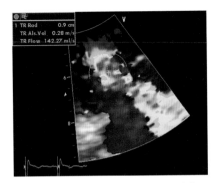

**Fig. 7.7.13** PISA measurement in an eccentric jet

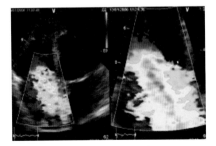

**Fig. 7.7.14** Massive TR with no real PISA

## 3D vena contracta (VC)—PISA in TR

- ◆ VC area calculation assumes a circular or elliptical orifice
- ◆ Complex geometry and various shapes of the VC (Fig. 7.7.15)
- ◆ 3D VC data are limited
- ◆ An EROA > 75 mm$^2$ seems to indicate severe TR

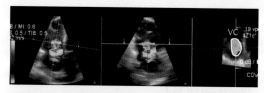

**Fig. 7.7.15** 3D imaging of the VC

## Hepatic vein flow

- ◆ Subcostal view (Fig. 7.7.16)
- ◆ Sample volume of PW places into the hepatic vein (Fig. 7.7.17)

### Usefulness/Advantages

- ◆ Simple

### Limitations

- ◆ Affected by RA pressure
- ◆ Affected by atrial fibrillation

### Interpretation

- ◆ Systolic flow reversal is specific for severe TR

### Peak E velocity

- ◆ Apical 4CV
- ◆ Sample volume of PW places at tricuspid leaflet tips (Fig. 7.7.18)

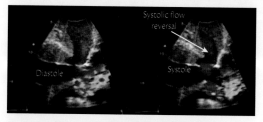

**Fig. 7.7.16** Colour Doppler showing systolic hepatic flow reversal

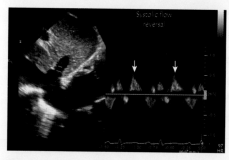

**Fig. 7.7.17** PW Doppler showing systolic hepatic flow reversal

## Usefulness/Advantages

- Simple, easily available
- Usually increased in severe TR

## Limitations

- Affected by
  - RA pressure
  - atrial fibrillation
- RV relaxation

## Interpretation

- Usually increased ($\geq 1$ m/s) in severe TR

## TR jet—CW Doppler (Fig. 7.7.21)

- A full CW Doppler envelope indicates more severe TR than a faint signal
- A triangular CW contour with an early peak velocity indicates elevated RA pressure or prominent pressure wave in the RA due to severe TR
- The velocity of TR does not reflect the severity of TR
  - **Mild/trivial TR** represents a common finding in healthy subjects (65–75%) and typically has a short colour jet, a low velocity = 1.7–2.3 m/s, with normal TV appearance and normal RV (Fig. 7.7.19)

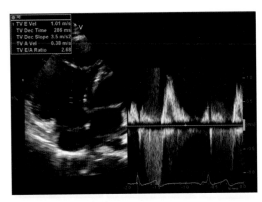

**Fig. 7.7.18** Tricuspid inflow

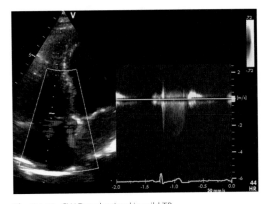

**Fig. 7.7.19** CW Doppler signal in mild TR

- ◆ Massive TR: often associated with a low jet velocity = near equalization of RA and RV pressure (< 2 m/s) (Fig. 7.7.20)
- ◆ Mild TR + severe pulmonary hypertension: possible high velocity jet
- ◆ Complete CW Doppler signal difficult to obtain in eccentric jet

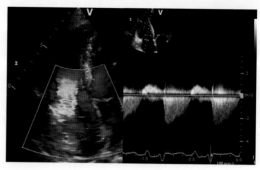

**Fig. 7.7.20** CW Doppler signal in massive TR

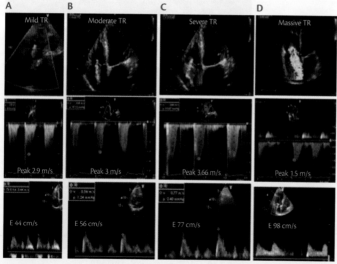

**Fig. 7.7.21** Examples of various degrees of TR (A: mild; B: moderate; C: severe; D: massive or free flow)

# Consequences of TR

## 2D tricuspid annulus dimensions (Fig. 7.7.22, Box 7.7.2)

### Tricuspid Annulus Diameter (TAD)

N: 28 ± 5 mm (4CV)

| Box 7.7.2 Tricuspid annulus dilatation |
| --- |
| TAD diast > 35 mm (> 21 mm/m$^2$) |

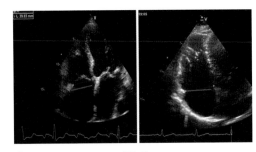

**Fig. 7.7.22** Measurement of TA diameter

## Estimation of RV systolic pressure (RVSP) (Box 7.7.3)

- ◆ Limitations
  - ◆ Underestimation of pressure if inadequate envelope
  - ◆ Enhanced signal by injecting agitated saline solution
  - ◆ Simplified Bernoulli equation: not applicable

| Box 7.7.3 Formulas to calculate RVSP (Fig. 7.7.23) |
| --- |
| RVSP = RA pressure + RV–RA max gradient<br>PASP = RAP + 4 V$^2$ max CW TR jet |

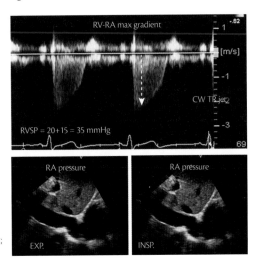

**Fig. 7.7.23** Estimation of RVSP (A: CW TR jet; B: measure of IVC diameter)

## RV size and function

- RV enlargement is measured by LV diameters (2D diameters, apical 4CV) and/or volumes with 3D-echo when imaging is of high quality
  - dilatation sensitive for chronic significant TR
  - normal size almost excludes significant chronic TR
- RV dysfunction is evaluated
  - by fractional area change (a value < 32% indicates RV dysfunction)
  - RV end-systolic area > 20 cm$^3$ is a marker of poor outcome
- RV ejection fraction is load dependent, often overestimates RV systolic performance and is not recommended
- Other parameters of RV dysfunction
  - TAPSE < 14 mm indicates RV dysfunction (Fig. 7.7.24)
  - Peak tissue Doppler tricuspid annulus systolic velocity (s') < 11 cm/s (Fig. 7.7.25)
  - → TAPSE and Peak Tr s' are less accurate in severe TR

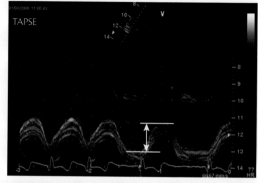

**Fig. 7.7.24** Measure of TAPSE

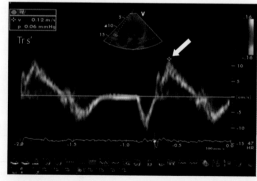

**Fig. 7.7.25** Measure of Tr s'

# Integrating indices of TR severity (Table 7.7.1)

**Table 7.7.1** Integrating indices of TR severity

| | Mild | Moderate | Severe |
|---|---|---|---|
| **Qualitative structural and Doppler parameters** | | | |
| Valve morphology (2D/3D) | Normal or abnormal | Normal or abnormal | Abnormal/flail/large coaptation defect |
| Colour-flow TR jet | Small, central jets | Intermediate | Very large central jet or eccentric wall impinging jet |
| Jet density (CW) | Faint/parabolic | Dense/parabolic | Dense/triangular with early peaking (peak < 2 m/s in massive TR) |
| **Semi-quantitative parameters** | | | |
| Vena contracta width, mm (colour flow) | Not defined | < 7 | > 7 |
| PISA radius (mm) | ≤ 5 | 6–9 | > 9 |
| Hepatic vein flow | Systolic dominance | Systolic blunting | Systolic flow reversal |
| Tricuspid inflow | Normal | Normal | E wave ≥ 1 m/s |
| **Quantitative parameters** | | | |
| EROA, cm$^2$ | Not defined | Not defined | ≥ 40 |
| Regurgitant volume, ml | Not defined | Not defined | ≥ 45 |
| | + RA/RV/IVC dimension | | |

# Persistent or recurrent TR after left-sided valve surgery (Box 7.7.4)

**Box 7.7.4** Persistent or recurrent TR after left-sided valve surgery

- ◆ TR severity/primary aetiology
- ◆ RV dysfunction (RV hypokinesia) (Fig. 7.7.26AB)
- ◆ Tr annulus dilatation (TAD diast > 40 mm or > 21 mm/m$^2$)
- ◆ Reduced TA fraction of shortening (< 25%)
- ◆ TV deformation
- ◆ Tenting area > 1.63 cm$^2$
- ◆ Coaptation distance > 0.76 cm

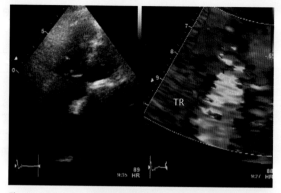

**Fig. 7.7.26A** Recurrent TR after MV repair

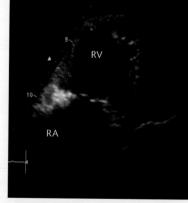

**Fig. 7.7.26B** Severe RV dilatation in a patient with severe MR

# 7.8 Pulmonary regurgitation (PR)

## Role of echo

**Imaging of PR patients should evaluate the aetiology**

- severity of regurgitation
- consequences

## Definition

Backflow of blood from pulmonary artery (PA) to right ventricle (RV) during diastole

## Aetiology

- Mild or trivial PR (physiologic) can be found in 40–78% of patients with normal PV and RV
- **Congenital PR (more frequent):**
  - morphologic PV anomalies (quadricuspid or bicuspid PV, PV hypoplasia, etc.)
  - post-repair of tetralogy of Fallot
  - PV prolapse
- **Acquired PR:**
  - normal PV: pulmonary hypertension with PA dilation
  - structural PV abnormalities: after valvulotomy/valvuloplasty, carcinoid, rheumatic, endocarditis, myxomatous degeneration, tumours, etc.

# Pulmonary valve (PV) anatomy/imaging (Figs. 7.8.1-3)

◆ The PV is a three-cusped structure, anatomically similar to the aortic valve, however it is thinner because of the lower pressures in the right than in the left heart system

◆ PV cusps are: anterior, right (closest to the right coronary cusp), and left (closest to the left coronary cusp)

◆ PV cusps are inserted on a crown-like annulus, demarcate shallow sinuses, and may have fibrous nodules (Morgagni nodules) on their free edge

◆ TTE, TOE, or 3D echo could provide useful information regarding anomalies of cusp number (bicuspid or quadricuspid valves), motion (doming or prolapse), or structure (hypoplasia, dysplasia, absence of pulmonary valve)

## Assessment of PR severity

### Pulmonary valve morphology

◆ Visual assessment
◆ Multiple views

**Usefulness/Advantages**

◆ Flail valve is specific for significant PR

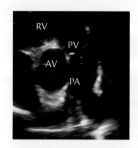

**Fig. 7.8.1** PTSAX view

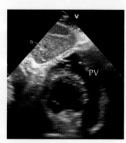

**Fig. 7.8.2** Subcostal view

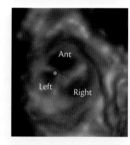

**Fig. 7.8.3** 3D view of the PV

## Limitations

- Other abnormalities are non-specific of significant PR

## Colour-flow imaging in TR

- Optimize colour gain/scale
- Evaluate in parasternal short-axis view

### Usefulness/Advantages

- Ease of use
- Evaluates the spatial orientation of PR jet
- Good screening test for mild vs severe PR

### Limitations

- Influenced by technical and haemodynamic factors

## Proximal jet width or the cross-sectional jet area to RVOT diameter ratio

Jet width > 50–65% of PV annulus is a sensitive sign of severe PR, but has rather low specificity (Fig. 7.8.4)

## Diastolic flow reversal in main pulmonary artery (PA)

100% sensitivity to detect severe PR, but has low specificity (Fig. 7.8.5)

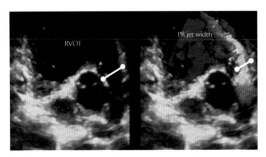

**Fig. 7.8.4** Evaluation of the PR severity using proximal jet width to RVOT ratio

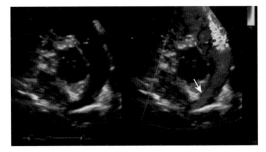

**Fig. 7.8.5** Flow reversal originating in the right branch of PA

### Diastolic flow reversal in PA branch

More specific for severe PR, especially if holodiastolic (Fig. 7.8.6)

### Vena contracta width in PR

◆ Probably a more accurate method than the jet width to evaluate PR severity by colour Doppler (Fig. 7.8.7)

◆ It lacks validation studies

◆ Limitations are similar to other valves

◆ The shape of the VC is complex in most cases

◆ The value of 3D echo has not yet been defined

### PISA method in PR

◆ In some patients, the flow convergence zone can be assessed (Fig. 7.8.8)

◆ However, no studies have examined the clinical accuracy of this method in quantifying the severity of PR

### Pressure half-time (PHT) (Fig. 7.8.9)

◆ Parasternal short-axis view

◆ PHT < 100 ms is a fairly sensitive index to predict severe PR

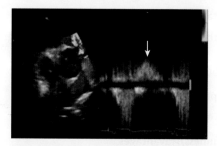

**Fig. 7.8.6** Holodiastolic flow reversal in the right branch of PA (PW Doppler)

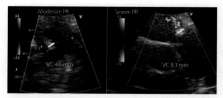

**Fig. 7.8.7** PR VC width assessment

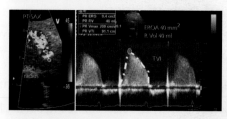

**Fig. 7.8.8** PISA method in PR

- Although less sensitive than PA diastolic flow reversal or PR jet width
- If RV has a restrictive physiology, PHT is 'falsely reduced'

## PR index = 100 * PR/diastole duration ratio

- PR index < 77% suggests haemodynamically significant PR
- When combined with the presence of diastolic flow reversal in PA branch, a PR index < 77% is 100% sensitive for severe PR

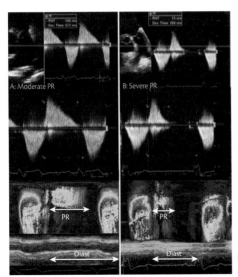

**Fig. 7.8.9** Measurement of the PHT (top) and colour M-mode evaluation of the PR jet (bottom)

# Integrating indices of PR severity (Table 7.8.1)

**Table 7.8.1** Integrating indices of PR severity

|  | Mild | Moderate | Severe |
|---|---|---|---|
| **Qualitative structural and Doppler parameters** | | | |
| Valve morphology (2D/3D) | Normal | Normal or abnormal | Abnormal |
| Colour-flow PR jet width | Small, usually < 10 mm in length with a narrow origin | Intermediate | Large, with a wide origin; may be brief in duration |
| Reversal flow in pulmonary arteries | Absent | Absent | Present |
| CW signal of PR jet | Faint/Slow deceleration | Dense/Variable | Dense/steep deceleration, early termination of diastolic flow |
| Pulmonic vs aortic flow by PW | Normal or slightly increased | Intermediate | Greatly increased |
| **Semi-quantitative parameters** | | | |
| Vena contracta width, mm (colour flow) | Not defined | Not defined | Not defined |
| Pressure half-time | Not defined | Not defined | < 100 ms |
| Jet width ratio | Not defined | Not defined | > 50–65% |
| **Quantitative parameters** | | | |
| EROA, cm$^2$ | Not defined | Not defined | Not defined |
| Regurgitant volume, ml | Not defined | Not defined | Not defined |
| + RV size | | | |

# 7.9 Multiple and mixed valve disease

## Role of echo

**Imaging of patients with multiple and/or mixed valve disease should evaluate the aetiology, the mechanism(s) of dysfunction, the severity, the consequences, and the possibility of repair, as with any single valve–single lesion disease**

### Main aetiologies of multivalvular disease

- Cardiac diseases
  - rheumatic heart disease
  - degenerative calcific
  - infective endocarditis
  - cardiac remodelling/dilatation (functional)
- Adverse effects of treatment
  - thoracic/mediastinal radiation therapy
  - ergot-derived agonists, anorectic agents
- Non-cardiac systemic diseases
  - end-stage renal disease/haemodialysis
  - carcinoid heart disease
- Congenital
  - connective tissue disorders (including Marfan syndrome, Ehler–Danlos syndrome
  - other rare congenital disorders (Trisomy 18,13,15, etc.)

# Diagnostic caveats and preferred methods for severity assessment (Table 7.9.1)

**Table 7.9.1** Main diagnostic caveats in multiple and mixed valve disease

| | | ...the diagnosis of the following lesion might be impaired | | | |
|---|---|---|---|---|---|
| | | AS | AR | MS | MR |
| In the presence of... | **AS** | | Pressure half-time method unreliable | Low-flow, low-gradient MS<br>Pressure half-time method unreliable | High RV; increased area of mitral regurgitant jet using CF mapping<br>ERO less affected |
| | **AR** | Simplified Bernoulli equation may be inapplicable<br>Gorlin formula using thermodilution invalid | | AR jet should not be mistaken for the MS jet<br>Continuity equation unreliable<br>Pressure half-time method unreliable | Doppler volumetric method inapplicable |
| | **MS** | Low-flow, low-gradient AS | MS may blunt the hyperdynamic clinical picture | | Not significantly affected |
| | **MR** | Low-flow, low-gradient AS<br>MR jet should not be mistaken for the AS jet | Doppler volumetric method inapplicable<br>Pressure half-time method may be unreliable | Continuity equation unreliable<br>Pressure half-time method unreliable<br>Gorlin formula using thermodilution invalid | |

## Aortic stenosis (AS) and mitral regurgitation (MR)

◆ AS jet should not be mistaken for the MR jet (AS: lower velocity, later onset (Fig. 7.9.1)
◆ Low-flow, low-gradient AS is not infrequent
◆ High intraventricular pressure may result in higher regurgitant volume and colour-flow jet planimetry of MR; mitral effective regurgitant volume less affected

### Preferred methods

◆ Continuity equation for AVA calculation
◆ EROA (and/or vena contracta) for MR assessment

## Aortic stenosis and mitral stenosis (MS)

◆ Low-flow, low-gradient AS and/or low-flow, low-gradient MS (paradoxical or not) is not infrequent
◆ Pressure half-time method for mitral valve area assessment is unreliable

### Preferred methods

◆ Continuity equation is accurate for MVA calculation in the absence of MR/AR ($MVA = ((\pi(D/2)^2) \times TVI_{LVOT})/TVI_{mitral}$)
◆ Direct planimetry of mitral valve orifice is the best method for rheumatic MS

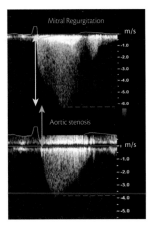

**Fig. 7.9.1** AS and MR CW Doppler

# Aortic regurgitation and mitral regurgitation

◆ LV may be severely dilated

◆ Doppler volumetric method (using Doppler mitral inflow and LVOT stroke volume) cannot be used

◆ Pressure half-time of AR jet may be shortened if increased left ventricular diastolic pressure

◆ If acute AR, the presence of diastolic MR (a marker of premature mitral valve closure) should be assessed (Fig. 7.9.2)

**Preferred methods**

◆ PISA method and vena contracta for MR assessment

◆ For AR assessment, consider multi-parametric evaluation including PISA method if feasible, vena contracta width assessment, demonstration of holodiastolic flow

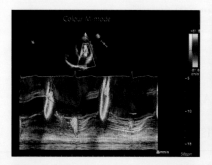 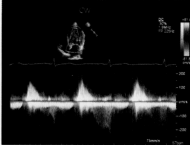 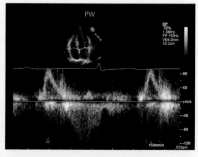

**Fig. 7.9.2** Premature mitral valve closure and diastolic MR in severe acute AR, assessed by colour M-mode (left panel), continuous-wave Doppler (CW, middle panel), and pulsed-wave Doppler (PW, right panel) modalities

reversal in the descending aorta and of a dense continuous-wave retrograde Doppler signal across the aortic valve

## Aortic regurgitation and mitral stenosis

◆ MS jet should not be mistaken for the AR jet (MS has a lower velocity and a later onset (Fig. 7.9.3)

◆ For the assessment of MS, continuity equation is invalid: because of increased anterograde aortic flow, mitral valve area may be overestimated

◆ For the assessment of MS, mitral valve pressure half-time may be shortened, and thus mitral valve area may be overestimated

### Preferred methods

◆ Direct planimetry of mitral valve orifice should be used if rheumatic MS

◆ Consider multi-parametric evaluation of AR, including calculation of regurgitant volume and fraction, PISA method if feasible, and vena contracta assessment

## Tricuspid and mitral valve disease

◆ Secondary tricuspid regurgitation (TR) is more frequent than primary

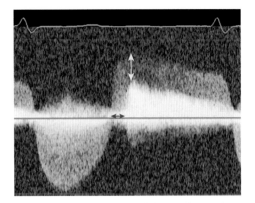

**Fig. 7.9.3** CW Doppler showing the lower velocity and later onset of MS as compared to AR jet

◆ Tricuspid annuloplasty should be considered when tricuspid annulus is dilated (> 40 mm or > 21 mm/m$^2$ as measured from the middle of the septal annulus to the middle of the anterior annulus in the four-chamber view)

## Tricuspid and pulmonic valve disease

◆ Severe TR may cause underestimation of PS severity by decreasing pulmonary pressure gradient ('low-flow, low-gradient' PS)
◆ Severe TS may aggravate TR

## Aortic stenosis and aortic regurgitation

◆ AR pressure half-time may be prolonged in the presence of left ventricular hypertrophy with impaired relaxation, or shortened if there is AS-induced elevation in LV diastolic pressure
◆ For pressure gradient assessment, simplified Bernoulli equation is not applicable if LVOT velocities are increased

### Preferred methods

◆ If severe AR, proximal velocity is frequently > 1 m/s and cannot be ignored for transaortic pressure gradient determination. The following formula should be used:
  ◆ pressure gradient = $(V2^2 – V1^2)$, where V2 = transvalvular velocities obtained with CW Doppler and V1 = LVOT velocities obtained with PW Doppler
  ◆ continuity equation is accurate for AVA calculation

- consider multi-parametric assessement of AR
- maximal anterograde transaortic velocity reflects both AS and AR severity in patients with ≥ moderate AS and ≥ moderate AR and preserved LV function

## Mitral stenosis and mitral regurgitation

- For the assessment of MS, continuity equation using LVOT diameter and flow invalid: the increased trans-mitral flow may induce mitral valve area underestimation
- For the assessment of MS, pressure half-time method is unreliable

### Preferred methods

- Direct planimetry of mitral valve orifice

# 7.10 Prosthetic valves (PrV)

## Classification of PrV

### Biological valves (Fig. 7.10.1ABC)

- ◆ Homografts: cadaveric valves
- ◆ Autografts: PrV implanted in aortic position (Ross procedure)
- ◆ Xenografts: the more used: stented, sutureless, stentless

### Transcatheter valves TAVI (Fig. 7.10.2AB)

### Mechanical valves (Fig. 7.10.3ABC)

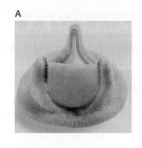
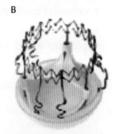
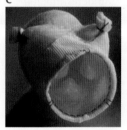

**Fig. 7.10.1** Examples of biological prosthetic valves A: Stented valve, B: Sutureless valve, C: Stentless valve

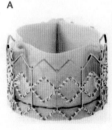
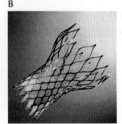

**Fig. 7.10.2** Examples of TAVI A: Edwards SAPIEN, B: CoreValve (Medtronic)

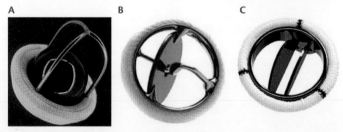

**Fig. 7.10.3** Examples of mechanical valves A: Caged ball valve, B: Tilting disc valve, C: Bileaflet valve

# Evaluation of PrV function (Table 7.10.1)

**Table 7.10.1** Essential parameters in the comprehensive evaluation of PrV function

|  | Parameters |
|---|---|
| **Clinical information** | ◆ Date of valve replacement<br>◆ Type and size of the prosthetic valve<br>◆ Height, weight, and body surface area<br>◆ Symptoms and related clinical findings<br>◆ BP and heart rate |
| **Imaging of the valves** | ◆ Motion of leaflets or occluder<br>◆ Presence of calcification on the leaflets or abnormal densities on the various components of the prosthesis<br>◆ Valve sewing ring integrity and motion |
| **Doppler echocardiography of the valve** | ◆ Contour of jet velocity signal<br>◆ Peak velocity and gradient<br>◆ Mean pressure gradient<br>◆ VTI of the jet<br>◆ DVI<br>◆ Pressure half-time in MV and TV<br>◆ EOA<br>◆ Presence, location, and severity of regurgitation |
| **Other echocardiographic data** | ◆ LV and RV size, function, and hypertrophy<br>◆ LA and right atrial size<br>◆ Concomitant valvular disease<br>◆ Estimation of pulmonary artery pressure |
| **Previous post-operative studies when available** | ◆ Comparison of above parameters in suspected prosthetic valvular dysfunction |

# Echo imaging of PrV (Fig. 7.10.4)

◆ Valves should be imaged from multiple views, with attention to:
  ◆ specific morphologic characteristics (different acoustic properties, increased reflectivity, acoustic shadowing)
  ◆ opening and closing motion of the moving parts (leaflets for bioprosthesis and occluders for mechanical ones)
  ◆ presence of leaflet calcification or abnormal echo density attached to the sewing ring, occluder, leaflets, stents, or cage

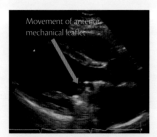
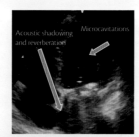
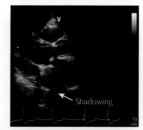
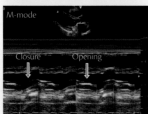
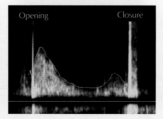
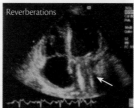

**Fig. 7.10.4** Example of echo imaging of MV PrV

- appearance of the sewing ring, including careful inspection for regions of separation from native annulus and for abnormal rocking motion during the cardiac cycle
  - different orientation of the valve according to its position
- Mild thickening is often the first sign of primary failure of a biologic valve
- Occluder motion of a mechanical valve may not be well visualized by TTE because of artefact and reverberations or in case of low-profile bileaflet valves

## Doppler echocardiography

- Doppler recordings should be performed at a sweep speed of 100 mm/s
- Measurements should be taken over one to three cycles in sinus rhythm
- In atrial fibrillation, Doppler measurements should be performed when possible during periods of physiologic heart rate (65–85 beats/min). Averaging from 5 to 15 beats in atrial fibrillation has been suggested
- In cases in which the derivation of a parameter requires measurements from different cardiac cycles (i.e. EOA by the continuity equation, DVI), matching of the respective cycle lengths to within 10% is advised
- For prosthetic aortic EOA calculation, the preceding intervals of LVOT velocity and prosthetic valve flow should be matched, whereas for mitral valves, the cycle length of mitral inflow should be matched with the preceding interval of LVOT velocity, if this is an acceptable site for stroke volume measurement (Tables 7.10.3, 7.10.4)

# Determination of gradients across the PrV

- PW, CW, colour Doppler, multiple views and angulations
- Blood velocity across a prosthetic valve is dependent on several factors, including flow and valve size and type
- **Simplified Bernoulli equation** non-invasive calculation of pressure gradients across prosthetic valves. $\Delta P = 4V^2$; P = pressure gradient; V = the velocity of the jet in m/s
- In aortic prostheses with high cardiac output or narrow LV outflow: velocity proximal to the prosthesis may be elevated and therefore not negligible (velocity > 1.5 m/s)
- In these situations, estimation of the pressure gradient is more accurately determined by considering the velocity proximal to the prosthesis as $P = 4\,(V_2^2 - V_1^2)$
- In bileaflet prostheses and caged-ball valves, overestimation of the gradient may occur, particularly with smaller valves and high cardiac output

# Effective orifice area (EOA) (Tables 7.10.2-4)

- Usually the reported size of the prosthesis refers to the outer diameter of the valve ring in millimetres. Functionally, only the inner diameters must be considered (Fig. 7.10.5)
- Furthermore, comparison of the different valve type is difficult because of major variations in sizing convention!

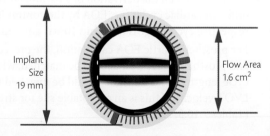

Implant Size 19 mm

Flow Area 1.6 cm$^2$

**Fig. 7.10.5** Example of mechanical valve sizing

The EOA of a prosthesis is obtained by the continuity equation (Fig. 7.10.6)

- $EOA = SV/VTI_{PrV} = (CSA_{LVOT} \times TVI_{LVOT}/TVI_{PrV})$
- Where $TVI_{PrV}$ is the velocity integral through the prosthesis obtained by CW echo-Doppler

**Table 7.10.2** Normal reference values of effective orifice areas for PV

| | Prosthetic aortic valve size, mm | | | | | | Prosthetic mitral valve size, mm | | | | |
|---|---|---|---|---|---|---|---|---|---|---|---|
| | 19 | 21 | 23 | 25 | 27 | 29 | 25 | 27 | 29 | 31 | 33 |
| **Stented bioprosthetic valves** | | | | | | | | | | | |
| Medtronic Intact | 0.85 | 1.02 | 1.27 | 1.40 | 1.66 | 2.04 | | | | | |
| Medtronic Mosaic | 1.20 | 1.22 | 1.38 | 1.65 | 1.80 | 2.00 | 1.5 ± 0.4 | 1.7±0.4 | 1.9 ± 0.5 | 1.9 ± 0.5 | – |
| Hancock II | ... | 1.18 | 1.33 | 1.46 | 1.55 | 1.60 | 1.5 ± 0.4 | 1.8±0.5 | 1.9 ± 0.5 | 2.6 ± 0.5 | 2.6 ± 0.5 |
| Carpentier–Edwards Perimount | 1.10 | 1.30 | 1.50 | 1.80 | 1.80 | ... | 1.6 ± 0.4 | 1.8±0.5 | 2.1±0.5 | | |
| St Jude Medical X-cell | ... | ... | ... | ... | ... | ... | | | | | |
| **Stentless bioprosthetic valves** | | | | | | | | | | | |
| Medtronic freestyle | 1.15 | 1.35 | 1.48 | 2.00 | 2.32 | ... | | | | | |
| St Jude Medical Toronto SPV | ... | 1.30 | 1.50 | 1.70 | 2.00 | 2.50 | | | | | |
| **Mechanical valves** | | | | | | | | | | | |
| St Jude Medical Standard | 1.04 | 1.38 | 1.52 | 2.08 | 2.65 | 3.23 | 1.5 ± 0.3 | 1.7±0.4 | 1.8±0.4 | 2.0±0.5 | 2.0±0.5 |
| St Jude Medical Regent | 1.50 | 2.00 | 2.40 | 2.50 | 3.60 | 4.80 | | | | | |
| MCRI On-X | 1.50 | 1.70 | 2.00 | 2.40 | 3.20 | 3.20 | 2.2±0.9 | 2.2±0.9 | 2.2±0.9 | 2.2±0.9 | 2.2±0.9 |
| Carbomedics | 1.00 | 1.54 | 1.63 | 1.98 | 2.41 | 2.63 | | | | | |
| Björk–Shiley CC | ... | ... | ... | ... | ... | ... | | | | | |

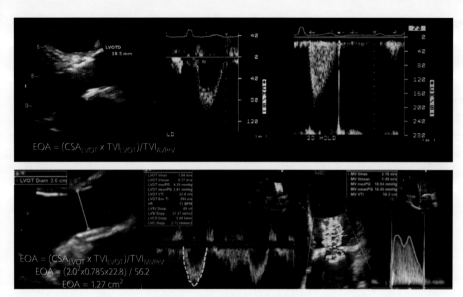

**Fig. 7.10.6** Continuity equation to calculate PrV EOA (Top: AV; Bottom: MV)

- SV is usually derived as the cross-sectional area (CSA = $\pi D^2/4$) just proximal to the prosthesis (in AV and PV) multiplied by TVI of the flow by CW Doppler at the site
- Direct measurement of LVOT diameter (D) is preferable to use, since valve size relates to the external diameter of the sewing ring, not the effective diameter of the subvalvular flow region

**Table 7.10.3** Recordings and measurements based on PrV positions

| Doppler measurements | |
| --- | --- |
| **Aortic position:**<br>peak velocity, mean gradient, TVI, DVI, and EOA by the continuity equation | ◆ DVI (DVI = TVILVOT/TVIPrAV) is helpful measure to screen for valve dysfunction, particularly when the CSA of the LVOT cannot be obtained or valve size is unknown (DVI is always < 1)<br>◆ DVI < 0.25 is highly suggestive of significant obstruction<br>◆ DVI is **not** affected by high flow conditions through the valve, including AR |
| **Pulmonary position:**<br>peak velocity mean pressure difference | ◆ EOA and DVI could be calculated for a prosthetic pulmonary valve, but little experience exists with these parameters |
| **Mitral and tricuspid positions:**<br>peak velocity, mean pressure gradient, TVI, pressure half-time | ◆ Heart rate reporting is essential<br>◆ PHT (220/PHT) to estimate orifice area in prosthetic valves is valid only for moderate/severe stenosis with EOA < 1.5 cm²<br>◆ For larger valve areas, PHT reflects atrial and ventricular compliance characteristics and loading conditions and has no relation to valve area<br>◆ The constant of 220 has not been validated for tricuspid prosthesis (Table 7.10.10)<br>◆ EOA can be calculated but few data exist for the TV |
| **Other pertinent echo-Doppler parameters** | ◆ **AV PrV: LV size**, function and hypertrophy, RV size, function, PAP<br>◆ **MV PrV: LV size**, LV size and function, LA size, RV size and function, PAP, hyperdynamic LV (i.e. severe MR (Table 7.10.8)) |

**Table 7.10.4** Doppler measurements based on AV and MV PrV positions

| Doppler measurements | |
|---|---|
| **Aortic position** | Doppler velocity recordings across normal PrVs usually resemble those of mild native aortic stenosis<br>Maximal velocity usually > 2 m/s, with **triangular shape** of the velocity contour<br>Occurrence of maximal velocity in early systole (AT: time from the onset of flow to maximal velocity **(< 80 ms)**)<br>With increasing stenosis, a higher velocity and gradient are observed, with longer duration of ejection and more delayed peaking of the velocity during systole |
| **Mitral position** | Heart rate reporting is essential<br>Pressure half-time formula (220/pressure half-time) to estimate orifice area in prosthetic valves is valid only for moderate or severe stenosis with orifice areas < 1.5 cm²<br>For larger valve areas, the pressure half-time reflects atrial and LV compliance characteristics and loading conditions and has no relation to valve area |

# Physiologic regurgitation/mechanical valves
## (Fig. 7.10.7, Table 7.10.6)

◆ Mild regurgitations, central or perivalvular are frequent, sometimes transient, and rarely progressive

◆ Mechanical prostheses usually show small regurgitation due to normal closure backflow (from the closing movements of the occluding device) and leakage backflow (after the valve is fully closed)

◆ Mitral regurgitation may be underestimated by TTE due to acoustic shadowing: look for indirect signs

◆ Severity: use same criteria as for native valves. If significant regurgitation suspected, look for underlying pathology → TOE

- ◆ Features
- ◆ Regurgitant area < 2 cm$^2$ and jet length < 2.5 cm in MV
- ◆ Regurgitant jet area < 1 cm$^2$ and jet length < 1.5 cm for AV
- ◆ Characteristic flow pattern
  - ◆ One central jet for Medtronic Hall
  - ◆ Two curved side jets for Starr–Edwards
  - ◆ Two unequal side jets for Björk–Shiley
  - ◆ Two side and one central jet for St Jude Medical

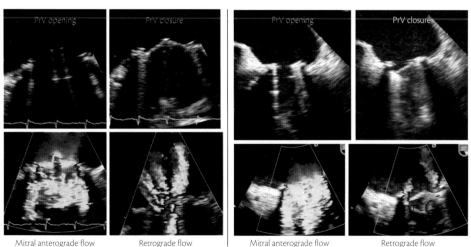

Mitral anterograde flow    Retrograde flow    Mitral anterograde flow    Retrograde flow

**Fig. 7.10.7** Examples of physiological regurgitation in tilting disk MV PrV

# Pathologic regurgitation in PrVs (Fig. 7.10.8ABC; Box 7.10.2)

- Eccentric or large jet
- Marked variance on the colour-flow display
- A jet that originates around the valve sewing ring (rarely transvalvular)
- Visualization of a proximal flow acceleration region on the LV side of the MV

## Severe aortic prosthetic regurgitation

- PHT of regurgitant jet > 250 msec
- Restrictive mitral inflow pattern (in acute aortic regurgitation)
- Holodiastolic reversal in the descending thoracic aorta
- Regurgitant fraction > 55%

## Severe mitral prosthetic regurgitation

- Increased mitral inflow peak velocity (> 2.5 m/s) and normal mitral inflow PHT (< 150 ms)
- Dense mitral regurgitant continuous-wave Doppler signals
- Regurgitant fraction > 55%
- Effective regurgitant orifice > 0.35 cm$^2$
- Systolic flow reversal in the pulmonary vein

**Fig. 7.10.8ABC** Examples of pathologic regurgitation in PrVs

**Fig. 7.10.8B** Mitral bioprosthesis dehiscence

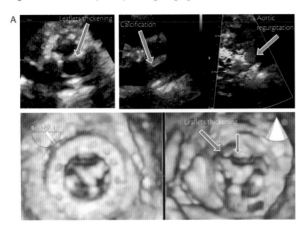

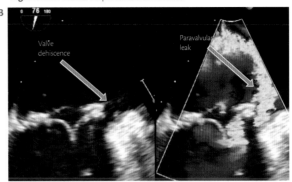

**Fig. 7.10.8A** Degenerative AV bioprosthesis with significant AR (with leaflet thickening, calcifications, limited opening)

**Fig. 7.10.8C** 3D recordings of a significant paravalvular leak. 3D echo is the method of choice in this case. It is very severe when > 30% of the circumference

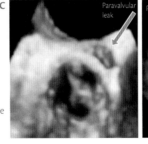

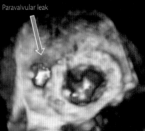

# Aetiology of high Doppler gradients in PrVs (Figs. 7.10.11 and 7.10.12)

- Central localized high velocity jet in bileaflet prosthesis
- Prosthesis-patient mismatch (i.e. too small a prosthesis in too large a patient (Table 7.10.7, Table 7.10.9))
- Prosthesis dysfunction due to an acute (i.e. thrombus, (Fig. 7.10.9), subacute (i.e. endocarditis), or chronic process (i.e. pannus, calcific degeneration in bioprosthesis) or entrapment (rope)
- Occult mitral prosthesis regurgitation
- High cardiac output conditions

Note: Pannus formation correspond to a fibroblastic hyperplasia originating from the periannular area and growing until interposition between leaflet and the ring with obstruction (Fig. 7.10.10, Box 7.10.1, Table 7.10.5)

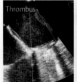 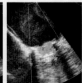 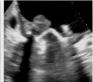 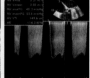

**Fig. 7.10.9** PrV thrombosis

**Table 7.10.5** Pannus vs thrombosis

|  | **Pannus** | **Thrombosis** |
|---|---|---|
| Chronology | Minimum 12 months, commonly 5 years from surgery date | Occurs at any time (if late usually associated with pannus) |
| Relation to anticoagulation (low INR) | Poor relationship | Strong relationship |
| Location | MV > AV | MV = AV |
| Morphology | ◆ Small mass<br>◆ Mostly involve suture line (Ring)<br>◆ Centripetal growth<br>◆ Confined to the disc plane<br>◆ Grow beneath disc | ◆ Larger mass than pannus<br>◆ Independent motion common<br>◆ Thin outer ring may be visible<br>◆ Project into LA<br>◆ Mobile elements |
| Echo density (video intensity ratio) | More > 0.7 (100% specific) | Less (< 0.4) |
| Impact on gradient | AV > MV | MV > AV |
| Impact on valve orifice | AV > MV | MV > AV |

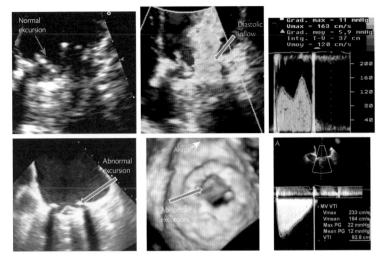

**Fig. 7.10.10** MV PrV pannus. Top: TTE, Bottom: TOE

**Box 7.10.1** TTE diagnosis of obstruction/stenosis

♦ Reduced occluder mobility or leaflet
♦ Presence of thrombotic material (mobile or immobile)
♦ Abnormal antegrade colour Doppler transprosthetic flow (orientation, eccentric jet)
♦ Central prosthetic regurgitation
♦ Elevated transprosthetic gradient
♦ Reduced effective EOA

**Table 7.10.6** Doppler parameters of prosthetic AV function in mechanical and stented biologic valves in conditions of normal stroke volume

| Parameter | Normal | Possible stenosis | Suggests significant stenosis |
|---|---|---|---|
| Peak velocity (m/s) | < 3 | 3–4 | > 4 |
| Mean gradient (mmHg) | < 20 | 20–35 | > 35 |
| DVI (TVI$_{AV}$/TVI$_{LVOT}$) | ≥ 0.30 | 0.29–0.25 | < 0.25 |
| EOA (cm$^2$) | > 1.2 | 1.2–0.8 | < 0.8 |
| Contour of jet velocity in PV | Triangular, early peaking | Triangular to intermediate | Rounded, symmetrical |
| AT (ms) | < 80 | 80–100 | > 100 |

**Table 7.10.8** Doppler parameters of prosthetic MV function

| Parameter | Normal | Possible stenosis | Suggests significant stenosis |
|---|---|---|---|
| Peak velocity (m/s) | < 1.9 | 1.9–2.5 | ≥ 2.5 |
| Mean gradient (mmHg) | ≤ 5 | 6–10 | > 10 |
| DVI (TVI$_{MV}$/TVI$_{LVOT}$) | < 2.2 | 2.2–2.5 | > 2.5 |
| EOA (cm$^2$) | ≥ 2 | 1–2 | < 1 |
| PHT (ms) | < 130 | 130–200 | > 200 |

**Table 7.10.7** Category of patient—prosthesis mismatch for AV PrV

| Category of PPM | Indexed EOA (cm$^2$/m$^2$) |
|---|---|
| Mild (haemodynamically insignificant) | > 0.85 |
| Moderate | 0.65–0.85 |
| Severe | < 0.65 |

**Table 7.10.9** Category of patient—prosthesis mismatch for MV PrV

| Category of PPM | Indexed EOA (cm$^2$/m$^2$) |
|---|---|
| Mild (haemodynamically insignificant) | > 1.2 |
| Moderate | 0.9–1.2 |
| Severe | < 0.9 |

**Table 7.10.10** TTE evaluation of prosthetic tricuspid valve stenosis

| Severe TV PrV stenosis | |
|---|---|
| Peak velocity | > 1.7 m/s |
| Mean gradient | ≥ 6 mmHg |
| PHT | ≥ 230 ms |
| Indirect, non-specific signs | Enlarged RA Dilated IVC |

**Box 7.10.2** TTE evaluation of prosthetic pulmonary valve stenosis

- Cusp or leaflet thickening or immobility
- Narrowing of foward colour map
- Peak velocity > 3 m/s or 2 m/s through an homograft
- Increase in peak velocity on serial studies
- Impaired RV function or elevated RV systolic pressure

Likewise, if you have a high gradient in the late follow-up, what do you do? In the late postoperative period, you can generally get a reliable measurement of the EOA by Doppler echocardiography. The first step would be to compare the EOA measured by Doppler echo to the normal reference value of EOA for the type and size of prosthesis that has been implanted in the patient. If the measured EOA is lower than normal and, moreover, it has decreased over time during follow-up, then you can suspect an intrinsic prosthesis dysfunction. One potential pitfall here is the presence of localized high gradient that may occur in bileaflet mechanical valves. If, on the other hand, the EOA is within normal range and has been relatively stable during follow-up, you should then calculate the indexed EOA and if is is lower than 0.85, you can conclude that this is probably patient–prosthesis mismatch.

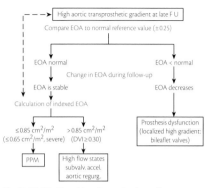

**Fig. 7.10.11** Algorithm for evaluation of abnormally high transvalvular gradient

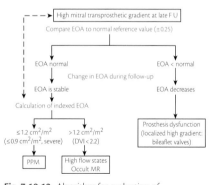

**Fig. 7.10.12** Algorithm for evaluation of abnormally high transvalvular gradient

## Associated features

### Strands (Fig. 7.10.13)

♦ Filamentous strands of varying length attached to valve prostheses have been described in patients undergoing TOE, but the frequency and clinical significance of these strands remain controversial

♦ For some authors, there is a significant correlation between the presence of strands and embolic rate: they suggest an aggressive anticoagulation

## Aortic valve prosthesis

♦ In the early post-operative period, the aortic root may be thickened as a result of haematoma or oedema after insertion particularly with a stentless valve included inside the aortic root, or after a Bentall procedure

♦ This appearance, which can be initially mistaken for an aortic root abscess, usually resolves over three to six months

## Follow-up transthoracic echocardiogram

♦ **First visit, two to four weeks** after hospital discharge, when the chest wound has healed, ventricular function has improved, and anaemia with its attendant hyperdynamic state has abated

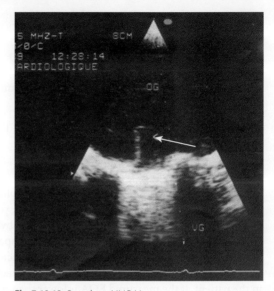

**Fig. 7.10.13** Strands on MV PrV

- before hospital discharge if the patient is being transferred and may not return
- the values obtained serve as reference for that patient
- **Routine annual clinical visit after valve replacement**, and perform an **echocardiography only if** there is a change in clinical status
- **Routine echocardiography after a first post-operative** study is not indicated in normally functioning prosthetic valve in the absence of:
  - other indications for echocardiography (i.e. follow-up of LV dysfunction)
  - clinical symptoms suggestive of valvular dysfunction
  - other cardiac pathology
- **Annual echocardiography after the first five years**
  - for patients with **bioprosthetic valves** (not for mechanical prosthetic valve) in the absence of a change in clinical status

# 7.11 Infective endocarditis (IE)

## Role of echo

- ◆ To diagnose IE and its complications
- ◆ To assess prognosis, including embolic risk
- ◆ To determine the indication and optimal timing for surgery
- ◆ To follow patients with IE during and after treatment, including surgery

## Definition

- ◆ Infective endocarditis (IE) is an inflammation of the endocardium, caused by an infection with a microorganism, and generally localized on cardiac valves

## The Duke echographic criteria (Fig. 7.11.1ABC)

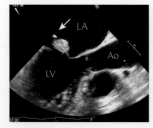

**Fig. 7.11.1A** Vegetation

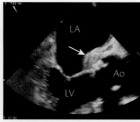

**Fig. 7.11.1B** Abscess

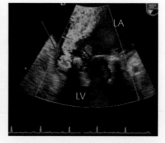

**Fig. 7.11.1C** New dehiscence of prosthetic valve

# Anatomic and echo findings (Table 7.11.1)

**Table 7.11.1** Surgery/necropsy and echocardiography findings in IE

|  | Surgery/necropsy | Echocardiography |
|---|---|---|
| **Vegetation** | Infected mass attached to an endocardial structure, or on implanted intracardiac material | Oscillating or non oscillating intracardiac mass on valve or other endocardial structures, or on implanted intracardiac material |
| **Abscess** | Perivalvular cavity with necrosis and purulent material not communicating with the cardiovascular lumen | Thickened, non-homogeneous perivalvular area with echodense or echolucent appearance |
| **Pseudoaneurysm** | Perivalvular cavity communicating with the cardiovascular lumen | Pulsatile perivalvular echo-free space, with colour Doppler flow detected |
| **Perforation** | Interruption of endocardial tissue continuity | Interruption of endocardial tissue continuity traversed by colour Doppler flow |
| **Fistula** | Communication between two neighbouring cavities through a perforation | Colour Doppler communication between two neighbouring cavities through a perforation |
| **Valve aneurysm** | Saccular outpouching of valvular tissue | Saccular bulging of valvular tissue |
| **Dehiscence of a prosthetic valve** | Dehiscence of the prosthesis | Paravalvular regurgitation identified by TTE/TOE with or without rocking motion of the prosthesis |

# Diagnosis of vegetation (Boxes 7.11.1, 7.11.2)

♦ Vegetations are typically attached on the low pressure side of the valve structure, but may be located anywhere on the components of the valvular and subvalvular apparatus (Fig. 7.11.2)

♦ When large and mobile, vegetations are prone to embolism and less frequently to valve or prosthetic obstruction

♦ Typical echocardiographic appearance is an oscillating mass attached on a valvular structure, with a motion independent to that of this valve

♦ Difficult situations (Fig. 7.11.3)

   ♦ very small (< 2 mm) vegetation

   ♦ non-vegetant endocarditis

   ♦ prosthetic and pacemaker endocarditis

   ♦ mitral valve prolapse with thickened valves

   ♦ vegetation not yet present or already embolized

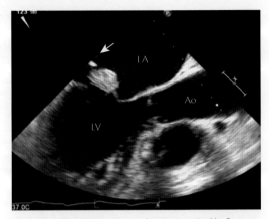

**Fig. 7.11.2** Typical vegetation on the anterior mitral leaflet

| **Box 7.11.1** Respective sensitivity to diagnose vegetation | **Box 7.11.2** Normal TOE |
|---|---|
| Sensitivity:    TTE = 60% <br> TOE = 90% | A normal TOE does not rule out endocarditis |

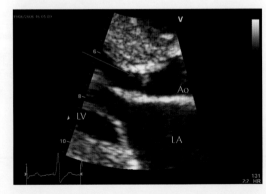

**Fig. 7.11.3** Atypical vegetation localized on the interventricular septum (arrow) in a patient with hypertrophic cardiomyopathy (TTE)

# Diagnosis of abscess (Box 7.11.3)

- They represent the second major echocardiographic criterion for IE
- They are more frequently observed in aortic valve IE and in prosthetic valve IE (Fig. 7.11.4)
- Abscess typically presents as a perivalvular zone of reduced echo density, without colour flow detected inside
- Difficult situations (Fig. 7.11.5ABC)
  - small abscesses
  - mitral annulus abscess
  - early thickening of the aortic root
  - post-operative aortic root abscess
  - prosthetic valve endocarditis

| Box 7.11.3 | Diagnosis |
|---|---|
| Sensitivity: | TTE = 30%<br>TOE = 85% |

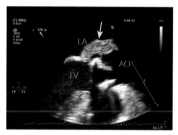

**Fig. 7.11.4** Aortic root abscess

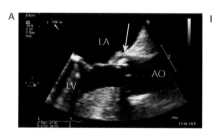

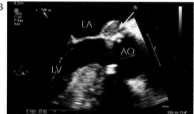

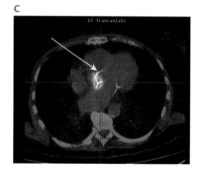

**Figs. 7.11.5AB** (A) Initial normal bioprosthetic aortic valve—doubtful thickening of the posterior aortic root (arrow); (B) Follow-up: typical posterior abscess

**Fig. 7.11.5C** Positive PET/CT intense uptake on the bioprosthesis

## Role of 3D echocardiograpy (Fig. 7.11.6ABC)

- ◆ 3D echocardiography has a limited additional role for the diagnosis of IE
- ◆ 3D echocardiography is particularly useful for the diagnosis of valve perforation
- ◆ 3D echocardiography is useful for the evaluation of perivalvular lesions
- ◆ 3D echocardiography allows an ideal presentation of valve lesions for comparison with anatomical findings

## Indications for echocardiography (Fig. 7.11.7, Box 7.11.6)

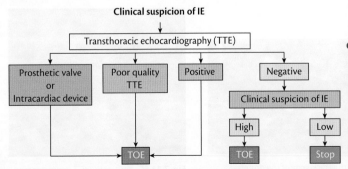

**Fig. 7.11.7** If initial TOE is negative but persistent suspicion of IE: repeat TOE within five to seven days

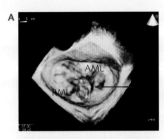

**Fig. 7.11.6A** 3D echo imaging of a large mitral vegetation (arrow)—3D TOE atrial view

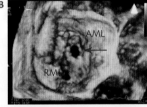

**Fig. 7.11.6B** 3D echo imaging of an anterior mitral valve perforation (arrow): 3D TOE atrial view

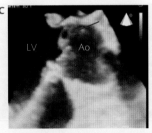

**Fig. 7.11.6C** 3D echo imaging of a perforation of the non coronary aortic leaflet: 3D TOE

LV: left ventricle, Ao: aorta, AML: anterior mitral leaflet, PML: posterior mitral leaflet

> **Box 7.11.4  Key points: diagnosis**
>
> 1. Both TTE and TOE are mandatory in the majority of patients with suspected or definite IE
> 2. The sensitivity and specificity of echocardiography are reduced in some subgroups, including PVE and patients with intracardiac devices
> 3. Echocardiography must be performed early, as soon as the diagnosis of IE is suspected and must be repeated in case of persisting high level of clinical suspicion
> 4. All echographic results must be interpreted taking into account the clinical presentation of the patient

## Echocardiographic prognostic markers
(Boxes 7.11.4, 7.11.5)

- Mortality is still high in IE (in-hospital mortality 20–25%)
- Several factors have been associated with an increased risk of death in IE including patients' characteristics (diabetes, comorbidity), presence or not of complications (heart failure, stroke, renal failure), and type of microorganism
- Several echocardiographic features have also been associated with worse prognosis

> **Box 7.11.5  Key points**
>
> 1. Periannular complications
> 2. Severe left-sided valve regurgitation
> 3. Low left ventricular ejection fraction
> 4. Pulmonary hypertension
> 5. Large vegetations
> 6. Severe prosthetic valve dysfunction
> 7. Premature mitral valve closure and other signs of elevated diastolic pressures

# Echocardiography in IE: follow-up (Table 7.11.2)

**Table 7.11.2** Recommendations

|  | Class | Level |
|---|---|---|
| A. Follow-up under medical therapy:<br>   Repeat TTE and TOE is recommended as soon as a new complication of IE is suspected | I | B |
| B. Repeat TTE and TOE should be considered during F U of uncomplicated IE: time and mode depend on the initial findings, type of microorganisms, and initial response to treatment | IIa | B |
| C. Intra-operative echocardiography<br>   Recommended in all cases of IE requiring surgery | I | C |
| D. Following completion of treatment:<br>   TTE is recommended at completion of antibiotic treatment for evaluation of cardiac and valve morphology and function | I | C |

# Indications for surgery—native IE (Table 7.11.3, Fig. 7.11.8ABC)

**Table 7.11.3** Indications for surgery in native IE

|  | Timing | Class | Level |
|---|---|---|---|
| **A. HEART FAILURE** | | | |
| Aortic or mitral IE with severe acute regurgitation or valve obstruction causing refractory pulmonary oedema or cardiogenic shock | Emergency | I | B |
| Aortic or mitral IE with fistula into a cardiac chamber or pericardium causing refractory pulmonary oedema or cardiogenic shock | Urgent | I | B |
| Aortic or mitral IE with severe acute regurgitation and persisting HF or echocardiographic signs of poor haemodynamic tolerance | Urgent | I | B |
| **B. UNCONTROLLED INFECTION** | | | |
| Locally uncontrolled infection | Urgent | I | B |
| Persisting fever and positive blood culture > 5–7 days | Urgent | I | B |
| Infection caused by fungi or multiresistant organisms | Urgent/elective | I | B |
| **C. PREVENTION of EMBOLISM** | | | |
| Aortic or mitral IE with large vegetations (> 10 mm) following one or more embolic episodes, despite appropriate antibiotic treatment | Urgent | I | B |
| Aortic or mitral IE with large vegetations (10 mm) and other predictors of complicated course (HF, persistent infection, abscess) | Urgent | I | C |
| Isolated very large vegetations (> 15 mm) | Urgent | IIb | C |

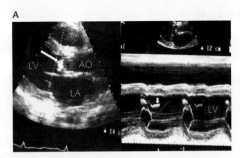

**Fig. 7.11.8A** Haemodynamic: Severe aortic IE with premature mitral closure

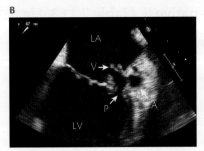

**Fig. 7.11.8B** Infectious: Mitral annular abscess with perforation into the LA

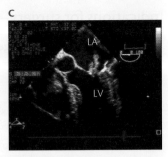

**Fig. 7.11.8C** Embolic: Huge and mobile mitral vegetation

## Infectious complications (Fig. 7.11.9ABC)

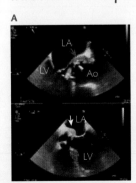

**Fig. 7.11.9A** Abscess: Thickened nonhomogeneous perivalvular area with echodense or echolucent aspect

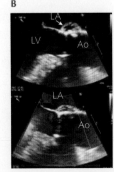

**Fig. 7.11.9B** Pseudoaneurysm: Pulsatile perivalvular echo-free space with colour Doppler flow detected

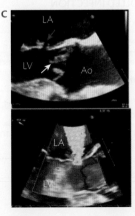

**Fig. 7.11.9C** Mitral aneurysm with perforation + saccular bulging of mitral valve with perforation into the LA
LA: left atrium, LV: left ventricle, Ao: aorta

# Prediction of embolic risk

- ◆ Embolism occurs in 20–40% of IE, but its incidence decreases to 10% after initiation of antibiotic therapy
- ◆ This risk is especially high during the first two weeks following the initiation of antibiotic therapy
- ◆ Embolism may be silent in about 20% of patients with IE and must be diagnosed by systematic non-invasive imaging
- ◆ Factors associated with an increased risk of embolism include the size and mobility of vegetation, its localization on the mitral valve, its increasing or decreasing size under antibiotic therapy, the type of microorganism, previous embolism, multivalvular endocarditis, and biological markers
- ◆ Patients with large vegetations (> 10 mm) have a higher risk of embolism (Figs. 7.11.10-7.11.11). Very large (> 15 mm) vegetations are associated with an increased mortality

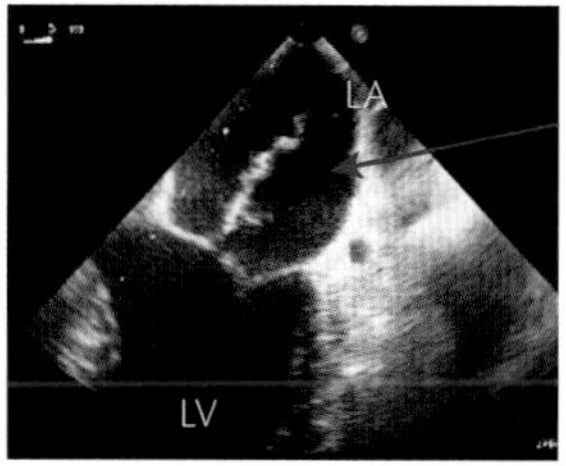

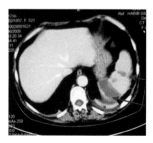

**Fig. 7.11.10** TOE: Huge vegetation on the anterior mitral valve (arrow)

---

**Box 7.11.6** Intra-operative echocardiography

1. Intra-operative TOE provides useful data for the planning of surgery, is essential for the immediate control of the surgical procedure, has the potential to improve surgical results, and is a reference for future studies

2. The impact of intra-operative TOE leads to recommend its routine and systematic use, especially in cases of conservative valve surgery and other complex procedures

3. Intra-operative TOE is recommended in all patients with IE undergoing cardiac surgery

**Fig. 7.11.11** Splenic embolism by CT-scan (arrows)

# IE: specific situations

- Prosthetic valve IE (PrVIE)
- Cardiac device-related IE (CDRIE)
- Right-sided IE

## Prosthetic valve IE (PrVIE) (Fig. 7.11.12)

- PrVIE is characterized by lower incidence of vegetations and higher incidence of abscesses and perivalvular complications
- TOE is mandatory in PrVIE because of its better sensitivity and specificity for the detection of vegetations, abscesses, and perivalvular lesions in this setting
- The value of both TTE and TOE is lower in PrVIE than in native IE
- Consequently, a negative echocardiography is relatively frequently observed in PrVE, and does not rule out the diagnosis of IE
- Repeat examination must be performed if clinical level of suspicion is still high

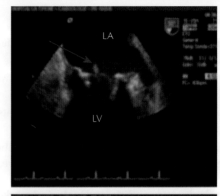

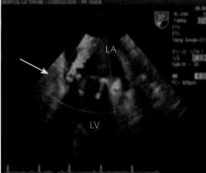

**Fig. 7.11.12** Mitral PrVIE
Vegetation (red arrow) and prosthetic dehiscence (white arrow) in a patient with bioprosthetic mitral valve IE

# Indications for surgery—PrVIE (Table 7.11.4)

**Table 7.11.4** Indications for surgery in PrVIE

|  | Timing | Class | Level |
|---|---|---|---|
| **A. HEART FAILURE** | | | |
| PrVIE with severe prosthetic dysfunction (dehiscence or obstruction) causing refractory pulmonary oedema or cardiogenic shock | Emergency | I | B |
| PrVIE with fistula into a cardiac chamber or pericardium causing refractory pulmonary oedema or cardiogenic shock | Emergency | I | B |
| PrVIE with severe prosthetic dysfunction and persisting heart failure | Urgent | I | B |
| Severe prosthetic dehiscence without heart failure | Elective | I | B |
| **B. UNCONTROLLED INFECTION** | | | |
| Locally uncontrolled infection (abscess, false aneurysm, enlarging vegetation) | Urgent | I | B |
| PrVIE caused by fungi or multiresistant organisms | Urgent/elective | I | B |
| PrVIE with persisting fever and positive blood culture > 5–7 days | Urgent | I | B |
| PrVIE caused by *Staphylocci* or Gram negative bacteria (most cases of early PrVIE) | Urgent/elective | I | C |
| **C. PREVENTION of EMBOLISM** | | | |
| PrVIE with recurrent emboli despite appropriate treatment | Urgent | I | B |
| PrVIE with large vegetations (10 mm) and other predictors of complicated course (HF, persistent infection, abscess) | Urgent | I | B |
| PrVIE with isolated very large vegetations (> 15 mm) | Urgent | IIb | C |

## Cardiac device-related IE (CDRIE) (Fig. 7.11.13)

- CDRIE, including permanent pacemaker and implantable cardioverter defibrillators, is a severe disease associated with high mortality
- CDRIE is defined by an infection extending to the electrode leads, cardiac valve leaflets, or endocardial surface
- Echocardiography plays a key role in CDRIE and is helpful both for the diagnosis of lead vegetation, tricuspid involvement, assessment of tricuspid regurgitation, sizing of vegetations, as well as follow-up after lead extraction
- Careful examination of the entire leads is mandatory, from the superior vena cava to the apex of the right ventricle
- Although TOE is superior to TTE, both are mandatory in suspected or definite CDRIE
- However, both TTE and TOE may be falsely negative in CDRIE
- The sensitivity of echocardiography is lower in CDRIE than in native valve IE

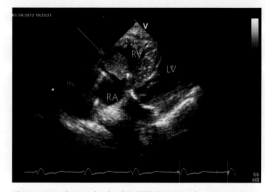

**Fig. 7.11.13** Pacemaker lead IE. TTE showing a huge vegetation (arrow) on a pacemaker lead

# Indications for surgery—CDRIE (Table 7.11.5)

**Table 7.11.5** Recommendations

|  | Class | Level |
|---|---|---|
| **A. PRINCIPLES of TREATMENT** | | |
| Prolonged antibiotic therapy and device removal are recommended in definite CDRIE | I | B |
| Device removal should be considered when CDRIE is suspected on the basis of occult infection without other apparent source of infection | IIa | C |
| In patients with native or prosthetic valve IE and an intracardiac device with no evidence of associated device infection, device extraction must be considered | IIb | C |
| **B. MODE of DEVICE REMOVAL** | | |
| Percutaneous extraction is recommended in most patients with CDRIE even those with large (> 10 mm) vegetations | I | B |
| Surgical extraction shoud be considered if percutaneous extraction is incomplete or impossible or when severe destructive tricuspid IE is associated | IIa | C |
| Surgical extraction may be considered in patients with very large (> 25 mm) vegetations | IIb | C |
| **C. REIMPLANTATION** | | |
| After device extraction, reassessment of the need for reimplantation is recommended. | I | B |
| When indicated, reimplantation should be postponed if possible to allow a few days or weeks of antibiotic therapy | IIa | B |
| Temporary pacing is not recommended | IIb | C |

# Right-sided IE (Fig. 7.11.14)

- ◆ TOE is not mandatory in isolated right-sided native valve IE with good quality TTE examination and unequivocal echocardiographic findings
- ◆ The size of the tricuspid vegetation and the severity of the tricuspid regurgitation must be evaluated by echocardiography, because these measurements have the potential to influence the therapeutic strategy

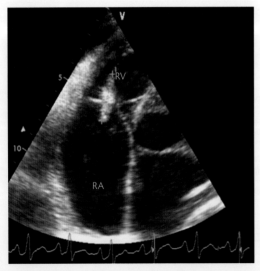

**Fig. 7.11.14** Tricuspid valve IE. TTE showing a large tricuspid vegetation in an intravenous drug user

# CHAPTER 8

# Cardiomyopathies

# Introduction

## Primary cardiomyopathies aetiologies

- **Genetic**
    - hypertrophic cardiomyopathy (HCM), arrhythmogenic right ventricular cardiomyopathy (ARVC), left ventricular non-compaction (LVNC), glycogen storage, mitochondrial myopathies, others
- **Acquired**
    - myocarditis, peripartum, Takotsubo, tachycardia-induced, infant of insulin-dependent mothers
- **Mixed**
    - dilated cardiomyopathy (DCM), restrictive (non-hypertrophied and non-dilated)

# 8.1 Dilated cardiomyopathy (DCM)

## Role of echocardiography

- Establish diagnosis
- Define aetiology
- Detect associated cardiac abnormalities such as valve disease
- Identify high-risk features
- Guide therapy

## Diagnostic findings

- LV dilatation—assessed by M-mode/2D/3D (Fig. 8.1.1)
- LVEDV > 112 mL/m$^2$ corrected for age and body surface area
- EF < 45% or fractional shortening < 25%
- LV wall thinning is a common finding in DCM (Fig. 8.1.2)

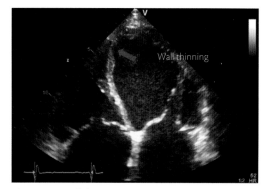

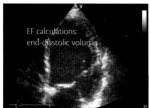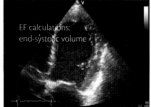

**Fig. 8.1.1** LV dilatation and EF measurements

**Fig. 8.1.2** LV wall thinning in DCM

## Associated findings

- LV spherical remodelling (Fig. 8.1.3)
  - typical for DCM
  - long-axis diameter (L) preserved and transverse diameter (l) increased
- LV systolic dyssynchrony (Fig. 8.1.4)
- LV thrombus (Fig. 8.1.5)
- Dilated atria
- Dilated RV (Fig. 8.1.6)
- Mitral regurgitations often due to dilated mitral annulus
- Pulmonary hypertension (Fig. 8.1.7)
- Diastolic dysfunction

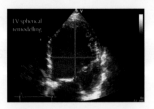

**Fig. 8.1.3** Remodelling of the LV: l/L (sphericity index) increased

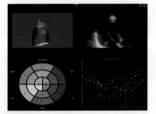

**Fig. 8.1.4** Extreme dyssynchrony

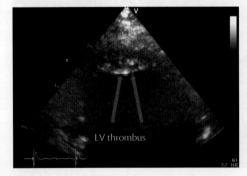

**Fig. 8.1.5** Apical thrombus

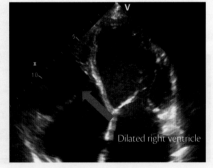

**Fig. 8.1.6** RV dilatation

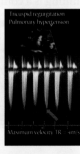

**Fig. 8.1.7** CW TR jet velocity in a patient with pulmonary hypertension

# Prognostic role of echocardiography

- ◆ Severity of systolic dysfunction
- ◆ LV filling pattern (Fig. 8.1.8)
- ◆ Coexistence of RV dysfunction
- ◆ Severity of LV dilatation
- ◆ Systolic dyssynchrony

## Echocardiographic role in CRT

- ◆ LVEF (2D Simpson's biplane, 3D)
- ◆ Dyssynchrony study—correct technique and further evidence needed (Fig. 8.1.9AB)
- ◆ Visual (apical rocking)
- ◆ Quantitative
  - ◆ interventricular dyssynchrony
  - ◆ atrioventricular dyssynchrony
  - ◆ intraventricular dyssynchrony
- ◆ Stress echo for viability and dyssynchrony assessment
- ◆ CRT optimization

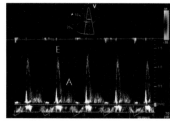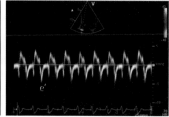

**Fig. 8.1.8** Restrictive mitral inflow pattern or pseudonormalization of mitral inflow. High filling pressures indicated by E/e' ratio > 15. Indicator of bad prognosis

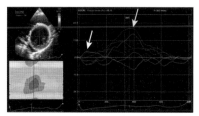

**Fig. 8.1.9A** Typical pattern as seen from radial view. The time difference between white and yellow arrow has been used as a measure of dyssynchrony

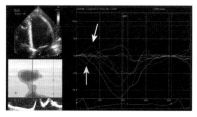

**Fig. 8.1.9B** Typical pattern as seen from longitudinal view. White arrow indicates early stretch from the lateral LV wall. Yellow arrow mark septal flash

# 8.2 Hypertrophic cardiomyopathy (HCM)

◆ Primary myocardial disease: inadequate hypertrophy, independent of loading conditions; + often other affected structures: mitral valve apparatus, small coronary arteries, cardiac interstitium (Boxes 8.2.1, 8.2.2 and 8.2.3)

## Diagnostic findings (Fig. 8.2.1ABCD)

◆ **LV hypertrophy → wall thickness (WT) ≥ 15 mm** (or > 2SD for age, gender, and height), lower in first relatives of patients, from one to all LV segments
◆ **ASH**: Asymmetrical septal hypertrophy: IVS/PWT > 1.3 in normotensive patients (or > 1.5 in HT)
  ◆ Frequent but non-specific, can be seen in
    ◆ early systemic hypertension (HT)
    ◆ RV hypertrophy
    ◆ inferior MI with previous LVH
◆ **Interventricular septum morphology** (IVS) and probability of positive genetic test
  ◆ reverse IVS: high probability of a positive genetic test
  ◆ apical or neutral IVS: moderate probability
  ◆ 'sigmoid' IVS = low probability of a positive genetic test

**Exclusion criteria** Cardiac/systemic causes of LV hypertrophy (aortic stenosis, long-standing systemic HT, other phenocopies, similar disorders with different causes)

**Box 8.2.1  First-degree relatives**

In first-degree relatives, lower cut-off values are used, and a WT ≥ 13 mm in the anterior septum or posterior wall suggests the diagnosis

**Box 8.2.2  Classical distribution types**

- I (anterior septum)
- II (anterior + inferior septum)
- III (anterior + inferior septum + lateral wall)
- IV (apical, etc.)

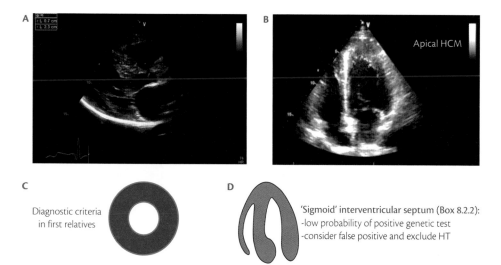

Apical HCM

C
Diagnostic criteria in first relatives

D
'Sigmoid' interventricular septum (Box 8.2.2):
-low probability of positive genetic test
-consider false positive and exclude HT

**Fig. 8.2.1**  LVH in HCM: ASH = IVS/PW = 23/7 = 3.2 (A); apical HCM, apical wall thickness 15 mm (B); diagnostic criteria in first relatives (C) (Box 8.2.1); 'sigmoid' IVS and genetic test (D)

# Associated findings (Fig. 8.2.2ABC)

- **Mitral valve:** <u>leaflets</u>: anterior leaflet elongation; dysplasia, MVP; <u>chordae</u>: elongation, laxity, hypermobility; <u>papillary muscles</u>: hypertrophy, bifidity, abnormal anterior position, abnormal insertion in the anterior leaflet
- **Left atrium:** dilation and dysfunction
- **LV:** typically non-dilated
- **Mitral regurgitation (MR):** more severe and frequent in HOCM (SAM-related); if SAM-related: eccentric posteriorly directed MR (in organic disease: central or anterior jet)

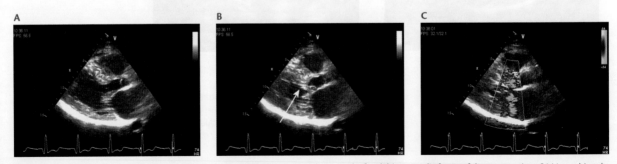

**Fig. 8.2.2** The mitral valve in HCM (A) early systolic frame, dysplastic, elongated anterior leaflet; (B) late systolic frame of the same patient, SAM touching the IVS; (C) late systolic frame, colour Doppler: posteriorly directed MR with aliasing in the LVOT (LVOT obstruction)

# Obstruction

## Obstructive HCM (HOCM)

- intraventricular gradient with CW Doppler, 'dagger-shaped' (late systolic peak)
- peak gradient > 30 mmHg at rest or after provocative manoeuvres: exercise, Valsalva, standing

## Level of obstruction

- **Left ventricular outflow tract (LVOT) obstruction**
  - Aortic valve mid-systolic partial closure (M-mode) (differential diagnosis: subaortic membrane) (Fig. 8.2.3A)
  - Mitral SAM (systolic anterior motion): non-specific (hypovolaemia, inotropes, LVH, etc.) (Fig. 8.2.3B)
  - Abnormal leaflets, chordae, papillary muscles, predisposing to obstruction (Fig. 8.2.3C)

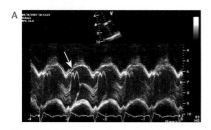 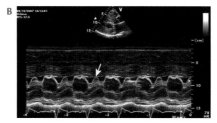 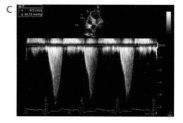

**Fig. 8.2.3** LVOT obstruction in HCM (A) aortic valve mid-systolic partial closure; (B) mitral SAM; (C) typical CW 'dagger-shaped' Doppler signal (late systolic peak)

## Mid-cavitary/apical obstruction (Fig. 8.2.4AB)

# Myocardial function in HCM

## Systolic function (Fig. 8.2.5AB)

- Normal EF and FS, reduced stroke volume
- Abnormal longitudinal function (DMI mitral annulus s' < 9 cm/s, DMI-derived strain, 2D- speckle tracking), usually preserved circumferential and rotational–twist–torsion mechanics

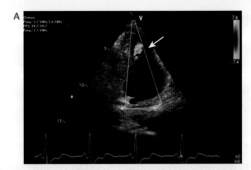

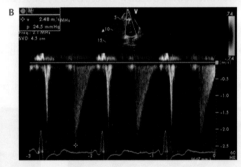

**Fig. 8.2.4** Paradoxical diastolic colour Doppler flow in the sequestered area (A) + paradoxical apex to base diastolic gradient (B)

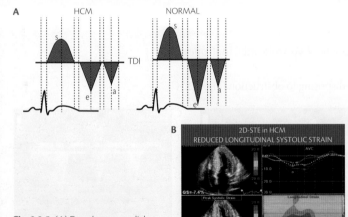

**Fig. 8.2.5** (A) Doppler myocardial imaging in HCM; (B) 2D- speckle tracking in HCM

## Diastolic function (Figs. 8.2.5A, 8.2.6, and 8.2.7)

- Global LV diastolic dysfunction → PW Doppler LV inflow profiles
  - classic patterns have poor correlation with LV filling pressures
  - 'bizarre diastolic patterns' (positive isovolumic relaxation flow, triphasic trans-mitral flow) → no prognostic impact
- LV subendocardial diastolic dysfunction
  - DMI: low e' velocities (e' < 7 cm/s; e'/a' < 1) in hypertrophic and non-hypertrophic segments, high heterogeneity of velocities
  - 2D speckle tracking: delayed LV untwist, occupying > 25% of diastole (normal: occurs in the first 25% of diastole)

## Increased filling pressures in HCM

- E/e' lateral ≥ 10
- Ar-A ≥ 30 ms
- LA indexed volume ≥ 34 ml/m² 
- PASP > 35 mmHg

➡ High LV filling pressures

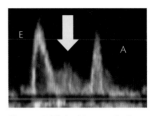

**Fig. 8.2.6** Triphasic trans-mitral flow in a HCM patient, without prognostic impact

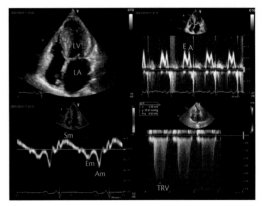

**Fig. 8.2.7** EACVI recommendations: high LV filling pressures in HCM (Courtesy of Pacileo)

**Box 8.2.3** Echocardiographic check list in HCM

- Presence of hypertrophy and its distribution; report should include measurements of LV dimensions and wall thickness (septal, posterior, and maximum) + IVS/PWT ratio
- LV global systolic function (EF) + comments on regional wall motion
- RV hypertrophy and whether RV dynamic obstruction is present
- LA volume indexed to body surface area
- LV diastolic function (comments on LV relaxation and filling pressures)
- Parameters of regional systolic and diastolic function
- Pulmonary artery systolic pressure
- Dynamic obstruction at rest and with Valsalva manoeuvre or exercise; report should identify the site of obstruction and the gradient
- Mitral valve and papillary muscle evaluation, including the direction, mechanism, and severity of mitral regurgitation

## Differential diagnosis

**HCM vs athlete's heart** (Table 8.2.1, Fig. 8.2.8AB)

**Table 8.2.1** EACVIs updated Maron's criteria to distinguish hypertrophic cardiomyopathy from athlete's heart

| HCM | Echo criteria | Athlete's heart |
|---|---|---|
| + | Atypical patterns of LVH | − |
| − | LVH regression after deconditioning | ++ |
| + | Small LV cavity (< 45 mm) | − |
| − | Big LV cavity (> 55 mm) | + |
| + | RV hypertrophy (right ventricular subcostal thickness > 5 mm) | − |
| + | LA dilatation (> 45 mm or ≥ 34 ml/m$^2$) | − |
| + | MV apparatus abnormalities | − |
| + | Dynamic obstruction (> 30 mmHg) | − |
| + | MR > mild | − |
| + | LV subendocardial systolic dysfunction<br>Pulsed DMI: mitral annulus velocities (average four sites): s'< 9 cm/s; 2S-STE peak regional strain ≤ −15% | − |
| + | Abnormal global diastolic function<br>Impaired LV relaxation | − |
| + | LV subendocardial diastolic dysfunction<br>Pulsed DMI: mitral annulus velocities (average four sites): e'< 7 cm/s; e'/a'< 1 in any site | − |
| + | Delayed LV untwist (LV untwist extending beyond 25% of diastole) | − |

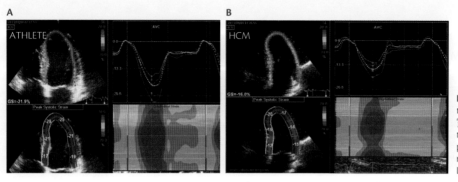

**Fig. 8.2.8AB** 2D- speckle tracking: two athletes with mild LVH in the 'grey zone' range: in opposition to the healthy athlete (A), the HCM patient (B) shows mildly reduced regional longitudinal strain in several LV segments

## HCM vs hypertensive heart disease (Table 8.2.2)

**Table 8.2.2** Differential diagnosis between HCM and hypertensive heart disease

| Echo data | HCM | Hypertensive heart disease |
|---|---|---|
| LVH | Severe, asymmetric, IVS/PW > 1.3 (1.5) | Moderate (< 15 mm—except chronic renal failure and blacks), concentric or mildly asymmetric IVS/PW < 1.3 (1.5) |
| LVOT obstruction | Frequent | Rare |
| 'Sigmoid septum' | Rare | Frequent |
| Severe longitudinal systolic dysfunction | Frequent | Rare (strain often supranormal) |
| Inhomogeneity (velocities and strain) | High | Low |
| Asynchrony (time intervals) | High | Low |
| Diastolic dysfunction | Present (impaired relaxation) | Absent |

## HCM vs cardiac amyloidosis (Table 8.2.3, Fig. 8.2.9)

**Table 8.2.3** Differential diagnosis between HCM and cardiac amyloidosis

| Echo data | HCM | Cardiac amyloidosis |
|---|---|---|
| LVH | Severe, asymmetric | Moderate, concentric, sparkling |
| LVOT obstruction | Frequent | Rare (may exist in early stage) |
| Global LV systolic function (EF) | Normal/moderately impaired | Normal or severely decreased in late stage |
| Global LV diastolic function (EF) | Impaired relaxation | Pseudonormal/restriction |
| LV subendocardial systolic dysfunction | +++ | +++ |
| LV longitudinal diastolic dysfunction | +++ | +++ |
| Apical sparing | Rare | Frequent |
| Pericardial effusion | Rare | Frequent |
| Interatrial septum hypertrophy | Rare | Frequent |

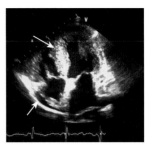

**Fig. 8.2.9** Amyloid heart disease: sparkling myocardial LVH + pericardial effusion + interatrial septum hypertrophy

# Diagnostic accuracy

- **False negatives:** anterior and/or lateral wall hypertrophy may be missed by echo in patients with poor acoustic window
- **False positives**
  - **False LVH:** foreshortened/oblique views; poor acoustic windows or poor technique, inclusion in measurement of other structures (tricuspid chordae, RV papillary muscles, false tendons, trabeculae, moderator band, etc.)
  - **Non-HCM hypertrophies (hypertension, AS, others)**

# Risk stratification

- **Sudden cardiac death predictors** (Fig. 8.2.10AB)
  - **conventional risk factor:** Massive LVH (> 30mm), LVOT gradient (> 30 mmHg)
  - **non-conventional risk factors:** LV aneurysms, systolic dysfunction, LV obstruction, LA dilation ≥ 34 mL/m², low mitral s' (< 4 cm/s), low septal e', intraventricular dyssynchrony (DMI delay > 45 ms), reduced regional systolic strain < −10%

# Clinical profiles and evolution: role of echo

## 'Heart failure' profile: evolution phases

- **Genotype +, phenotype negative**—completely normal echo study, including DMI and speckle tracking
- **Early phenotype–pre-hypertrophic stage**—no hypertrophy, myocardial crypts, mitral dysplasia, abnormal DMI data (lateral s' < 13 cm/s and reduced e' velocities), low regional longitudinal 2D-STE

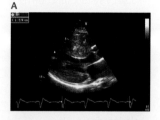

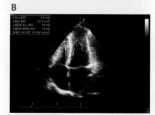

**Fig. 8.2.10** (A): massive LVH (IVS = 39 mm) (B): left atrial dilation (LA indexed volume 41 ml/m²)

- ◆ **Classical phenotype**
- ◆ **Adverse remodelling** (LVH regression, regression of obstruction, LA dilation, decreased EF /global strain, s'< 4 cm/s)
- ◆ **Overt dysfunction** restrictive hypokinetic type—more common; dilated hypokinetic type—more rare

**Obstructive—MR profile: greater morbidity and mortality, worse prognosis**

**'AF and stroke' profile: LA indexed volume ≥ 34 mL/ m² → prognostic impact; LA dysfunction (2D speckle tracking)**

## Echo treatment guidance

- ◆ **Medical treatment:** Assessment of gradient reduction, follow-up of systolic and diastolic function, gradient, MR
- ◆ **Alcohol septal ablation** (Fig. 8.2.11ABCD)
  - ◆ Patient selection (LVOT gradient > 50 mmHg + symptoms) and procedure guidance (myocardial contrast echo for location of the target septal branch: septal perfusion at the level of SAM contact and no remote segments/papillary muscles perfusion)
    - ◆ assessment of efficacy, detection of complications, follow–up

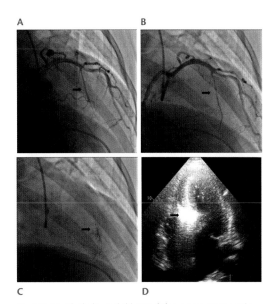

**Fig. 8.2.11** Alcohol septal ablation. (A) coronary angiography (cranial right oblique incidence) of the left coronary artery showing the target septal perforator; (B) selective catheterization of the target artery and balloon positioning; (C) selective angiography of the target artery; (D) transthoracic contrast (SonoVue) echocardiography, 4CV hyperechogenic basal septum, no perfusion of remote territories (Courtesy of Fiarresga A)

## Surgical myectomy (Fig. 8.2.12AB)

- Patient selection, surgical planning, and **intraprocedure TOE** guidance (definition of septal and mitral morphology, MR, and obstruction mechanisms)
- Assessment of efficacy and adequacy of repair, detection of complications, follow-up

## DDD pacing

- Patient selection and procedure guidance (lead positioning)
- Assessment of efficacy, detection of complications
- Follow–up: optimization of the A—V interval according to diastolic filling and/or aortic TVI

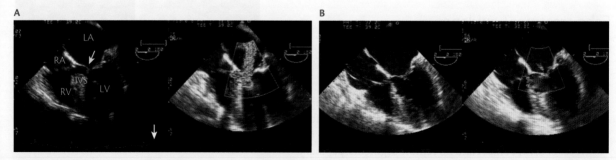

**Fig. 8.2.12** Intra-operative TOE, mid-oesophageal 4CV (A) pre-myectomy: hypertrophic septum, mitral SAM, colour aliasing in the LVOT and moderate to severe MR; (B) post-myectomy—truncated basal septum, no mitral SAM, no aliasing in the LVOT, mild MR (courtesy of F Santos Siva)

# 8.3   Arrhythmogenic RV cardiomyopathy (ARVC)

**Fatty or fibro-fatty infiltration of the RV with apoptosis and hypertrophied trabeculae of the RV** (Table 8.3.1)

## Diagnostic findings (Box 8.3.1)

- RV systolic dysfunction (global or regional) with or without LV dysfunction
- Early stage of ARVC: structural changes may be absent or subtle and confined to a localized region of the RV, typically the inflow tract, outflow tract, or apex of the RV, the 'triangle of dysplasia', (contrast echo may be helpful)
- Progression to more diffuse RV disease and LV involvement, typically affecting the posterior lateral wall, is common (Fig. 8.3.1)

**Table 8.3.1**  Taskforce criteria 2010 for ARVC

| Factor | Major criteria | Minor criteria |
| --- | --- | --- |
| Global or regional dysfunction and structural alterations | Severe dilatation of the RV and reduced RVEF, severe segmental dilatation of the RV, localized RV aneurysms (akinetic or dyskinetic areas with diastolic bulging) | Mild dilatation of the RV or reduced RVEF, mild segmental dilatation of the RV, regional RV hypokinesia |
| Tissue characterization | Fibro-fatty replacement of RV | |

**Box 8.3.1** Echocardiography

- ◆ Regional RV akinesia, dyskinesia, or aneurysm and one of the following findings (end diastole)
- ◆ PTLAX RVOT ≥ 32 mm (corrected for body size (PTLAX/BSA) ≥ 19 mm/m²)
- ◆ PTSAX RVOT ≥ 36 mm (corrected for body size (PTSAX/BSA) ≥ 21 mm/m²) (Fig. 8.3.2) = **major criteria** or fractional area change ≤ 33% = **major criteria**
- ◆ Dilated RV
- ◆ RV aneurysms, outpouchings (at RV inflow, apex, infundibulum)
- ◆ Focal RV wall thinning (Fig. 8.3.3)
- ◆ Abnormal global/regional RV systolic wall motion
- ◆ Potential LV involvement

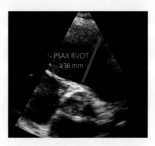

**Fig. 8.3.2** RV cardiomyopathy

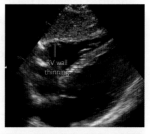

**Fig. 8.3.3** Focal RV wall thinning

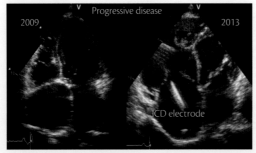

**Fig. 8.3.1** Illustration of progression of RV dilatation over time in ARVC

# 8.4 Left ventricular non-compaction (LVNC)

**Previously 'spongy heart syndrome', absence of involution of LV trabeculae during embryogenic process**

## Diagnostic findings

- Multiple trabeculations with deep endomyocardial recesses (Fig. 8.4.1A)
- Two-layer myocardial structure with a thin compacted (C) and a thick non-compacted (NC) layer (contrast may be helpful)
- Colour Doppler evidence of perfused intertrabecular recesses
- Systolic NC:C ratio > 2 (PTSAX view) (Fig. 8.4.1B)
- No associated heart disease
- Evolutive disease
- LV function can be preserved or severely decrease

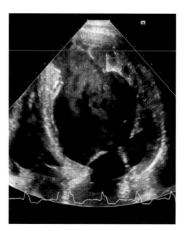

**Fig. 8.4.1A** LVNC with multiple trabeculations and deep recesses. Note the dilatation of the LV and decrease in ejection fraction

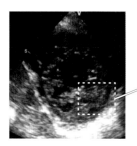
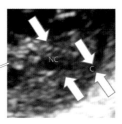

**Fig. 8.4.1B** PTSAX view for end-systolic measurement of NC/C ratio. An end-diastolic measurement can also be useful

# 8.5 Myocarditis

◆ Myocardial inflammation (infectious or not)

## Diagnostic findings

### Acute phase

◆ Global or regional transient wall thickening (oedema)
◆ Regional wall motion abnormalities (eyeball, DMI, 2D STE) (Fig. 8.5.1)
◆ Global ventricular systolic dysfunction
◆ Pericardial effusion (myopericarditis)

or

◆ Completely normal echocardiogram

### Follow-up

LV systolic function assessment → may evolve to dilated cardiomyopathy

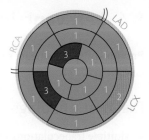

**Fig. 8.5.1** Regional LV function in myocarditis: abnormal WMSI, 'patchy distribution', without CAD distribution

# 8.6 Takotsubo cardiomyopathy

**Broken heart syndrome or stress cardiomyopathy**

## Diagnostic findings

- Hypokinesia/akinesia which does not follow a coronary territory of distribution
- No scar in the myocardium with hypokinesia/akinesia, no coronary artery lesions nor plaque rupture (angiography)
- Hypokinetic apex with hyperkinetic basal segments— typical Takotsubo (apical ballooning, light bulb-like LV) (Figs. 8.6.1, 8.6.2) or apical RV (Fig. 8.6.3)
- Variant form—sparing apex (Fig. 8.6.4)
- Typical complete recovery in a few weeks

## Complications

- LV thrombus
- Apical rupture
- RV involvement

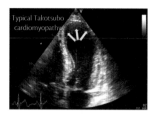

**Fig. 8.6.1** Hypokinetic apex with hyperkinetic basal segments

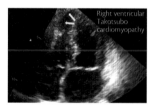

**Fig. 8.6.3** RV apical Takotsubo

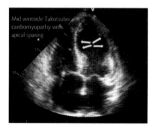

**Fig. 8.6.4** Variant form of Takotsubo

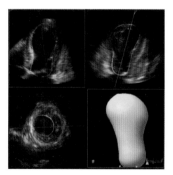

**Fig. 8.6.2** 3D view of typical Takotsubo

# 8.7 Restrictive cardiomyopathy (RCM)

**Restrictive ventricular physiology + normal or reduced diastolic volumes (one or both ventricles) + normal or reduced systolic volumes + normal wall thickness**

## Diagnostic findings (Fig. 8.7.1)

◆ Normal wall thickness, with small to normal LV cavity size

◆ Normal/mildly decreased LV systolic function

◆ Dilated atria (typical appearance: big atria + small ventricles)

◆ Abnormal diastole (usually > grade 2 diastolic dysfunction with increased filling pressures)

◆ Low myocardial velocities with regional function inhomogeneity

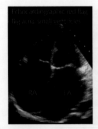 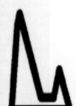 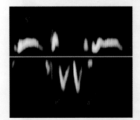 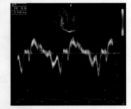

**Fig. 8.7.1** Morphological and functional features of RCM: Dilated atria, small ventricles, E/A > 1, short deceleration time, E/e' > 15, low myocardial systolic and diastolic velocities

# Specific causes

♦ Amyloidosis (RV and LV hypertrophy, granular sparkling, apical sparing with deformation imaging) (Fig. 8.7.2)

♦ Löffler syndrome (hypereosinophilic syndrome, wall thickening, thrombotic/fibrotic obliteration of the apex, etc.)

## Differential diagnosis with constrictive pericarditis

(see Chapter 10, Pericardial disease)

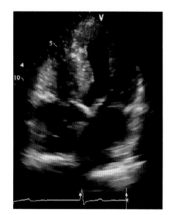

**Fig. 8.7.2** Cardiac amyloidosis

# Suggested reading

1. McKenna W, Spirito P, Desnos M, et al. Experience from clinical genetics in hypertrophic cardiomyopathy: Proposal for new diagnostic criteria in adult members of affected families. *Heart* 1997;77:130–32.

2. Bos J, Towbin JA, Ackerman MJ. Diagnostic, prognostic and therapeutic implications of genetic testing for hypertrophic cardiomyopathy. *J Am Coll Cardiol* 2009;54:201–11.

3. Nagueh S, Appleton CP, Gillebert TC, et al. Recommendations for the evaluation of left ventricular diastolic function by echocardiography. *Eur J Echocardiogr* 2009;10:165–93.

4. Elliot P. Diagnosis and management of dilated cardiomyopathy. *Heart* 2000;84:106–12

5. Pasotti M, Klersy C, Pilotto A, et al. Long-term outcome and risk stratification in dilated cardiomyopathies. *J Am Coll Cardiol* 2008;52:1250–60.

# CHAPTER 9

# Right Heart Function and Pulmonary Artery Pressure

# 9.1  RV function

## Right-chamber imaging and views

♦ Apical 4CV, RV-focused apical 4CV, and modified apical 4CV, left PTLAX and PTSAX, left parasternal RV inflow, and subcostal views

♦ To measure the RV, a dedicated view focused on RV should be used (Fig. 9.1.1)

♦ When feasible, using 3DE should complement the basic 2DE (Fig. 9.1.2)

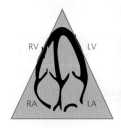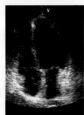

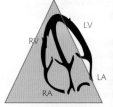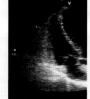

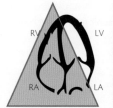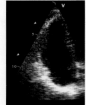

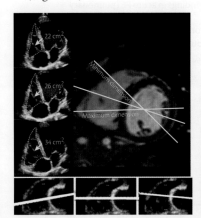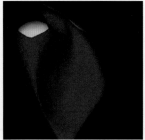

**Fig. 9.1.2**  3DE for guiding 2D measurements and volumes measurements

**Fig. 9.1.1**  Apical 4CV, modified, and RV-focused view

# RV measurements

## RV linear dimensions

**Inflow** (RVOT prox) = **linear** dimension measured from the anterior RV wall to the interventricular septal–aortic junction (in PTLAX) or to the aortic valve (in PTSAX) at end-diastole. Distal RV outflow diameter (RVOT distal) = linear transversal dimension measured just proximal to the pulmonary valve at end-diastole (Fig. 9.1.3AB). Maximal transversal dimensions mid and basal in RV focused view (Fig. 9.1.4). RV longitudinal length measurement in 4CV is not recommended

## RV areas

Tracing of RV endocardial border from the lateral tricuspid annulus along the free wall to the apex and back to medial tricuspid annulus, along the interventricular septum at end-diastole and at end-systole (Fig. 9.1.5)

## 3D RV volumes

Dedicated multi-beat 3D acquisition, with minimal depth and sector angle (for a temporal resolution > 20–25 vps) that encompasses entire RV cavity (Fig. 9.1.6)

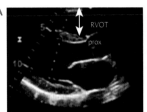

**Fig. 9.1.3** RV linear dimensions

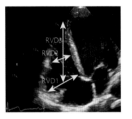

**Fig. 9.1.4** Maximal transversal dimensions mid and basal in RV focused view

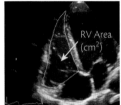

**Fig. 9.1.5** Tracing of RV endocardial border from the lateral tricuspid annulus

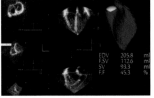

**Fig. 9.1.6** Dedicated multi-beat 3D acquisition

## RV wall thickness

Below the tricuspid annulus at a distance approximating the length of anterior tricuspid leaflet, when it is fully open and parallel to the RV free wall (Fig. 9.1.7)

## RV function

♦ The function of the RV is to generate pressure to facilitate blood flow against the resistive forces of the pulmonary vasculature
♦ RV function is particularly influenced by loading conditions (Fig. 9.1.8)
♦ Estimates of load (especially pulmonary artery pressures) should be included in RV assessment

## Causes of RV dysfunction

♦ Increased RV afterload
    ♦ pulmonary hypertension (due to pulmonary vascular and/ or left heart disease)
    ♦ pulmonary valve stenosis (uncommon)
♦ Increased RV preload
    ♦ atrial septal defect
    ♦ tricuspid regurgitation

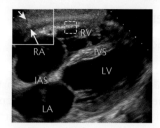

**Fig. 9.1.7** Below the tricuspid annulus

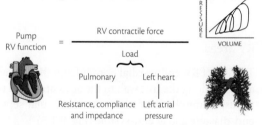

**Fig. 9.1.8** RV function is proportional to contractility and inversely to load

- Primary myocardial pathology
  - RV infarct
  - dilated cardiomyopathy
  - arrhythmogenic cardiomyopathy, sarcoidosis, etc.

## Measures of RV function

- **RV systolic function** comprises longitudinal and radial (free wall and septum moving and thickening inwards)
- Although much of RV function can be attributed to longitudinal function, changes in radial function may be important in some pathologies
- A comprehensive assessment of RV function should include measures describing different components of RV function and a global measure of function (Fig. 9.1.9)

**Diastolic RV function** can be assessed using measures derived from LV experience (tricuspid inflow ratio and E/e') but measures have not been adequately validated for routine clinical use

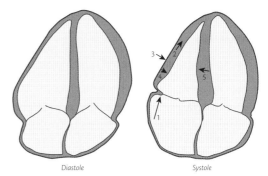

*Diastole*  *Systole*

**Fig. 9.1.9** Measures of normal RV function (legend right)
1. Longitudinal motion
   - tricuspid annular plane motion (TAPSE)
   - tricuspid annular systolic velocity (s')
2. RV free wall longitudinal deformation
   - systolic strain and strain rate
3. RV radial free wall motion
4. RV free wall thickening (radial)
5. IV septal shift and thickening
   - eccentricity index

**Combined functional measures**
- RV fractional area change (RVFAC)
- RV ejection fraction (RVEF)

**Timing measures**
- Myocardial performance index (MPI )
- Isovolumic acceleration time (IVA)
- Isovolumic relaxation time (IVRT)

# Measures of RV function—longitudinal measures

## Tricuspid annular plane systolic excursion (TAPSE)

- **Advantages:** simple, highly reproducible
- **Disadvantages:** moderate accuracy, limitations in more advanced RV pathologies, inaccurate when there is apical displacement ('rocking')
- **Technique:** M-mode cursor placed at the lateral annulus parallel to the free wall (Fig. 9.1.10, Box 9.1.1)

| Box 9.1.1  TAPSE measurement |
|---|
| Abnormal TAPSE > 17 mm |

## Tricuspid annular plane systolic velocity (s')

- **Advantages:** simple, reproducible
- **Disadvantages:** moderate accuracy, dependent on alignment
- **Technique:** Pulse-wave Doppler: ROI placed in the lateral annulus parallel to the free wall (Fig. 9.1.11, Box 9.1.2)

| Box 9.1.2  Velocity |
|---|
| Abnormal s' > 9.5 cm/s |

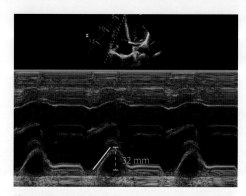

**Fig. 9.1.10** M-mode cursor

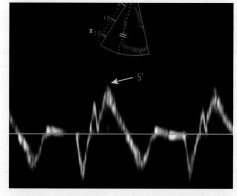

**Fig. 9.1.11** PW Doppler

## Longitudinal strain (ε) and systolic strain rate (SRs)

- **Advantages:** less geometry and load-dependent
- **Disadvantages:** more complex analysis, less reproducible, not yet sufficiently robust for routine clinical use
- **Technique:** colour-coded DMI or 2D speckle tracking of the free wall (usually in three equally spaced regions) (Fig. 9.1.12, Box 9.1.3)

## Measures of RV function—combined measures

### RV fractional area change (RVFAC)

- **Advantages:** single measure, summary of multiple RV dimensions
- **Disadvantages:** less reproducible due to variation in identifying max RV dimension
- **Technique:** apical 4CV through the apex and crux of the AV plane. Rotate the probe until maximum RV dimension (Fig. 9.1.13A)
- 'Stroke area' (RVAD–RVAS) can be expressed to the ratio of diastolic area (RVFAC Fig. 9.1.13B, Box 9.1.4) → Analogous to ejection fraction

| Box 9.1.4 'Stroke area' |
| --- |
| Abnormal RVFAC > 35% (or < 0.35) |

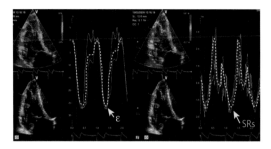

**Fig. 9.1.12** Colour-coded DMI or 2D speckle tracking of the free wall

| Box 9.1.3 Values |
| --- |
| Abnormal ε > 20%;<br>SR < 0.9/s (absolute values) |

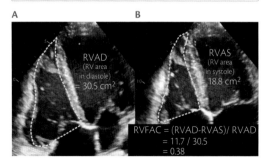

**Fig. 9.1.13** Apical 4CV through the apex and crux of the AV plane (A). Rotate the probe until maximum RV dimension (B)

## RV ejection fraction (RVEF%)

- **Advantages:** three dimensions of complex geometry (Fig. 9.1.14, Box 9.1.5)
- **Disadvantages:** difficult to acquire the full volume of the RV, especially when RV is dilated
- **Technique:** acquire in modified apical 4CV (slightly laterally through the LV apex)
- Gated multi-beat acquisition usually required for larger RVs

## Timing measures

- **Myocardial performance index (Tei index)**
- **Advantages:** less load-dependent, independent of ventricular geometry
- **Disadvantages:** less reproducible, requires stable rhythm
- **Technique:** acquire: 1) CW Doppler of TR and 2) PW Doppler of RVOT; then subtract ejection time (ET) from tricuspid regurgitant time (TR) and divide difference by ET

Fig. 9.1.15AB demonstrating abnormal MPI in a patient with pulmonary hypertension. See Box 9.1.6

| Box 9.1.5  RV ejection fraction |
| --- |
| Abnormal RV EF < 45% |

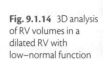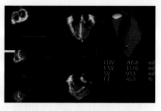

**Fig. 9.1.14** 3D analysis of RV volumes in a dilated RV with low–normal function

| Box 9.1.6  Demonstrating abnormal MPI |
| --- |
| Abnormal RV MPI < 0.4 |

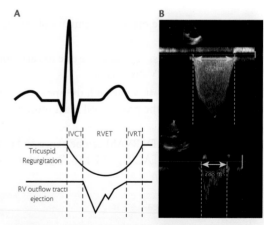

A

B

IVCT   RVET   IVRT

Tricuspid Regurgitation

RV outflow tract ejection

**Fig. 9.1.15** CW Doppler of TR (A) and PW Doppler of RVOT (B)

## Isovolumic relaxation time (IVRT)

- **Advantages:** an excellent single measure that is simpler than RV MPI, relatively easy to acquire, somewhat binary (any appreciable IVRT may be abnormal)
- **Disadvantages:** strongly influenced by pulmonary pressures
- **Technique:** usually by DMI of tricuspid annulus. Doppler of RV inflow/outflow can also be used but is more difficult

Fig. 9.1.16 compares a prolonged IVRT in a patient with pulmonary hypertension with a healthy subject. See Box 9.1.7

## Isovolumic acceleration (IVA)

- **Advantages:** perhaps the most load independent measure (may quantify RV function even when PA pressures are elevated)
- **Disadvantages:** small dynamic range, poor reproducibility, ill-defined normal range
- **Technique:** pulse-wave or colour-coded DMI of tricuspid annulus

Fig. 9.1.17 Reduced IVA and prolonged IVRT in a patient with RV failure. See Box 9.1.8

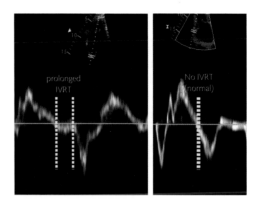

**Fig. 9.1.16** Prolonged IVRT in a patient with pulmonary hypertension and a healthy subject

| Box 9.1.7 Prolonged IVRT |
|---|
| Abnormal RV IVRT > 30 ms |

| Box 9.1.8 Reduced IVA and prolonged IVRT |
|---|
| Abnormal IVA < 1.1 m/s$^2$ |

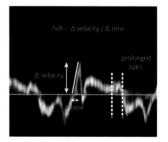

**Fig. 9.1.17** Reduced IVA and prolonged IVRT in a patient with RV failure

# Right atrial (RA) measurements

- **Linear dimensions:** The minor axis of the RA measured in the apical 4CV (distance between the lateral RA wall and inter-atrial septum, at the mid-atrial level defined by half of RA long-axis) (Fig. 9.1.18)
- **Area:** Measured in the apical 4CV at end-systole, on the frame just prior to tricuspid valve opening, by tracing the RA blood–tissue interface, excluding the area under the tricuspid valve annulus (Fig. 9.1.19)
- **Volume**
  - 2D tracings of the blood–tissue interface on the apical 4CV. At the tricuspid valve level, the contour is closed by connecting the two opposite sections of the tricuspid ring with a straight line (Fig. 9.1.20)
  - volumes can be computed by using either the single-plane area length or the discs summation technique
  - 3D datasets are usually obtained from the apical approach using a full-volume acquisition (Fig. 9.1.21)

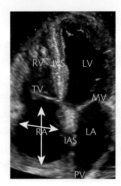

**Fig. 9.1.18** The minor axis of the RA measured in the apical 4CV

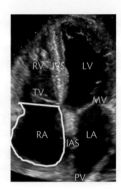

**Fig. 9.1.19** Apical 4CV at end-systole

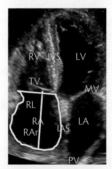

**Fig. 9.1.20** 2D tracings of the blood-tissue interface on the apical 4CV

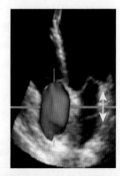

**Fig. 9.1.21** Right atrial measurements

# 9.2 RV volume overload

The concept of a pure volume and pressure overload dichotomy is somewhat artificial. A volume overload often causes increased pulmonary flow and pressures and secondary pressure overload. Conversely, pressure load causes RV dilation (as a means of harnessing 'free' Starling recoil forces), thereby causing some volume overload. Most RV pathologies involve a degree of both pressure and volume overload

## Aetiology

- Left to right shunts—atrial septal defects most commonly
- Tricuspid regurgitation
    - functional: secondary to RV dilation; secondary to atrial fibrillation and atrial dilation ('TRAAF' tricuspid regurgitation associated with AF)
    - primary: intrinsic valve pathology; valve disruption due to pacing leads; rare: carcinoid, rheumatic, congenital
- Pulmonary regurgitation—mostly in context of repaired congenital heart disease

## Specific echocardiographic findings

- RV dilation
- Increased R → L septal shift during diastole (which can be quantified using the LV eccentricity index)
- Hyperdynamic RV, functional measures early in disease process but normalization and then decreased RV function with chronicity

Illustration of specific echocardiographic findings (Figs. 9.2.1 and 9.2.2)

40 y male with an atrial septal defect

- RV dilated
- Eccentricity index increased (below) in diastole and not systole
- RVFAC normal or mildly decreased
- TAPSE, s', strain, and strain rate mildly increased
- A reduction in RV functional measures implies a failing RV with reduced contractility

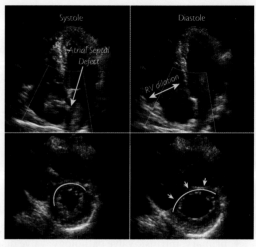

**Fig. 9.2.1** Patient with an atrial septal defect seen on colour Doppler flow in systole (above left) causing RV dilation and diastolic septal flattening resulting in an increase in eccentricity index

$$\text{Eccentricity Index} = \frac{\text{antero-posterior diameter } (x)}{\text{septo-lateral diameter } (y)}$$

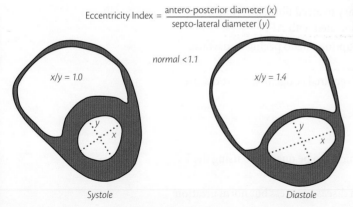

*normal < 1.1*

x/y = 1.0

x/y = 1.4

*Systole*

*Diastole*

**Fig. 9.2.2** Eccentricity index in systole and diastole

# 9.3 RV pressure overload

## Aetiology

◆ Pulmonary hypertension (PH) secondary to left heart disease ('post-capillary' or group 2 PH), the most common cause of RV pressure overload

◆ Pulmonary arterial hypertension (PAH) due to pulmonary vascular disease ('pre-capillary')

◆ PH associated with lung disease 'Cor pulmonale'

◆ PH associated with pulmonary emboli or chronic thromboembolism

◆ Pulmonary valve stenosis (uncommon in adults)

## How to measure RV pressures

◆ RV systolic pressure equals pulmonary artery systolic pressure (PASP) in the absence of pulmonary stenosis and can be approximated with the formula derived from the Bernoulli equation (Fig. 9.3.1, Box 9.3.1, Box 9.3.2)

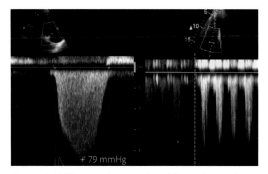

**Fig. 9.3.1** CW Doppler determination of TR velocity to estimate PASP in this patient with pulmonary hypertension
N.B. The TR Doppler signal can be enhanced using agitated contrast (saline or colloid bubble solution)

| Box 9.3.1 Measuring RV pressures |
|---|
| **Normal** PASP < 37 mmHg |

| Box 9.3.2 Using the Bernoulli equation |
|---|
| $PASP = 4v^2 + RAP$ where: $v$ is the maximal tricuspid regurgitation velocity, **RAP** is the estimated right atrial pressure |

# RV pressures

Alternative measures of increased RV pressures are:

♦ Raised RVEDP calculated from the pulmonary regurgitation velocity on CW Doppler (Fig. 9.3.2)

♦ Short pulmonary acceleration time (time from start of ejection to peak flow) (Fig. 9.3.3)

♦ Notched RV outflow through pulmonary valve by PW Doppler (Fig. 9.3.4)

## Echocardiographic findings in acute PE (pulmonary embolism)

♦ A range of pulmonary vascular and RV findings may be observed. Normal PASP/RV function does not exclude PE

♦ PASP may be elevated and RV function may be impaired. Most frequently, reduced RV contraction occurs with little or no RV dilation

♦ McConnell's sign (akinesis of the mid RV free wall) and other regional RV dysfunction are common and may be identified qualitatively or with strain/strain rate

♦ Combination of PAT < 60 ms and PASP < 60 mmHg ('60/60 sign') is relatively specific for PE

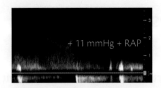

**Fig. 9.3.2**  Raised RVEDP

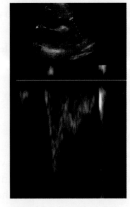

**Fig. 9.3.3**  Short pulmonary acceleration time

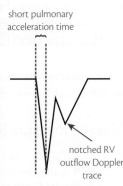

short pulmonary acceleration time

notched RV outflow Doppler trace

**Fig. 9.3.4**  Notched RV outflow through pulmonary valve by PW Doppler

- RV function usually normalizes following small PEs but chronic changes may follow large or repeated PEs (chronic thromboembolic pulmonary hypertension)

## Echo findings in chronic PAH and secondary PH

- RV hypertrophy and dilation are common
- Increased R → L septal shift during systole (Figs. 9.3.5 and 9.3.6)
- Reduced RV function
  - ↓ TAPSE, ↓ RVFAC, ↓ RV EF, ↓ strain
  - ↑ RV MPI, ↑ IVRT

## Exercise testing for pulmonary hypertension

- Exercise testing is not recommended for the diagnosis of PH but there is increasing understanding of what represents an abnormal PASP response to exercise

Importantly

- Pulmonary pressures increase with exercise in **normal physiology** (Fig. 9.3.7)
- There is more data for invasive mean PAP than echo-derived PASP
- An increase in mean PAP > 3 mmHg for each 1 L/min of cardiac output may be abnormal
- **Pulmonary artery pressure must be considered relative to workload or cardiac output**

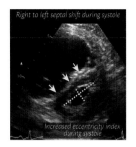

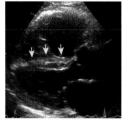

**Fig. 9.3.5** Increased eccentricity index

**Fig. 9.3.6** Increased eccentricity index 'D-shape LV' during systole in a patient with pulmonary hypertension and RV dilation

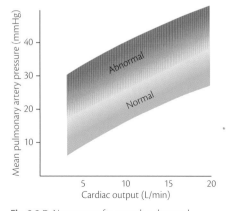

**Fig. 9.3.7** Normogram for normal vs abnormal increases in PAP estimates during exercise

# Reference values

| RV dimensions | Mean value (95% CI) | Normal limit (95% CI) |
|---|---|---|
| RV basal diameter (mm) | 33 (32–34) | 41 (39–43) |
| RV mid diameter (mm) | 27 (24–30) | 35 (32–38) |
| RV longitudinal diameter (mm) | 71 (67–74) | 83 (79–88) |
| RVOT PLAX diameter (mm) | 25 (23–27) | 30 (32–35) |
| RVOT proximal diameter (mm) | 28 (27–30) | 35 (31–39) |
| RVOT distal diameter (mm) | 22 (17–26) | 27 (22–32) |
| RV wall thickness (mm) | 3 (3–4) | 5 (4–6) |

**RVOT EDA (cm²)**

| | Mean value (95% CI) | Normal limit (95% CI) |
|---|---|---|
| Overall | 17 (17–18) | 25 (24–26) |
| Men | 17 (17–18) | 24 (23–26) |
| Women | 14 (13–14) | 20 (19–20) |

**RV EDA indexed to BSA (cm²/m²)**

| | Mean value (95% CI) | Normal limit (95% CI) |
|---|---|---|
| Overall | 9.8 (9.0–10.5) | 13.7 (12.8–14.7) |
| Men | 8.8 (8.6–9.0) | 12.6 (12.0–13.2) |
| Women | 8.0 (7.8–8.2) | 11.5 (10.9–12.0) |

**RV ESA (cm²)**

| | Mean value (95% CI) | Normal limit (95% CI) |
|---|---|---|
| Overall | 9 (8–10) | 14 (14–15) |
| Men | 9 (9–10) | 15 (14–15) |
| Women | 7 (6–7) | 11 (11–12) |

**RV ESA indexed to BSA (cm²/m²)**

| | Mean value (95% CI) | Normal limit (95% CI) |
|---|---|---|
| Overall | 5.6 (3.0–8.3) | 8.8 (5.8–11.7) |
| Men | 4.7 (4.6–4.8) | 7.4 (7.2–7.5) |
| Women | 4.0 (3.9–4.1) | 6.4 (6.2–6.5) |

**RV EDV indexed to BSA (ml/m²)**

| | Mean value (95% CI) | Normal limit (95% CI) |
|---|---|---|
| Overall | 64 (55–74) | 86 (76–97) |
| Men | 61 (55–67) | 87 (80–94) |
| Women | 53 (47–58) | 74 (68–80) |

**RV ESV indexed to BSA (ml/m²)**

| | Mean value (95% CI) | Normal limit (95% CI) |
|---|---|---|
| Overall | 26 (20–32) | 40 (32–47) |
| Men | 27 (21–33) | 44 (38–50) |
| Women | 22 (15–30) | 36 (30–43) |

| RV function | Lower normal limit (95%CI) | Upper normal limit (95%CI) |
|---|---|---|
| TAPSE (mm) | 17 (16–18) | |
| Pulsed Doppler S wave (cm/s) | 9.5 (9.0–10.0) | |
| Colour Doppler S wave (cm/s) | 6.0 (5.3–6.9) | |
| RV fractional area change (%) | 35 (33–37) | |
| RV free wall 2D strain (%) | 20 (19–22) | |
| RV 3D ejection fraction (%) | 45 (42–49) | |
| Pulsed Doppler MPI | | 0.42 (0.39–0.46) |
| Tissue Doppler MPI | | 0.54 (0.48–0.61) |
| E wave deceleration time (ms) | 119 (104–133) | 242 (227–256) |
| E/A | 0.8 (0.7–0.9) | 2 (2.0–2.1) |
| E/e' | 6.0 (5.7–6.4) | |

| RA dimensions | Women | Men |
|---|---|---|
| RA minor axis dimension (cm/m²) | 1.9±0.3 | 1.9±0.3 |
| RA major axis dimension (cm/m²) | 2.5±0.3 | 2.4±0.3 |
| 2DE right atrial volume (ml/m²) | 21±6 | 25±7 |

# Suggested reading

1. Triffon D, Groves BM, Reeves JT, et al. Determinants of the relation between systolic pressure and duration of isovolumic relaxation in the right ventricle. *JACC* 1988;11:322–9.

2. Vogel M, Schmidt MR, Kristiansen SB, et al. Validation of myocardial acceleration during isovolumic contraction as a novel noninvasive index of right ventricular contractility: comparison with ventricular pressure-volume relations in an animal model. *Circulation* 2002;105:1693–9.

3. Ryan T, Petrovic O, Dillon JC, et al. An echocardiographic index for separation of right ventricular volume and pressure overload. *JACC* 1985;5:918–27.

4. Hatle L, Angelsen BA, Tromsdal A. Non-invasive estimation of pulmonary artery systolic pressure with Doppler ultrasound. *Br Heart J* 1981;45:157–65.

5. Himelman RB, Stulbarg M, Kircher B, et al. Noninvasive evaluation of pulmonary artery pressure during exercise by saline-enhanced Doppler echocardiography in chronic pulmonary disease. *Circulation* 1989;79:863–71.

6. Jeon DS, Luo H, Iwami T, et al. The usefulness of a 10% air–10% blood–80% saline mixture for contrast echocardiography: Doppler measurement of pulmonary artery systolic pressure. *JACC* 2002;39:124–9.

7. McConnell MV, Solomon SD, Rayan ME, et al. Regional right ventricular dysfunction detected by echocardiography in acute pulmonary embolism. *AJC* 1996;78:469–73.

8. Kurzyna M, Torbicki A, Pruszczyk P, et al. Disturbed right ventricular ejection pattern as a new Doppler echocardiographic sign of acute pulmonary embolism. *AJC* 2002;90:507–11.

9. Lewis GD, Bossone E, Naeije R, et al. Pulmonary vascular hemodynamic response to exercise in Cardiopulmonary Diseases. *Circulation* 2013;128:1470–9.

# CHAPTER 10

# Pericardial Disease

# Introduction

- ◆ Echocardiography is the first-line examination for the diagnosis of suspected pericardial disease
- ◆ The cause of pericardial disease may also be determined at the same time
- ◆ In various clinical scenarios, a rapid assessment of pericardial disease may be of critical importance for the management of the patients:
  - ◆ acute pericarditis
  - ◆ pericardial effusion and cardiac tamponade
  - ◆ constrictive pericarditis
  - ◆ post-traumatic cardiovascular injury
  - ◆ acute coronary syndromes
  - ◆ associated with specific diseases (systemic autoimmune diseases, renal failure, neoplastic disease, drug- and toxin-related diseases, infectious diseases, etc.)
  - ◆ aortic dissection
  - ◆ post-cardiac or thoracic surgery
  - ◆ post-cardiac interventional procedures
- ◆ Moreover, echocardiography may be very helpful for the follow-up of pericardial disease and for guiding treatments like pericardiocentesis

# 10.1 Pericardial effusion

## Pericardial effusion

### Normal findings

◆ Small amount of fluid can be detected in normal conditions and can be identified as a small echo-free space in the posterior atrioventricular junction, increasing in size during systole (Fig. 10.1.1)

### Semi-quantification

◆ Small: < 0.5 cm (< 100 mL);
◆ Moderate: ≤ 1 cm (100–500 mL);
◆ Large: > 1 cm (> 500 mL)

### Differential diagnosis

◆ Pleural effusion
  ◆ effusion behind the left atrium is more likely pleural than pericardial (Fig. 10.1.2)

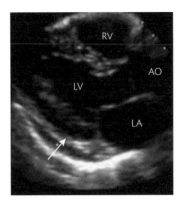

**Fig. 10.1.1** Physiological amount of pericardial fluid (arrow)

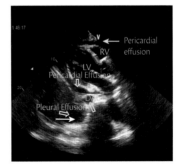

**Fig. 10.1.2** Pleural effusion behind the left atrium and decending aorta (DA)

- Epicardial fat
  - epicardial fat increases with age and obesity. Fat is usually observed at the level of the anterior part of the heart without any pathologic significance. It can be differentiated from effusion by a higher density (white echoes) with ultrasound compared to fluid (Fig. 10.1.3)

## Echocardiographic findings in pericardial effusion

### Presence

- 2DE/M-mode: echo-free space external to myocardial wall increasing in size with systole. Its absence doesn't exclude the diagnosis of pericarditis

### Location

- Can be localized or circumferential (3D echo helpful in case of loculated effusion)

### Content

- Can present with adherences and/or contain fibrinous material (potential factors for future constriction)

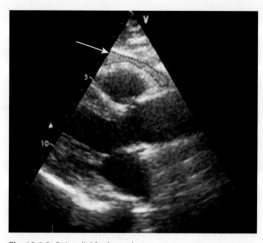

**Fig. 10.1.3** Epicardial fat (arrow)

- Haematoma shows similar density similar to that of myocardium (Fig.10.1.4)

## Amount

- Variable (can be semi-quantified)
- Less important than the rate of accumulation

## Haemodynamic consequences

- Using all echo modalities, assessment of potential tamponade, or constriction physiology

## Associated lesions

- Masses and tumours, aortic dissection, rupture of ventricular wall, myocarditis, etc.

# Cardiac tamponade

## Definition

- Life-threatening clinical condition related to elevated intrapericardial pressure above normal filling pressure of the heart
- A pulsus paradoxus may be present (> 10 mmHg decrease of systolic blood pressure with inspiration)

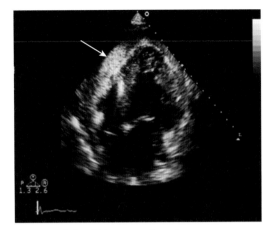

**Fig. 10.1.4** Pericardial haematoma (arrow)

## Physiology

- Compression when the filling pressures are lower during the phases of the cardiac cycle (systole for atria and diastole for ventricles)
- Decrease ventricular filling and subsequently of the stroke volume
- With tamponade, the decrease in pressure with inspiration (Fig. 10.1.5, Box 10.1.1) will be less at the level of the pericard compared to intrathoracic level, decreasing the left ventricle filling gradient (Fig. 10.1.6A)
- Pericardial constraint will exaggerate the respiratory variations in filling, the ventricular interdependence, outflow tract, and hepatic veins velocities (Fig. 10.1.6BC)

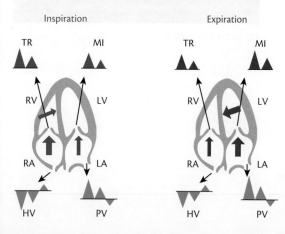

**Fig. 10.1.5** Normal respiratory variations of the filling and ventricular interdependence (HV = hepatic veins, LA = left atrium, LV = left ventricle, MI = mitral valve, PV = pulmonary veins, RA = right atrium, RV = right ventricle, TR = tricuspid

**Box 10.1.1** Normal conditions

In normal conditions, these variations never exceed 30%

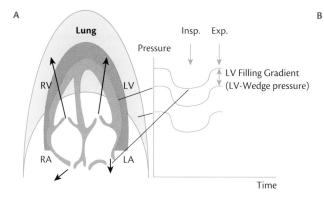

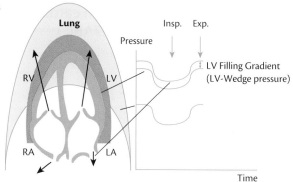

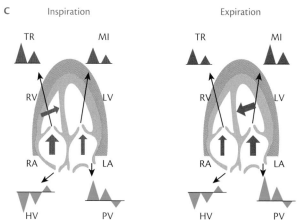

**Figs. 10.1.6** Respiratory variations of the filling and ventricular interdependence (HV = hepatic veins, LA = left atrium, LV = left ventricle, MI = mitral valve, PV = pulmonary veins, RA = right atrium, RV = right ventricle, TR = tricuspid) Fig. 10.1.6A. Normal conditions; Fig. 10.1.6BC. Tamponade

# Echocardiographic findings in cardiac tamponade
## (Box 10.1.2, 10.1.3, Fig. 10.1.7ABC)

**Box 10.1.2** How to assess

- All 2D standard views (+3D if available)
- **Use of a respirometer**
- M-mode to assess cyclic variations of the effusion size with systole, respiratory changes of the inferior vena cava, timing of wall compression, and abnormal ventricular septum motion
- PW Doppler at the tip of the mitral leaflet, at the level of pulmonary veins, and of the hepatic veins. Sweep speed at **25 mm/s** (see respiratory variations)
- Colour-flow Doppler to identify wall rupture and aortic regurgitant flow in case of aortic dissection

**Box 10.1.3** Parameters to evaluate

1. Right atrial collapse during systole (and time of collapse:time of cardiac cycle; ratio > 0.34) (Fig. 10.1.7A)
2. Right ventricular diastolic collapse (PTLAX/PTSAX usually best views) (Fig. 10.1.7B)
3. Swinging heart (four chambers free-floating in phasic manner)
4. Compression of the left atrium or left ventricle
5. Reciprocal changes in ventricular volumes and septum motion toward left ventricle with inspiration and toward right ventricle during expiration
6. Dilatation of the inferior vena cava and blunted respiratory changes (Fig. 10.1.7C)
7. Mitral and tricuspid Doppler velocity profiles with respiratory variation exceeding 30%

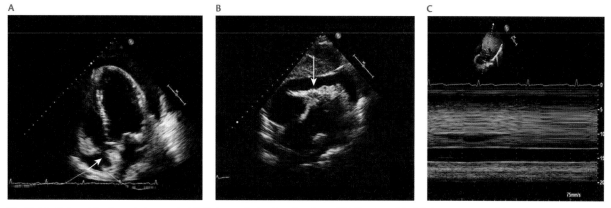

**Fig. 10.1.7** Right atrial collapse during systole (A). Right ventricular diastolic collapse (B). Dilatation of the inferior vena cava and blunted respiratory changes (C)

# 10.2 Constrictive pericarditis

## Constrictive pericarditis

### Definition

**Constrictive pericarditis is characterized by impaired cardiac diastolic function due to a thickened, inflamed, or adherent, frequently calcified pericardium**

**Often post-surgery, radiotherapy, or as evolution of effusive pericarditis**

### Physiology

- Although the physiopathology is different from tamponade, the haemodynamics chararcteristics in regard to respiratory variation are similar (Fig. 10.2.1)
- In constrictive pericarditis, the early filling is preserved and very rapid (atrial pressures are elevated)
- When the relaxing ventricle meets the non-compliant pericardium, the left ventricle pressure declines by mid-diastole
- The increase in atrial afterload impairs atrial contraction

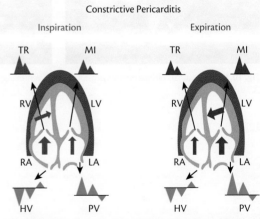

Constrictive Pericarditis

**Fig. 10.2.1** Respiratory variations of the filling and ventricular interdependence (HV = hepatic veins, LA = left atrium, LV = left ventricle, MI = mitral valve, PV = pulmonary veins, RA = right atrium, RV = right ventricle, TR = tricupsid) with thickened and constrictive pericard

- ◆ Illustration of septal bouncing in a 4C apical view (Fig. 10.2.2A)
- ◆ Doppler recordings of the mitral inflow with an increase > 25% with expiration (Fig. 10.2.2B)
- ◆ Tissue Doppler velocities of the septal and lateral mitral annulus (annulus reversus) (Fig. 10.2.2C)
- ◆ Differential diagnosis with restrictive cardiomyopathy (Table 10.2.1)

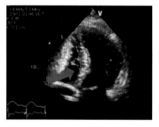

**A**

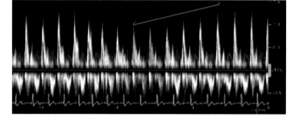

**B**

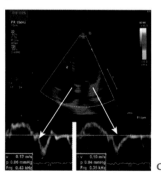

**C**

**Fig. 10.2.2** Illustration of septal bouncing in a 4-chamber apical view (A). Doppler recordings of the mitral inflow with an increase > 25 % with expiration (B). Tissue Doppler velocities of the septal and lateral mitral annulus (C)

**Table 10.2.1** Differential diagnosis with restrictive cardiomyopathy

| | Constriction | Restriction |
|---|---|---|
| Mitral inflow | respiratory Δ E ≥ 25% | no respiratory Δ E |
| | DT ≤160 ms | DT < 160 ms, E/A ≥ 2 |
| Tricuspid inflow | respiratory Δ E ≥ 40% | respiratory Δ E ≤ 15% |
| | DT ≤160 ms | DT < 160 ms, E/A ≥ 2 |
| Hepatic vein flow | ↓ expir. diastolic flow | systolic < diastolic flow |
| | ↑ inspir. diastolic flow | ↑ inspir. systolic and diastolic reversals |
| | ↑ expir. diastolic reversal | |
| Pulmonary vein flow | respiratory Δ ≥ 25% | – |
| Mitral annulus velocity | e' ≥ 8 cm/s | e' < 8 cm/s |

# Echocardiographic findings in constrictive pericarditis (Boxes 10.2.1, 10.2.2, 10.2.3)

**Box 10.2.1**  How to assess

- ◆ All 2D standard views
- ◆ **Use of a respirometer**
- ◆ M-mode to the thickness of the pericard, respiratory changes of the inferior vena cava, timing of wall compression, and abnormal ventricular septum motion
- ◆ PW Doppler at the tip of the mitral/ tricuspid leaflets, at the level of pulmonary veins, and of the hepatic veins. Sweep speed at **25 mm/s** (see respiratory variations). A measure of isovolumic relaxation time (IVRT) by placing the PW Doppler sample volume in between LV inflow and outflow to simultaneously display the end of aortic ejection and the onset of mitral E-wave velocity
- ◆ Colour-flow Doppler
- ◆ Colour Doppler M-mode to assess velocity of propagation of mitral inflow
- ◆ Tissue Doppler imaging to assess mitral and tricuspid annulus velocities
- ◆ Speckle tracking imaging to assess septal strain (and left ventricular twist) if available

**Box 10.2.2** Parameters to evaluate (Fig. 10.2.2ABC)

1. Thickening of the pericard (low sensitivity) > 3–5 mm

2. Abnormal interventricular septal motion (bouncing) or diastolic posterior wall flattening

3. Left ventricular inflow with a prominent E-wave with rapid early diastolic deceleration time (< 160 ms) and a small A-wave

4. An increase of left ventricular IVRT > 20% on first beat after inspiration

5. Dilatation of the inferior vena cava and blunted respiratory changes

6. Mitral Doppler velocity profiles with an inspiratory decrease exceeding 25% and tricuspid Doppler velocity profiles with inspiratory increase exceeding 30%

7. Increased reversal flow during expiration at the hepatic vein level

8. Septal e'> 7 cm/s; lateral e' < septal e' (annulus reversus); e' higher in expiration (to note that E/e' appears inversely proportional to wedge pressure (annulus paradoxus))

9. Septal strain usually normal

10. Velocity of propagation of mitral inflow determined in colour Doppler M-mode > 55 cm/s

**Box 10.2.3** Pitfalls

1. Absence of thickening or calcification doesn't exclude the diagnosis

2. Mitral inflow respiratory variations can also be present in acute heart dilatation, pulmonary embolism, RV infarct, pleural effusion, COPD

3. Respiratory variation of mitral inflow can be absent or revealed by head-up tilt test

# Echo-guided pericardiocentesis (Fig. 10.2.3AB)

- ◆ **Pre**
  - ◆ Determine distribution, depth of the effusion, optimal puncture site, and guide direction of needle
- ◆ **During**
  - ◆ Confirmation of pericardial access (visualization of tip of needle, eventually microbubbles injections), decrease of pericardial volume
- ◆ **Post**
  - ◆ Assess completeness of fluid removal and its haemodynamic consequences

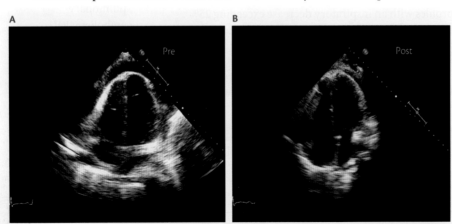

**Fig. 10.2.3** Echo before (A) and after pericardiocentesis (B)

# 10.3  Pericardial cyst

## Pericardial cyst

### Definition

♦ Benign lesion consisting of delineated insulated pericardial portion

### Echocardiographic findings

♦ Thin-walled structure located near the heart (> right anterior cardiophrenic angle) (Fig. 10.3.1)
♦ Echo-free (no colour Doppler flow)

## Congenital absence of pericard

♦ Total absence
♦ Partial absence (less common)

### Echocardiographic findings

♦ Extreme levorotation or shift to left chest with exaggerated cardiac motion
♦ Partial absence may lead to herniation and/or strangulation of a portion of the heart

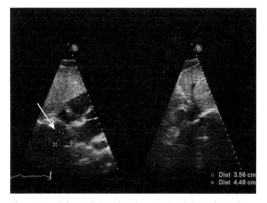

**Fig. 10.3.1** Subcostal view showing a pericardial cyst (arrow)

# 10.4  Congenital absence of pericardium

◆ Total absence (Fig. 10.4.1)
◆ Partial absence (less common)

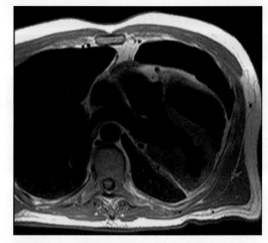

**Fig. 10.4.1**  Short-axis spin-echo MR image of extreme levorotation due to congenital absence of pericardium

# Suggested reading

1. Oh JK, Seward JB, Tajik JA. *The Echo Manual* 3rd edn. Baltimore, MD: Lippincott Williams and Wilkins, 2006.
2. Galiuto L, Badano L, Fox K, et al. *The EAE Textbook of Echocardiography*. Oxford: Oxford University Press, 2011.

## Suggested reading

1.

2.

# CHAPTER 11

# Cardiac Transplants

# Introduction

◆ Orthotopic when the recipient heart is excised and the donor's one placed in the correct anatomical position (biatrial or bicaval) (Fig. 11.1AB)

◆ Heterotopic when the donor's heart is placed in the right chest alongside the recipient heart. The anastomosis allows blood to pass through either or both hearts (Fig. 11.1C)

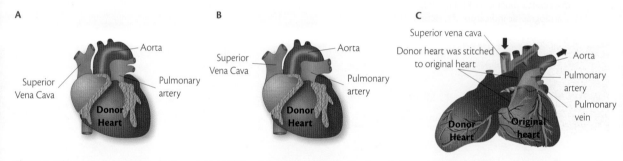

**Fig. 11.1** Schematic representation of orthotopic biatrial (A), orthotopic bicaval (B), and heterotopic (C) heart transplantation

# 11.1 Heart transplantation (HT)

## Role of echocardiography

Comprehensive baseline examination with normal findings assessment

Detect acute allograft rejection

Detect cardiac allograft vasculopathy

Guide endomyocardial biopsies and assess their complications (Fig. 11.1.1)

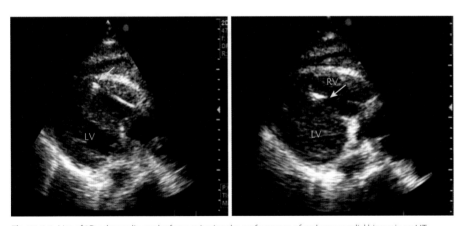

**Fig. 11.1.1** Use of 2D echocardiography for monitoring the performance of endomyocardial biopsy in an HT recipient. The arrow indicates the site of the biopsy. Left panel: at the apex of right ventricle; Right panel: at the level of the right side of the interventricular septum

# Normal echocardiographic findings
## (Boxes 11.1.1, 11.1.2)

**Box 11.1.1** Normal findings in transplanted heart

- Biatrial dilatation (Fig. 11.1.2)
- Hyperechogenicity at biatrial anastomosis (Fig. 11.1.2)
- Pericardial effusion (small or loculated)
- Abnormal (in systole) or flat interventricular septal motion
- Decreased interventricular thickening
- Increased LV posterior or septal thickness
- Increased LV mass (LVM) or LVM index
- Increased RV dimensions and thickness
- Beat to beat variation of the mitral inflow pattern
- Mild pulmonic, tricuspid, or mitral regurgitation

**Box 11.1.2** Recommendation

A baseline examination soon after the transplantation is strongly recommended for follow-up comparison

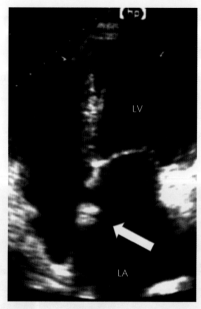

**Fig. 11.1.2** Atrial dilatation after orthotopic transplantation (arrow indicates atrial stitching)

# Echocardiographic indicators of rejection (Boxes 11.1.3, 11.1.4)

**Box 11.1.3  Echo indicators of rejection**

- Progressive increase in wall thickness > 4 mm (interventricular septum and posterior wall)
- Increased myocardial echogenicity (Fig. 11.1.3)
- Diastolic pattern indicating restriction
- New or increasing pericardial effusion
- New onset of mitral/tricuspid regurgitation
- A >10% decrease in LVEF
- A >10% decrease in e'
- A 20% decrease in IVRT
- Dobutamine stress echo to detect allograft vasculopathy
- Speckle tracking global/regional strain is promising

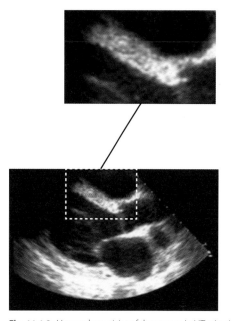

**Fig. 11.1.3** Hyperechogenicity of the septum in HT rejection

**Box 11.1.4  Rejection**

- A combination of two or more parameters may indicate rejection
- These indicators can be absent even in case of rejection proven by biopsies

# Suggested reading

1. Thorn EM, de filippi CR. Echocardiography in the cardiac transplant recipient. *Heart Failure Clin* 2007;3:51–67.
2. Sun JP, Abdalla IA, Asher CR, et al. Non-invasive evaluation of orthotopic heart transplant rejection by echocardiography. *J Heart Lung Transplant* 2005;24:160–65.
3. Al-Dadah AS, Guthrie Tj, Pasque MK, et al. Clinical course and predictors of pericardial effusion following cardiac transplantation. *Transplant Proc* 2007;39:1589–92.
4. Marciniak A, Eroglu E, Marciniak M, et al. The potential clinical role of ultrasonic strain and strain rate imaging in diagnosing acute rejection after heart transplantation. *Eur J Echocardiogr* 2007;8:213–21.
5. Derumeaux G, Redonnet M, Mouton–Schleifer D, et al. Dobutamine stress echocardiography in orthotopic heart transplant recipients. VACOMED Research Group. *J Am Coll Cardiol* 1995;25:1665–72.
6. Amitai ME, Schnittger I, Popp RL, et al. Comparison of three-dimensional echocardiography to two-dimensional echocardiography and fluoroscopy for monitoring of endomyocardial biopsy. *Am J Cardiol* 2007;99:864–86.

# CHAPTER 12

# Critically Ill Patients

# 12.1 Critically ill patients

## Acute dyspnoea (Table 12.1.1)

**Definition: subjective experience of acute breathing discomfort**

### Role of echo

- to help establish whether the dyspnoea is cardiogenic
- to help establish the aetiology of cardiogenic dyspnoea

### Lung ultrasound

- to help establish whether the dyspnoea is cardiogenic (by B-lines evaluation)
- to assess other pulmonary causes of dyspnoea (acute respiratory distress syndrome (ARDS), pneumothorax (PNX), lung consolidations, pleural effusion)

## How to perform lung ultrasound

- Lay your probe along intercostal spaces on anterior, lateral, or posterior chest (to exclude cardiogenic pulmonary oedema, check first for the dependent zones, i.e. posterior lung bases or axillary lines) (Fig. 12.1.1)
- Which probe? Convex: first choice; cardiac: second choice; vascular: for PNX

**Table 12.1.1** Main causes of acute dyspnoea

| Cardiac | Acute pulmonary oedema due to heart failure, cardiac tamponade |
|---|---|
| Pulmonary | COPD exacerbation, pulmonary embolism, PNX, pneumonia, ALI/ARDS, lung cancer, worsening interstitial lung disease, pulmonary hypertension |
| Other | Metabolic, psychogenic, anaemia |

COPD: chronic obstructive pulmonary disease

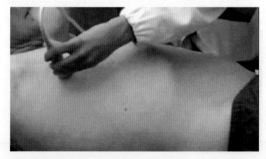

**Fig. 12.1.1** Lung ultrasound probe position

- Appreciate **lung sliding** → the depiction of a regular rhythmic movement synchronized with respiration, which occurs between the parietal and visceral pleura
- Check for **B-lines** → laser-like vertical hyperechoic artefacts that arise from the pleural line and move synchronously with lung sliding
- They are the sonographic sign of the pulmonary interstitial syndrome (Fig. 12.1.2AB)
    - B-lines are very sensitive for interstitial pulmonary oedema (close to 100%)
    - Specificity is lower: multiple, diffuse, bilateral B-lines can be present in cardiogenic pulmonary oedema, acute lung injury (ALI)/ARDS, and pulmonary fibrosis

# Acute cardiogenic pulmonary oedema

## 2D echo and colour Doppler

### Mainly systolic dysfunction

- Dilated cardiac chambers, poor global LV systolic function

A          B

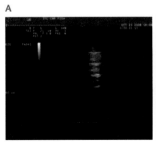

**No pulmonary interstitial syndrome**
(normal lung, COPD, psychogenic)

**Pulmonary interstitial syndrome**
(acute pulmonary oedema)

**Fig. 12.1.2** Lung ultrasound evaluation. A: No pulmonary interstitial syndrome. No B-lines are visible. B: Multiple B-lines in a patient with pulmonary oedema. This sonographic appearance should be present in more than one scan for each hemithorax, and bilaterally

- Exclude acute myocardial infarction in presence of regional wall motion abnormalities (compare with a previous exam and integrate in the clinical context)
- Functional mitral regurgitation (MR) and/or tricuspid regurgitation (TR)

**Mainly diastolic dysfunction**

- Normal left ventricular (LV) size and normal or near-normal global LV function
- LV hypertrophy, left atrium (LA) enlargement
- Doppler signs of high LV filling pressures

**Valvular heart disease**

- Worsening of chronic severe aortic stenosis (AS), mitral stenosis (MS), aortic regurgitation (AR), MR
- Acute severe MR (ischaemic ruptured papillary muscle, flail leaflet) or AR (aortic dissection, endocarditis)
- Prosthesis dysfunction (obstruction, leak, rocking)

N.B. In patients with hypertensive pulmonary oedema, LV systolic function is usually normal with diastolic dysfunction

## Lung ultrasound (Fig. 12.1.2AB)

- Multiple, diffuse, bilateral B-lines (lay a cardiac or convex probe in the intercostal spaces, start with dependent zones)
- Free pleural effusion can be present, generally bilateral, at lung bases
- → **if B-lines or pleural effusion are monolateral: it is likely NOT to be cardiogenic**

# Acute lung injury/acute respiratory distress syndrome (ALI/ARDS)

## 2D echo and colour Doppler

◆ LV function can be normal
◆ RV can be dilated/hypokinetic

## Lung ultrasound (Fig. 12.1.3ABC)

◆ Multiple diffuse B-lines, dishomogeneously distributed
◆ Subpleural alterations
◆ Pleural effusion mono- or bilateral

A        B        C

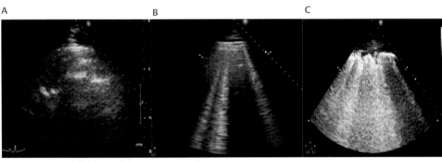

**Fig. 12.1.3** Lung ultrasound evaluation. A: no pulmonary interstitial syndrome. No B-lines are visible. B: multiple B-lines in a patient with pulmonary oedema. C: multiple B-lines and subpleural alterations in a patient with ARDS

**No pulmonary interstitial syndrome**
(normal lung, COPD, psychogenic)

**No pulmonary interstitial syndrome**
(acute pulmonary oedema)

**No pulmonary interstitial syndrome with subpleural consolidations**
(acute lung injury/acute respiratory distress syndrome)

# Pneumothorax (PNX)

## 2D echo and colour Doppler

- ◆ Cardiac window can be hampered by air in left PNX
- ◆ LV usually normal
- ◆ RV can be dilated/hypokinetic

## Lung ultrasound (Figs. 12.1.4 and 12.1.5)

- ◆ No lung sliding, no B-lines, no lung pulse
- ◆ Lung point pathognomonic of PNX

# Exacerbation of chronic obstructive pulmonary disease (COPD)

## 2D echo and colour Doppler

- ◆ LV function and dimensions can be normal
- ◆ Right chambers usually dilated with elevated pulmonary artery systolic pressure (PASP)

## Lung ultrasound

- ◆ Absence of multiple diffuse B-lines (only a few B-lines can be visualized)

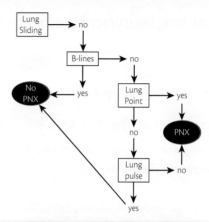

**Fig. 12.1.4** Flow chart with the four sonographic signs to rule out or in PNX

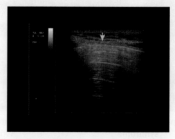

**Fig. 12.1.5** Lung point: the point where you can appreciate the transition from absence of lung sliding to reappearing of lung sliding. It represents the physical limit of PNX as mapped on the chest wall

# Pneumonia

## 2D echo and colour Doppler

- LV and RV function and dimensions can be normal

## Lung ultrasound (Figs. 12.1.4 and 12.1.5)

- Lung consolidation can be visualized (scan the site of chest pain) (Fig. 12.1.6)

# Pulmonary embolism

## 2D echo and colour Doppler

- Dilated and hypokinetic RV
- Variable increase in RV systolic pressure (depending also on RV function)
- Paradoxical motion of the IV septum and D-shape of the LV
- Significant tricuspid regurgitation
- McConnell sign (RV free-wall hypokinesis with sparing of the apex—may be present also in RV infarction)
- 60/60 sign (PASP < 60 mmHg and acceleration time < 60 ms)
- Direct visualization of the thrombus intracardiac or in the pulmonary artery is pathognomonic (Fig. 12.1.7)

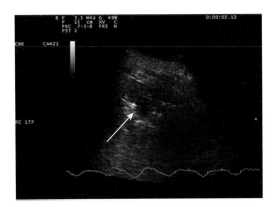

**Fig. 12.1.6** Lung ultrasound appearance of a subpleural consolidation, visualized in the site of chest pain, consistent with pneumonia

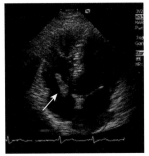

**Fig. 12.1.7** RA thrombus in a patient with acute pulmonary embolism

◆ TOE useful only in selected patients (RV dysfunction, hypotension/shock, cardiac arrest) to visualize the thrombus in the main pulmonary trunk

◆ Integration with peripheral venous Doppler echo increases accuracy

**Lung ultrasound**

◆ In presence of pulmonary infarction, a lung consolidation can be visualized (start scanning the site of chest pain), which typically has sharp margins and is triangular or wedge-shaped (Fig. 12.1.8)

## Specific problems in ventilated patients

◆ During mechanical ventilation, in contrast to spontaneous ventilation, venous return is decreased during inspiration and increased during expiration

◆ Positive end-expiratory pressure (PEEP) elevates right atrial pressures and makes it difficult to use them to assess volume status

◆ Inferior vena cava (IVC) diameter depends on ventilation parameters, therefore is not reliable to assess fluid responsiveness

◆ Recording of reliable images can be technically difficult

➡ In the ventilated patient TOE is less hampered by these limitations

## Shock/hypotension (Table 12.1.2)

**Cardiopulmonary ultrasound is useful to**

◆ Detect a life-threatening cause of shock

◆ Differentiate cardiac from non-cardiac causes

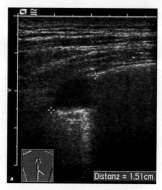

**Fig. 12.1.8** Subpleural triangular-shaped consolidation, consistent with pulmonary infarction in a patient with pulmonary embolism

**Table 12.1.2** Focused integrated ultrasound approach to shock/hypotension

| Type of shock | Organ | Ultrasound findings |
|---|---|---|
| **Hypovolaemic shock** (haemorrhagic shock, dehydration) | Heart | Hyperkinetic LV, small RV |
| | IVC | Small diameter + high collapsibility index |
| | Lung | No B-lines |
| | Abdomen | Free intraperitoneal fluids |
| **Cardiogenic shock** | Heart | Dilated, hypokinetic LV |
| | IVC | Large diameter + low collapsibility index |
| | Lung | Multiple, diffuse B-lines |
| **Distributive shock** (septic, neurogenic, anaphylactic) | Heart | Hyperkinetic LV or mildly reduced LV function |
| | IVC | Small diameter + high collapsibility index |
| | Lung | Multiple B-lines mono- or bilateral + consolidation |
| **Obstructive shock** (cardiac tamponade) | Heart | Pericardial effusion |
| | IVC | Large diameter + low/absent collapsibility index |
| **Obstructive shock** (pulmonary embolism) | Heart | RV dilation and dysfunction, paradoxical IV septum motion, pulmonary hypertension, thrombus |
| | IVC | Large diameter + low collapsibility index; sludge can be present |
| | Lung | No bilateral B-lines; consolidation in case of pulmonary infarction |
| | Peripheral veins | Deep-vein thrombosis |
| **Obstructive shock** (tension PNX) | Heart | Cardiac window hampered in left PNX. RV can be dilated/hypokinetic |
| | IVC | Large diameter + low collapsibility index |
| | Lung | No sliding, no lung pulse, no B-lines, no consolidations |

◆ **Assess fluid responsiveness**
   ◆ if stroke volume (SV) has significant respiratory variations, there is likely to be a fluid responsive circulation
   ◆ fluid responsiveness is defined by an increase in at least 15% of SV following a volume challenge or passive leg raising
   ◆ if the IVC is < 1 cm in diameter, there is a high probability of fluid responsiveness
   ◆ if the IVC is > 2.5 cm in diameter, there is a low probability of fluid responsiveness
   ◆ anterior multiple bilateral B-lines (without subpleural consolidations) is accurate for hydrostatic pulmonary oedema and might contraindicate further volume resuscitation

## Cardiogenic shock

◆ Severely impaired LV function
◆ Functional/organic mitral regurgitation
◆ RV dilation/dysfunction often present
◆ Pulmonary hypertension

## Hypovolaemic shock

◆ Hyperkinetic LV
◆ Small RV cavity
◆ Very small IVC with high or complete collapsibility

## Septic shock

- Hyperkinetic LV in the acute phase. LV systolic function can be also reduced (sign of poor prognosis), although LV filling pressure usually not elevated systolic dysfunction can be reversible
- RV systolic function often reduced and associated to pulmonary hypertension in patients with acute lung injury
- IVC evaluation and SV useful to assess fluid responsiveness

## Pulmonary embolism

(see specific section)

## Cardiac tamponade

- Pericardial effusion (usually large)
- RA collapse (in late diastole and early systole; low specificity) and RV collapse (in early diastole; low sensitivity, high specificity). Duration of collapse during cardiac cycle parallels the severity of haemodynamic compromise (Figs. 12.1.9 and 12.1.10)
- Dilated non-collapsible IVC during inspiration
- Exaggerated inspiratory increase in right-heart velocities and decrease of left-heart velocities
- Check for signs of aortic dissection, trauma, tumours

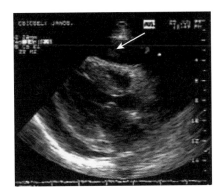

**Fig. 12.1.9** Circumferential pericardial effusion and RV free wall diastolic collapse are shown (white arrow)

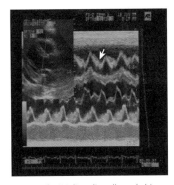

**Fig. 12.1.10** M-mode: RV diastolic collapse (white arrow) due to cardiac tamponade

Cardiac tamponade is a haemodynamic condition; the definitive diagnosis is clinical. TTE useful to guide pericardiocentesis and for the follow-up. TOE needed when acute aortic dissection is suspected and diagnosis is in doubt from TTE

## Echo in cardiorespiratory arrest and focused echo protocols (Table 12.1.3)

**Table 12.1.3** Focused echo protocols for critically ill patient, including cardiorespiratory arrest

|  | **FEEL** | **FATE** | **FAST** | **E-FAST** |
|---|---|---|---|---|
|  | Focused Echo Evaluation in Life Support | Focused Assessed Transthoracic Echocardiography | Focused Assessed Sonography in Trauma | Extended Focused Assessed Sonography in Trauma |
| **When** | Emergency life support, peri-arrest | Critically ill patient | Unstable patient with blunt thoraco-abdominal trauma | Unstable patient with blunt thoraco-abdominal trauma |
| **Where** | ◆ PLAX<br>◆ PSAX<br>◆ A4CV<br>◆ Subcostal | ◆ Subcostal<br>◆ A4CV<br>◆ PLAX<br>◆ PSAX<br>◆ Pleural | ◆ Subcostal<br>◆ RUQ<br>◆ LUQ<br>◆ Pelvis | ◆ Left anterior upper chest<br>◆ Right anterior upper chest<br>◆ Subcostal<br>◆ RUQ<br>◆ LUQ<br>◆ Pelvis |

**Table 12.1.3** Focused echo protocols for critically ill patient, including cardiorespiratory arrest (*continued*)

| | FEEL | FATE | FAST | E-FAST |
|---|---|---|---|---|
| **What** | ◆ Cardiac activity (identify true asystole, electromechanical dissociation)<br>◆ Gross left and right ventricular function<br>◆ Pericardial effusion (tamponade) | ◆ Pericardial effusion<br>◆ Left and right ventricular dimensions and function<br>◆ Pleural effusion | ◆ Pericardial effusion<br>◆ Free intraperitoneal fluid<br>◆ Pleural effusion | ◆ Pneumothorax<br>◆ Pericardial effusion<br>◆ Free intraperitoneal fluid<br>◆ Pleural effusion |

## Left ventricular assistance device

An LV assistance device (LVAD) is a continuous-flow device which unloads the LV of the blood by the presence of an inflow cannula, and pumps it to the aorta through an outflow cannula. It is used to treat patients with advanced HF

◆ Echocardiography is the most important imaging modality in the management of LVAD

◆ It should be performed:
  ◆ pre-implant (TTE, and if necessary TOE)
  ◆ during implant (TOE)
  ◆ post-implant (TTE, and if necessary TOE)
  ◆ long-term follow-up (mostly TTE, and if necessary TOE)

Specific echocardiographic considerations should be taken into account according to the LVAD model used

**Pre-LVAD implant assessment** is performed to:

- Establish the suitability of the patient's heart to LVAD implant
- Establish concurrent surgical procedures (e.g. aortic valve replacement)
- Detect cardiac abnormalities that could determine post-surgical complications

You should carefully evaluate:

- RV function
- AR (that may be underestimated due to high LV filling pressure) and MS
- Dimension of the LV
- Disease of the ascending aorta (plaque, calcification, dilation)
- Degree of pulmonary hypertension
- Cardiac abnormality that could lead to right to left shunt after VAD implant
- Intracardiac thrombi (IV contrast increases the accuracy of detecting an LV apical or LA appendage thrombus)

## Peri-LVAD implant assessment by TOE:

- Is performed to assess inflow cannula orientation
- The cannula should be aligned with the mitral valve opening, without contact with LV walls (Fig. 12.1.11AB)
- Turbulence and elevated Doppler velocity suggest obstruction of the inflow cannula (normal filling velocity about 100–200 cm/s depending on preload and intrinsic LV function → peak velocity > 230 cm/s can be used as indicative of obstruction)

- Assess outflow cannula
- PW sample volume about 1 cm proximal to the aortic anastomosis
- Normal peak velocity about 100–200 cm/s
- Assess AV patency
- Assess RV function
- Assist changes in the speed of the pump to unload the LV properly
- Detect air bubbles in the immediate post-LVAD implant, before the device is activated (preferential embolization to the right coronary artery and innominate artery), evaluating:
  - ascending and descending aorta
  - cannulas
  - anastomotic sites
  - LV apex

**Post-LVAD implant assessment** is performed to:

- Assess the surgical results of the implant, by evaluating:
  - LVAD dysfunction, most commonly due to thrombosis (risk of thrombosis 9–16%)
  - LV and RV dimensions and function
  - degree of MR and TR (persistence of significant MR or TR after VAD insertion may indicate inadequate LV unloading)
  - presence of interatrial shunts

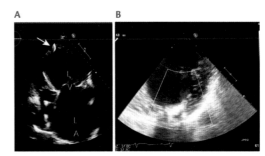

**Fig. 12.1.11** A: proper position of the inflow cannula (white arrow); B: malposition of the inflow cannula, located too close to the cardiac wall, with abnormally high velocity and turbulent flow as detected by Doppler within the cavity.

Courtesy of Dr Enrico Ammirati and Dr Benedetta De Chiara

- spontaneous echocardiographic contrast in the LA or LV (can be a sign of LVAD dysfunction)
- interventricular septal motion (Fig. 12.1.12AB)
    - neutral or slight leftward shift → adequate LV and LA compression
    - rightward shift → suspect inadequate LV decompression (device dysfunction, inlet obstruction)
    - leftward shift → suspect excessive LV decompression (high pump speed, significant TR, RV systolic dysfunction)
- Assess post–surgical complications and haemodynamics
    - acute RV dysfunction
    - cardiac tamponade (interventricular independence should not be considered)
    - hypovolaemia

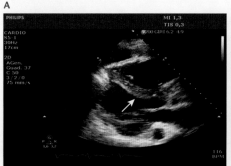
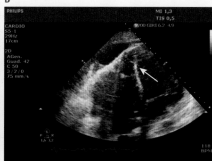

**Fig. 12.1.12** The interventricular septum is not neutrally positioned between the RV and the LV. This is indicative of an excessive unloading of the LV. Pericardial effusion and RV dysfunction are also present. Courtesy of Dr Benedetta De Chiara

- A normal LVAD function leads to reduced LV end-filling pressure and pulmonary pressures with intermittent opening of the AV, and adequate cardiac output through the LVAD

**Follow-up after LVAD implant by TTE** is performed to:

- Routinely evaluate LVAD function, by:
  - LV and RV dimensions and function
  - IVS motion
  - inflow and outflow cannula position and flow
  - LA volume and MR
  - degree of TR and of pulmonary pressure
  - degree of AV opening (M-mode to assess the duration of AV opening) and AR (Fig. 12.1.13AB)
  - thrombi

Evaluation of potential aetiologies of recurrent HF associated with LVAD dysfunction

- Low pump flow with increased power (due to increased LVAD afterload, as in systemic hypertension or device thrombosis)
- Low pump flow with normal power (due to reduced LVAD preload, as in RV failure or hypovolaemia)
- High pump flow with low cardiac output (due to futile cycle, as in severe AR)

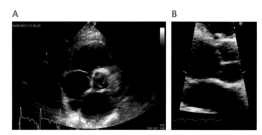

**Fig. 12.1.13** (A) normal aortic valve opening; (B) absence of aortic valve opening in axial flow device. An intermittent opening should be present.

Courtesy of Dr Benedetta De Chiara

# Suggested reading

1. Neskovic AN, Hagendorff A, Lancellotti P, et al. Emergency echocardiography: the European Association of Cardiovascular Imaging recommendations. *Eur Heart J Cardiovasc Imaging* 2013;14:1–11.

2. Volpicelli G, Elbarbary M, Blaivas M, et al. International evidence-based recommendations for point-of-care lung ultrasound. *Intensive Care Med* 2012;38:577–91.

3. Schmidt GA, Koenig S, Mayo PH. Shock: Ultrasound to guide diagnosis and therapy. *Chest* 2012;142:1042–8.

4. Ammar KA, Umland MM, Kramer C, et al. The ABCs of left ventricular assist device echocardiography: a systematic approach. *Eur Heart J Cardiovasc Imaging* 2012;13:885–99.

# CHAPTER 13

# Adult Congenital Heart Disease

# 13.1  Shunt lesions

## Atrial septal defects (ASD) (Fig. 13.1.1, Box 13.1.1)

---

**Box 13.1.1**  Atrial septal defects

**Four types**

◆ (Ostium) secundum

◆ (Ostium) primum

◆ Sinus venosus

◆ Coronary sinus

Transthoracic echo may not be enough to fully elucidate the type, location, and potential associated anomalies with ASDs

**Echocardiography role:**

◆ Identify defect is present (**2D + colour**)

◆ Define defect type

◆ Describe location and borders

◆ Assess haemodynamic effect

◆ Identify coexisting congenital cardiac abnormalities

◆ Assess if intervention is required and type

◆ Imaging for transcatheter closure of secundum ASD (Box 13.1.4)

◆ Imaging post-ASD repair/closure

---

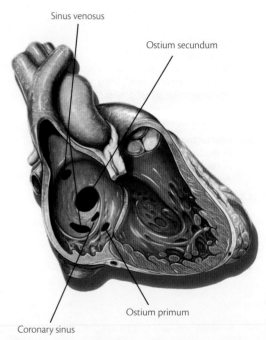

**Fig. 13.1.1** Schematic representation of the four ASD subtypes

## Ostium secundum ASD (Box 13.1.2)

---

**Box 13.1.2  Ostium secundum**

- ◆ Most common type
- ◆ Located in central portion of the interatrial septum
- ◆ Multiple defects may coexist (fenestrated IAS)
- ◆ Variable shape, therefore obtain multiple views

**Transthoracic echocardiogram (TTE)** (Figs. 13.1.2 and 13.1.3)

**Best views**: to find defect (with and without colour)

- ◆ Subcostal
- ◆ Modified apical 4CV
- ◆ Parasternal short-axis (PTSAX)

**Limitations of TTE**

- ◆ Accuracy of ASD size measurement is limited
- ◆ Superior and especially inferior rims are less well seen, thus limited accuracy of ASD size measurement and risk of misdiagnosing sinus venosus defects as secundum defects
- ◆ Transthoracic views of the pulmonary venous return in larger patients can be limited

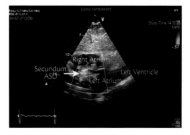

**Fig. 13.1.2**  TTE subcostal long-axis 4CV showing flow across the atrial septum

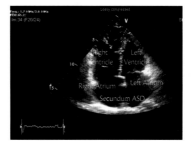

**Fig. 13.1.3**  TTE modified-apical 4CV showing a secundum ASD

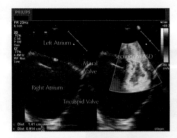

**Fig. 13.1.4** TOE with sizing on 2D and colour Doppler of a secundum ASD at 0° of rotation (Box 13.1.3)

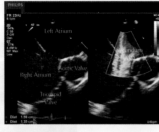

**Fig. 13.1.5** TOE with sizing on 2D and colour Doppler of a secundum ASD at ~45°

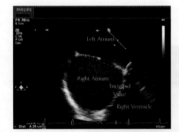

**Fig. 13.1.6** TOE showing the full atrial septal measurement at 0°

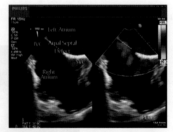

**Fig. 13.1.7** TOE with sizing on 2D and colour Doppler of a secundum ASD in the bicaval view (90°)

---

**Box 13.1.3  Ostium secundum TOE**

- Defect sizing (Figs. 13.1.4–13.1.7)
- Exclusion of other abnormalities, especially anomalous pulmonary venous return, is required for complete assessment

**Rims** (Figs. 13.1.8–13.1.11)

- Aortic (superoanterior)
- Atrioventricular (AV) valve (mitral or inferoanterior)
- Superior vena caval (SVC or superoposterior)
- Inferior vena caval (IVC or superoposterior)
- Pulmonary venous rim
- Posterior rim
- Views: move mid to low oesophagus in each view to fully review the septum
- Measure in 2D and on colour Doppler in each view the defect itself, septal margin (rim), and the total septal length

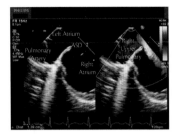

**Fig. 13.1.8** TOE ASD rim measurement to the right upper pulmonary vein at 0° rotation

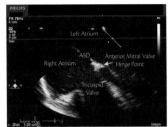

**Fig. 13.1.9** TOE ASD rim measurement to the aorta at ~45° rotation

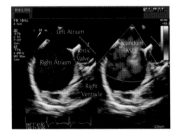

**Fig. 13.1.10** TOE ASD rim measurement to the mitral valve at 0° rotation

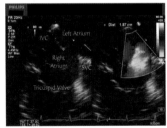

**Fig. 13.1.11** TOE ASD rim measurement to the IVC at 90°

**Box 13.1.3** Ostium secundum TOE *(continued)*

◆ 0° (transverse) for the pulmonary venous and mitral rims

◆ 30°–50° for the aortic and posterior rim

◆ ~90° to the right (longitudinal) for the SVC and IVC rim (N.B. IVC rim still can be difficult)

➔ **3D echo, either full–volume, multi-planar reconstruction, or real-time (live) mode is the best method of defining ASD position and shape and of device closure guidance**

**Box 13.1.4** Transcatheter ASD closure (Figs. 13.1.12–13.1.13)

- Same views but mainly the view preferred by the interventional operator

- ASD balloon sizing (if performed) is done at 0°, 45°, and at 90° views

- Alternatively, colour defect width may be used to guide device size

- 3D 'live' during closure allows device assessment from both left and right atrial positions

- Review septum capture between the device discs and adjacent structure function following device placement

- TTE several hours following the procedure to exclude device embolization and pericardial effusion is an accepted standard protocol—see post repair for ongoing assessment

## Ostium primum ASD

- Forms part of the spectrum of atrioventricular septal defects
- An abnormality of the AV junction not the septum primum itself
- There may be an additional secundum defect
- Predominantly associated with an abnormal left AV valve which is not of typical mitral valve morphology as it is trileaflet (see atrioventricular septal defects)

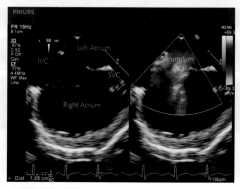

**Fig. 13.1.12** TOE ASD rim measurement to the SVC at 90° (Box 13.1.4)

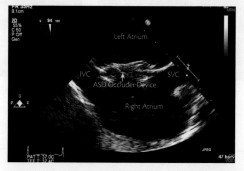

**Fig. 13.1.13** TOE showing ASD occluder device in position

- Significant left AV valve regurgitation is commonly associated in adults
- TTE and TOE assessment (see secundum ASD section)

## Coronary sinus defect (unroofed coronary sinus)

- Defect in the wall separating the coronary sinus from the left atrium
- Rarest type of atrial septal defect

### Four types

- I—completely unroofed + left superior vena cava (SVC)
- II—completely unroofed without left SVC
- III—partial unroofed mid portion
- IV—partial unroofed terminal portion

### TTE

- **Best views:** Apical 4CV posteriorly orientated + parasternal long axis
- Seen as an enlarged coronary sinus and loss of a clear border between the coronary sinus and the left atrium

### TOE

- Only used if poor TTE views so not commonly performed
- **Mid to low oesophagus 0°** 4CV + /- retroflex to see coronary sinus, **90°–100°** with aortic outflow, LA and coronary sinus in view, colour box over coronary sinus wall to LA
- **~120°–130°** oblique mid-oesophageal view can also show the defect

# Sinus venosus defect (Figs. 13.1.14 and 13.1.15)

- ◆ Predominantly superior (associated with the SVC)
- ◆ Inferior sinus venosus defects can extend towards fossa ovalis being easily mistaken for a secundum ASD
- ◆ The defect is located on the rightward septal surface adjacent to SVC or IVC drainage
- ◆ Anomalous drainage of the right sided pulmonary veins (usually right upper) is commonly associated
- ◆ **TTE**
  - ◆ in adults is **poor at differentiating these defects**
  - ◆ **Best views:** parasternal short axis and a sagittal subcostal view
- ◆ **TOE**
  - ◆ **0°** to posterior LA in mid-oesophageal view to review the right pulmonary veins can sometimes identify both the defect and the anomalous venous drainage
  - ◆ **Best view 90°** rotating the probe towards the right bicaval view with the right pulmonary artery in cross-section to see the defect (overriding of the SVC or IVC) and potentially anomalous veins moving up and down to view the SVC/IVC (for views of pulmonary venous return, see PAPVD section)

**Any doubt then consider other imaging by CT or MRI**

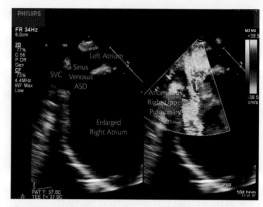

**Fig. 13.1.14** TOE view of a sinus venosus ASD with anomalous right upper pulmonary veins entering the RA at 0° rotation

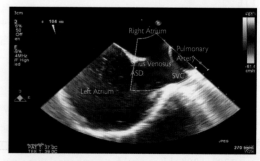

**Fig. 13.1.15** TOE view of sinus venosus ASD

## Haemodynamic effects of ASD

- Needs assessment in the decision to refer for intervention
- **Echocardiographic features of significant left to right shunt**
  - RA and RV dilatation
  - septal flattening during diastole on parasternal SAX
  - 'paradoxical' septal motion due to volume overload (M-mode in parasternal views helps identify this)
  - elevated RV systolic pressure: estimated from the peak TR velocity (if sufficient trace) with addition of the estimated RA pressure
  - RAP can be estimated by ($JVP_{cmH2O}$ + 5/1.3) or by assessing IVC collapse with inspiration ➜ **RVSP= (peak TR systolic velocity$^2$ × 4) + RAP**

**Estimation of left to right shunt: Qp:Qs = ($TVI_{RVOT}$ × $CSA_{RVOT}$)/($TVI_{LVOT}$ × $CSA_{LVOT}$)**
**Qp:Qs >1.5:1 with other parameters suggests a significant shunt**

## Echo post-ASD intervention

- Exclude residual shunt
- Review position of septal occluder device relative to structures and exclude impedance or obstruction to their function (same transthoracic views as preclosure)
- Assessment of RV size and function
- Review for presence of pulmonary hypertension
- Review AV valve function especially with primum ASDs
- Exclude pulmonary venous stenosis/hypertension where the pulmonary veins have been baffled to the left atrium

# Partial anomalous pulmonary venous drainage (PAPVD)
## (Fig. 13.1.16ABC, Boxes 13.1.5A, 13.1.5B)

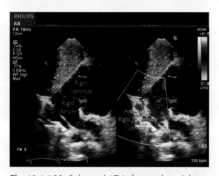

**Fig. 13.1.16A** Subcostal 4CV of anomalous right pulmonary veins

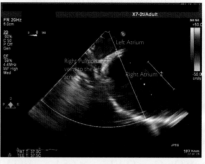

**Fig. 13.1.16B** TOE view of normal right pulmonary venous drainage to LA

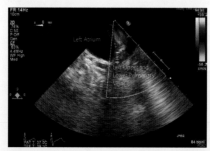

**Fig. 13.1.16C** TOE view of normal left pulmonary venous drainage to LA

## Box 13.1.5A Partial anomalous pulmonary venous drainage

Rare congenital abnormality in which some of the pulmonary veins drain into the right atrium or one of its venous tributaries

**N.B.** pulmonary venous drainage and connections can be challenging to establish on echo (see section on sinus venosus ASD as well)

### Role of TTE in PAPVD

+ **Suspicion:** dilated RA and RV, even with an ASD present (PAPVD and ASDs are commonly associated)

+ Echo evidence of pulmonary hypertension

+ Turbulent flow in SVC or IVC + /− dilated SVC or IVC

+ **Best views of pulmonary veins:** high left parasternal PTSAX, apical 4CV, subcostal sagittal

+ Look for an absent connection of one of the four pulmonary veins or reversed flow in the area of the usual location of pulmonary venous inflow

+ 3D echo of SVC/RA junction can identify anomalous pulmonary venous entry to the SVC

## Box 13.1.5B Role of TOE in PAPVD

### Role of TOE in PAPVD

+ Not always definitive—consider alternative imaging where there is doubt

### Right pulmonary venous return:

+ 0° rotate to right (clockwise) towards the posterior LA in mid-oesophageal view

+ 0° upper oesophageal view rotate to the bifurcation of pulmonary arteries and further rotate clockwise to view SVC and RUPV in cross section

+ 45°–60° oblique short axis rotate extreme right ('Y' shape as veins enter)

+ 90° rotating the probe towards the right bicaval view with the right pulmonary artery in cross section (potentially anomalous veins to SVC and IVC along with sinus venosus ASDs—see section)

### Left pulmonary venous return

+ 0° rotate to left (anti-clockwise) towards the posterior LA—upper pulmonary vein is parallel to the appendage and advancing slightly shows left lower pulmonary vein

+ 60° with upper pulmonary vein in view shows its long axis

# Ventricular septal defects (VSD) (Fig. 13.1.17, Box 13.1.6)

**Box 13.1.6** Ventricular septal defects

- The RV can be divided into three regions
  - **inlet**
  - **trabecular/muscular**
  - **outlet**
- Septal defects can occur anywhere within these areas
- VSD nomenclature is based on their position as viewed by the surgeons from the RV
- **Three types**
  - **perimembranous**
  - **muscular**
  - **doubly-committed**

**Role of echo**

- Identify defect (**2D and with colour Doppler**)
- Identify type and number of defect(s) by location and borders
- Assess the haemodynamic effect
- Look for coexistent congenital defects
- Assess if intervention is required
- Imaging post-VSD repair/closure

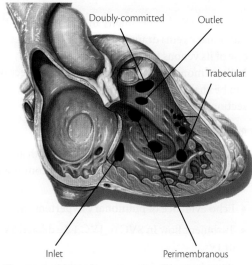

**Fig. 13.1.17** Schematic representation of the VSD subtypes

## Perimembranous VSD (Box 13.1.7)

> **Box 13.1.7** Perimembranous VSD
>
> ◆ Most common type
>
> ◆ Located in the membranous septum or on the border of it
>
> ◆ There is (fibrous) continuity via the defect between the leaflets of the aortic and tricuspid valves
>
> ◆ It may have extension from the subaortic area into the inlet, outlet, or trabecular portion of the right ventricle
>
> ◆ There can be deviation of the outlet septum causing sub-pulmonary (anterior deviation) or sub-aortic (posterior deviation) obstruction—thus look for further abnormalities
>
> ◆ The VSD can be partially closed by accessory tricuspid tissue (ideal)
>
> ◆ **Aortic sinus prolapse** into the VSD: an uncommon complication necessitating assessment of aortic valve function over time (see doubly-committed)
>
> **Role of TTE** (Figs. 13.1.18 and 13.1.19)
>
> ◆ **Best views:** for proximity of the defect to the tricuspid valve are an apical 4CV and parasternal short-axis

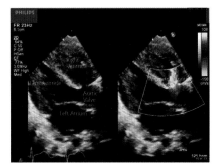

**Fig. 13.1.18** Parasternal long-axis view of perimembranous VSD

**Box 13.1.7  Perimembranous VSD** *(continued)*

- **Best views:** for proximity of the VSD to the aortic valve are parasternal and apical long-axis views
- **Inlet extension** is best explored in apical 4CV
- **3D views** help define VSD size and borders

**Role of TOE (helpful for 3D assessment)**

- **Mid oesophagus 5CV 0°** with aortic outflow shown
- **Mid oesophagus ~30°–45°** looking clockwise opening up tricuspid, RV, and pulmonary valve with aortic valve en face
- **Mid oesophagus ~130°** with aortic valve outflow and RVOT demonstrated

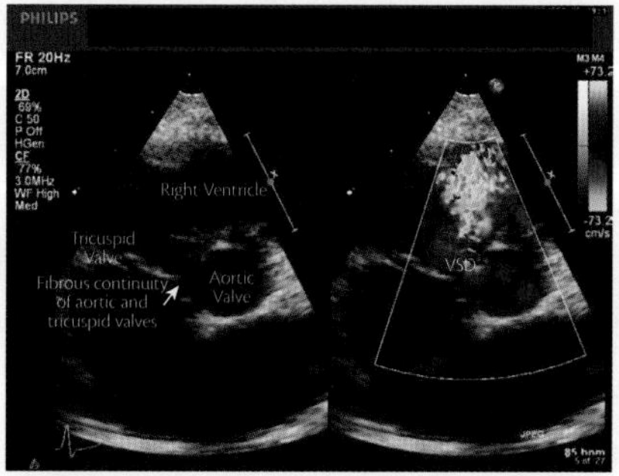

**Fig. 13.1.19** Parasternal short-axis view showing a classical perimembranous VSD

## Muscular VSD (Box 13.1.8)

**Box 13.1.8  Muscular VSD**

- Can be in the inlet, outlet, or trabecular area within the boundaries of the muscular septum
- Can be single or multiple

**Box 13.1.8** Muscular VSD (*continued*)

- Are easy to miss so the septum should be viewed at multiple levels from multiple angles (apical area especially)
- Ensure the whole septum is assessed with colour Doppler

**Role of TTE** (Figs. 13.1.20 and 13.1.21)

- **Best views:** apical 4CV, PTSAX at multiple levels down to the apex, subcostal sagittal
- **3D echo** imaging where windows are good is helpful to define VSD borders and estimate size

**Role of TOE** (Figs. 13.1.22 and 13.1.23)

- Still can be challenging to view this type of VSD
- **Best views:** are moving up and down the septum in
  - **Transgastric** view at mid short axis 0°
  - **Lower mid oesophageal** 0° 4CV
  - **Mid oesophageal** 130° moving left to right
- **3D review** of defects can be helpful where good window makes it possible to define size, borders, and location

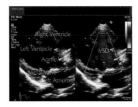

**Fig. 13.1.20** Parasternal long-axis view showing a muscular inlet VSD

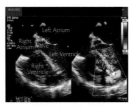

**Fig. 13.1.21** Parasternal short-axis view of muscular inlet VSD

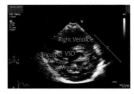

**Fig. 13.1.22** Apical muscular VSD

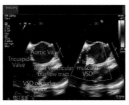

**Fig. 13.1.23** Inlet muscular VSD

## Doubly-committed/juxta-arterial VSD (Box 13.1.9)

> **Box 13.1.9** Doubly-committed /juxta-arterial VSD
>
> ◆ The least common type of defect with (fibrous) continuity via the defect between leaflets of the PV and AV
>
> ◆ Superiorly the defect has the arterial valves and the postero-inferior margin may be perimembranous or muscular septum
>
> ◆ ~50% of doubly-committed VSDs are complicated by **aortic sinus (coronary cusp) prolapse** which partially or completely closes the defect and commonly leads to aortic regurgitation
>
> ◆ Untreated larger defects cause **pulmonary hypertension** early in life due to direct flow via the VSD to the pulmonary artery
>
> **Role of TTE**
>
> ◆ **Best views:** PTLAX view rotated slightly clockwise or PTSAX
>
> ◆ Assessment for **pulmonary hypertension**
>
> **Role of TOE** (Figs. 13.1.24 and 13.1.25)
>
> ◆ **Mid oesophageal**
>
> ◆ **~130°** with both aortic and pulmonary outflows seen
>
> ◆ **~30°–45°** rotated rightwards with RVOT and PV in view and AV en face
>
> ◆ **Deep transgastric 0° or transgastric 110°–140°** shows aortic outflow to assess for AR

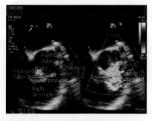

**Fig. 13.1.24** Doubly-committed VSD with AV right coronary cusp prolapse

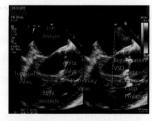

**Fig. 13.1.25** Doubly-committed VSD with AV right coronary cusp prolapse with AR

## VSD size and haemodynamic effect (Box 13.1.10A)

| |
|---|
| **Box 13.1.10A** VSD size and haemodynamic effect |
| Needs assessment in the decision to refer for intervention<br>**Size**<br><br>♦ Small < 5 mm<br><br>♦ Moderate 5–10 mm<br><br>♦ Large > 10 mm<br><br>**Echocardiographic features of a significant left to right shunt**<br><br>♦ Increased LA and LV size and volume<br><br>♦ Low instantaneous gradient < 25 mmHg with pure left to right flow<br><br>♦ + /− functional mitral regurgitation<br><br>Estimation of RV pressure by VSD gradient<br><br>$$RVSP = \text{Systolic BP} - 4 \times (\text{VSD peak velocity})^2$$<br><br>Estimation of left to right shunt Qp:Qs (See ASD section for full details)<br><br>**Echocardiographic features of a restrictive VSD**<br><br>♦ Normal LA and LV size and volume<br><br>♦ High instantaneous peak gradient > 64 mmHg<br><br>♦ No evidence of pulmonary hypertension<br><br>**Pulmonary vascular disease can be well established in patients with VSDs indicated by**<br>**bidirectional or right to left flow through the VSD with normalized LA and LV**<br>(see pulmonary hypertension section for full assessment) |

## Review post-VSD intervention (Box 13.1.10B)

**Box 13.1.10B** Review post-VSD intervention

VSDs remain predominantly managed via surgical closure

**Echocardiography aims:**

- Exclude a residual shunt
- Assessment of biventricular size and function
- Exclude pulmonary hypertension
- **AV function** especially where prolapse into the VSD was evident and aortic cusp resuspension has been undertaken
- Review MV function where regurgitation was evident
- Subaortic and subpulmonary stenosis (beware of the **double-chamber RV**)

# Atrioventricular septal defects (AVSD) (Boxes 13.1.11A, 13.1.11B, 13.1.12)

---

**Box 13.1.11A** Atrioventricular septal defects

- There is loss of the normal AV valve offset due to a common AV junction, guarded classically by five AV valve leaflets.
- Neither AV valve resembles a typical TV or MV, the left AV valve is trileaflet.

**Five leaflet configuration**

- Superior bridging leaflet spans across the ventricular septum superiorly
- Inferior bridging leaflet spans the gap across the ventricular septum inferiorly
- Two leaflets (anterosuperior and inferior) are exclusive to the right ventricular inlet
- One mural leaflet is exclusive to the left ventricular inlet

**Left ventricular outflow tract**

- The aorta is unwedged from its normal position between the inlet valves and is displaced anteriorly and to the left, leading to elongation and anterior deviation of the LVOT

**Classification** (Figs. 13.1.26 and 13.1.27)

- **Partial AVSD**—the bridging leaflets are tethered to crest of ventricular septum obliterating a VSD component. There is usually a large interatrial communication (ostium primum defect) above the bridging leaflets and the left AV valve is trileaflet
- **Complete AVSD**—a combination of a common AV valve, a primum ASD and an unrestricted VSD below the bridging leaflets

---

## Box 13.1.11B  Role of echo

### Role of echo

- Identify defect (**2D and with colour**)
- Define defect type
- Assess haemodynamic effect
- Assess for coexistent congenital cardiac abnormalities
- Imaging post AVSD repair

### Features of adult AVSD patients

- Most patients with a complete AVSD have had surgical repair in infancy or childhood
- Partial AVSD echo diagnosis—see the ASD section
- Un-operated AVSD with a large ventricular component
- Commonly results in irreversible pulmonary vascular disease (Eisenmenger)

### TTE best views

- Atrial and ventricular defects: apical 4CV, PTSAX, subcostal
- AV valves—apical 4CV, parasternal, subcostal
- LV outflow—apical 5CV, PTLAX

Require full assessment of ventricular size and function

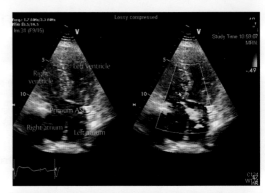

**Fig. 13.1.26**  TTE apical 4CV partial AVSD (Box 13.1.12)

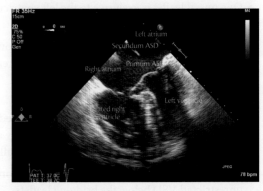

**Fig. 13.1.27**  TOE 4CV of partial AVSD

## Box 13.1.12  Role of TOE in AVSD

- Specific assessment of AV valves (especially the left) and shunt assessment (including **additional secundum ASDs**)

- **Mid oesophagus 0°** review ostium primum defect, assessment of the AV valves, (N.B. flexing helps to identify the three leaflet components of the left AV valve)

- Chordal attachments of the AV valves can be assessed scanning up and down in a **transverse plane 45°–60°**

- **Transgastric 0°** to assess AV valves en face

- The AV valves should be visualized from **0°–130°** for full assessment

- The crest of the septum should also be visualized from **0°–180°** to identify any ventricular communication +/– colour-flow mapping

- **3D assessment** of AV valves to assess the mechanism of regurgitation

**Haemodynamic effect in AVSD**

- The shunt level determines whether there is right- or left-heart loading

- For haemodynamic assessment see ASD and VSD section

**Echo post repair** (Figs. 13.1.28–13.1.30)

- Exclude a residual shunt at atrial or ventricular level

- Review AV valve function–particularly the left valve—and define mechanism of regurgitation as this may influence interventional timing (i.e.: is it an easily repairable issue?)

- Assessment of biventricular size and function

- Assessment for LVOT obstruction

- Assessment for pulmonary hypertension

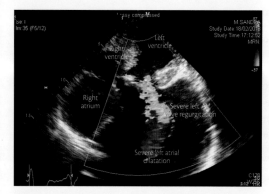

**Fig. 13.1.28** TTE apical 4CV of previously repaired AVSD with LAV valve regurgitation

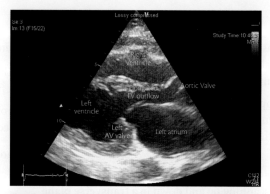

**Fig. 13.1.29** TTE PTLAX view of previously repaired AVSD

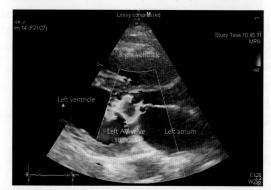

**Fig. 13.1.30** TTE PTLAX view of previously repaired AVSD with LAV valve stenosis

# Patent ductus arteriosus (PDA) (Figs. 13.1.31–13.1.33, Boxes 13.1.13A, 13.1.13B)

---

**Box 13.1.13A  Patent ductus arteriosus**

- Persisting communication between the descending aorta and the bifurcation of the main pulmonary trunk

- In a left aortic arch, the PDA usually arises from the descending aorta opposite the left subclavian artery origin connecting to the left pulmonary artery origin

- In right aortic arch, PDA most commonly between the left subclavian to the left pulmonary artery or from the descending aorta to the right pulmonary artery

### Role of echocardiography

- Identify patent duct and its location
- Assess the haemodynamic effect and flow pattern
- Identify coexistent congenital abnormalities

- Assess if intervention is required
- Imaging post PDA closure

### Role of TTE

- **Suspicion of PDA:** diastolic reversal in aorta without other cause, dilated pulmonary vasculature, pulmonary hypertension, dilated left heart in absence of other cause

- **Best views:** high modified left parasternal or left infraclavicular with slight clockwise rotation to outline both aortic and pulmonary ends

- **Assess with colour Doppler: a PDA can be easily missed**

- Helpful views for confirmation: suprasternal, subcostal, high parasternal sagittal and parasternal SAX

## Box 13.1.13B   Role of TOE

### Role of TOE

◆ To diagnose PDA is challenging, requiring high oesophageal views—alternative imaging modalities should be considered if transthoracic views are poor

### PDA flow dynamics and haemodynamic effect

### Size

◆ Small PDA has high velocity left to right shunt with continuous Doppler flow pattern

◆ Intermediate PDA without pulmonary vascular disease will have lower velocity left to right flow + left chamber enlargement

◆ Large PDA with elevated pulmonary vascular resistance will have low velocity left to right or bidirectional shunt + /− left chamber enlargement with echo evidence of pulmonary hypertension

### Echocardiographic features of significant left to right shunt

◆ Increased LA and LV size and volume

◆ + /− functional MR

◆ May have elevated RV systolic pressure (reflecting elevated pulmonary pressures)

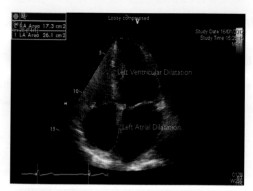

**Fig. 13.1.31**  Left heart dilatation due to PDA

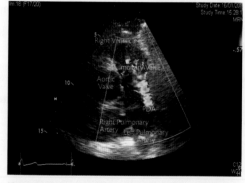

**Fig. 13.1.32**  Parasternal SAX showing PDA flow into the main pulmonary artery

## Echo review post PDA intervention (transcatheter or rarely surgical) (Box 13.1.13C)

<table>
<tr><td>

**Box 13.1.13C**  Echo review post PDA intervention

- ◆ Exclude residual shunt
- ◆ Review the position of occluder device/coil relative to pulmonary arteries and aorta and exclude obstruction to flow
- ◆ Assessment of LV size and function and any residual MR
- ◆ Review for pulmonary hypertension

</td></tr>
</table>

## Persistent left superior vena cava (SVC)

- ◆ Rare (0.5% general population)
- ◆ Generally benign, 80–90% also have a right SVC
- ◆ Implications for cannulation for cardiopulmonary bypass and transvenous pacing
- ◆ Increased prevalence in association with other congenital cardiac anomalies (3–4%) so all cardiac anatomy needs to be assessed
- ◆ Clinical implications in case of coexistence with a coronary sinus defect or when it directly drains to the left atrium

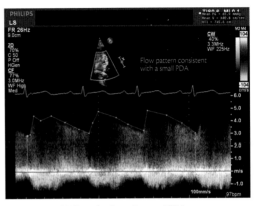

**Fig. 13.1.33**  CW Doppler through a small PDA

## Role of TTE (Fig. 13.1.34)

- **Suspicion:** dilated coronary sinus in the posterior atrioventricular groove in PTLAX
- **Best views:** PTSAX (anterior to left pulmonary artery), high parasternal sagittal (drainage to coronary sinus)
- **Confirmation:** an agitated saline injection into the left antecubital vein with parasternal LAX view scanning showing coronary sinus opacification before the RA and RV (or LA opacification if communication exists). (Confirmation of right SVC is confirmed by injection into the right antecubital vein with PTSAX view scanning)

## Role of TOE

- if transthoracic views are poor then a contrast study can be done profiling the coronary sinus with deep oesophageal + /– retroflexed apical view at 0° with contrast injection into a left arm vein

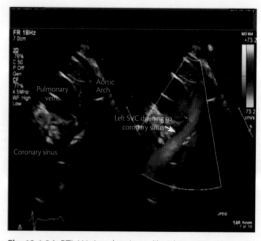

**Fig. 13.1.34** PTLAX view showing a dilated coronary sinus. High parasternal sagittal view showing left SVC to coronary sinus

# 13.2 Obstructive lesions

## LV outflow tract obstruction

### Subvalvular aortic stenosis

- Obstruction of the left ventricular outflow tract below the aortic valve
- Association with a variety of other cardiac anomalies in two-thirds of patients: coarctation of the aorta, VSD

### Echocardiographic findings

- Four basic anatomic variants
  - Thin discrete endocardial fold and fibrous tissue (Fig. 13.2.1)
  - Fibromuscular ridge on the crest of the interventricular septum
  - Fibromuscular ring or collar attached to the base of the LVOT and AML
  - Diffuse fibromuscular tunnel-like narrowing of the LVOT and aortic annular hypoplasia
- LVOT obstruction secondary to accessory tissue
- Anomalous chordal attachment of the mitral valve

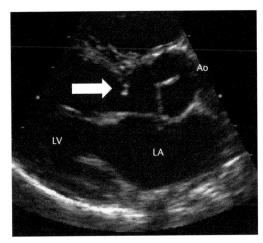

**Fig. 13.2.1** TTE PTLAX view of subvalvular aortic stenosis (arrow). LA = left atrium; LV = Left ventricle; Ao = aorta

## Supravalvular aortic stenosis

◆ Obstruction of the left ventricular outflow tract above the aortic valve

◆ Occurrence: sporadic, familial, Williams syndrome

◆ From localized (33%) to diffuse (15%) and symmetric to asymmetric

◆ Association with degenerative coronary artery disease and subvalvular left ventricular outflow tract obstruction (45%)

## Echocardiographic findings

Fibrous diaphragm

◆ The peak instantaneous pressure gradient across ≅ catheter-measured peak-to-peak gradient

◆ Hourglass deformity and diffuse hypoplasia (Fig. 13.2.2)

◆ The peak gradient measured by Doppler echocardiography > the peak-to-peak gradient measured by catheterization (pressure recovery)

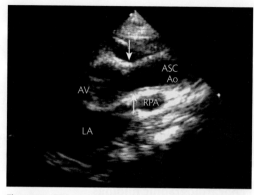

**Fig. 13.2.2** TTE parasternal LAX view of supravalvular hourglass type aortic stenosis (arrow). LA = left atrium; AV = aortic valve; ASC Ao = ascending aorta, RPA = right pulmonary artery

# Aortic stenosis (Box 13.2.1)

## Dysplastic/thickened valve leaflets and/or abnormal number of cusps

**Box 13.2.1   Aortic stenosis**

- ◆ The most common form of congenital heart disease
- ◆ Bicuspid valve (BAV) disease is the most frequent cause of aortic valve replacement in Europe
- ◆ Associated defects: left ventricle hypertrophy, dilated ascending aorta, coarctation of the aorta, Turner's syndrome, Williams syndrome

**Role of echo**

- ◆ Identify the valve abnormality
- ◆ In case of bicuspid valve, classify in subtype (Fig. 13.2.3ABC)
- ◆ Assess the severity of stenosis through Doppler quantification and planimetry (see aortic stenosis section)
- ◆ Review LV size, mass, and function
- ◆ Review for other potential congenital cardiac abnormalities (dilatation of the aorta, dissection of the aorta, coarctation of the aorta)
- ◆ 3D echo may be helpful

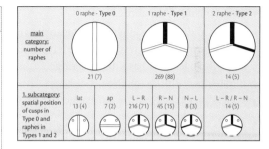

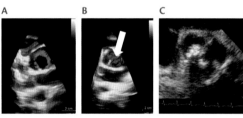

**Fig. 13.2.3**  Subtypes of BAV following Sievers classification; (A) Type 0; (B) Type I (arrow = raphe); (C) Type 2

# Aortic coarctation (Figs. 13.2.4–13.2.6, Boxes 13.2.2 and 13.2.3)

---

**Box 13.2.2** Aortic coarctation

- A narrowing of the aortic arch
- Almost always at the junction of the aortic arch and the descending aorta just below the left subclavian artery (in a left arch) as a discrete ridge
- Rarely more diffuse tubular hypoplasia
- Occasionally at the level of the abdominal aorta
- Adults may have well-developed collateral arterial supply making assessment of severity challenging

**Other potential associated features**

- Bicuspid aortic valve (very common)
- VSDs
- MV abnormalities
- Intracranial aneurysms

**Role of echo**

- Identify location, length, and nature of coarctation
- Where able, review supra-aortic arterial branches
- Assess the severity through Doppler quantification
- Review LV size, mass, and function
- Review RV size and function
- Review for other potential congenital cardiac abnormalities

---

### Box 13.2.3 Views

**TTE**

- **Best views:** for the descending thoracic aorta and branches are high parasternal, supraclavicular, or suprasternal long-axis positions (with and without colour)

- **Best views:** for the abdominal aorta subcostal (sagittal)

- **Transoesophageal echocardiogram** is of limited value

**Doppler assessment for aortic coarctation**

- Turbulent colour Doppler flow pattern at the site of coarctation helps define its location

- PW Doppler shows an increased velocity distal to the coarctation in descending aorta and blunted pulsatility with continuous flow on abdominal aortic Doppler

- CW Doppler defines the overall severity

- Characteristic Doppler trace = high-velocity systolic flow wave profile (peak pressure drop can be estimated) with continuous diastolic flow (diastolic tail)

- PW Doppler above the coarctation should be taken into account if it is above 1.0 m/s with the expanded Bernoulli equation used

Expanded Bernoulli equation = $4 \, (V2^2 - V1^2)$

- > 30 mmHg peak gradient across the descending aorta with a pan-diastolic tail supports a severe coarctation

- In extreme cases, the presence of large collaterals or a patent ductus will cause a reduced peak gradient

**N.B. CT or MRI give much better three-dimensional assessment pre- and post-coarctation intervention**

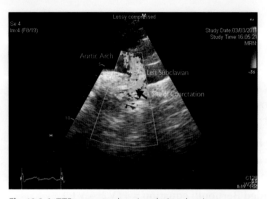

**Fig. 13.2.4** TTE suprasternal aortic arch view showing turbulent colour flow

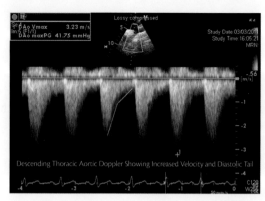

**Fig. 13.2.5** Descending thoracic aortic Doppler of a significant aortic coarctation

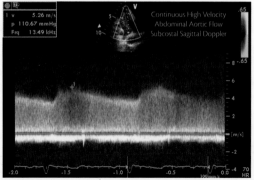

**Fig. 13.2.6** Abdominal aortic Doppler from a sagittal subcostal view showing loss of pulsatility in severe coarctation

# 13.3 Complex congenital lesions

## Segmental approach

### Position

- Left-sided: levocardia
- Right-sided: dextrocardia
- Mesocardia

### Orientation of the atria (Fig. 13.3.1)

- Situs solitus
- Situs inversus (thoracalis, abdominalis, totalis)
- Situs ambiguous
- Left atrial isomerism (associated with polysplenia)
- Right atrial isomerism (associated with asplenia)

### Aids to situs identification (Fig. 13.3.2)

- Position of the aorta and inferior vena cava at the diaphragm
- Bronchial morphology (position of the right bronchus)
- Atrial septal morphology: atrial strands
- Atrial appendage appearance
- Course of the descending aorta

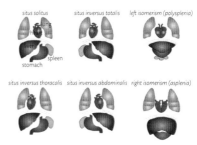

**Fig. 13.3.1** Schematic representation of orientation of atria

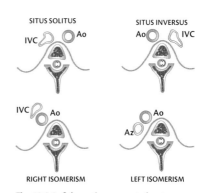

**Fig. 13.3.2** Schematic representation to facilitate situs identification

## Connection

### Atrioventricular connection

Concordance (left atrium to left ventricle, right atrium to right ventricle (Fig. 13.3.3A)

Discordance (left atrium to right ventricle, right atrium to left ventricle) (Fig. 13.3.3B)

Double inlet (two atria to one ventricle)

Single inlet (one atrium to one ventricle)

### Ventriculo-arterial connection

Concordance (left ventricle to aorta, right ventricle to pulmonary trunk)

Discordance (left ventricle to pulmonary trunk, right ventricle to aorta)

Single outlet (one ventricle to one great artery)

Double outlet (one ventricle to two great arteries) (Fig. 13.3.4)

## Orientation of the great vessels (aorta and pulmonary arteries)

Normal position (aorta posterior, pulmonary trunk anterior)

Transposition (aorta anterior, pulmonary trunk posterior) (Fig 13.3.5)

Malposition (left- or right-sided aorta arch)

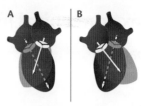

**Fig. 13.3.3** Schematic representation of atrio-ventricular connection

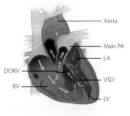

**Fig. 13.3.4** Schematic representation of ventriculo-arterial connection

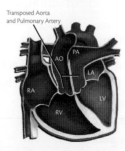

**Fig. 13.3.5** Schematic representation of transposition

# Tetralogy of Fallot (TOF) (Boxes 13.3.1A, 13.3.1B, 13.3.2A, 13.3.2B)

---

**Box 13.3.1A** Tetralogy of Fallot

**Four aspects** (Fig.13.3.6)

1. Anterior malalignment type VSD

2. RVOT obstruction (atresia at the extreme)

3. Rightward deviation of the aorta to override the two ventricles (and the VSD)

4. RV hypertrophy

**Other potential associated features**

◆ Right sided aortic arch

◆ ASD or PFO

◆ Atrioventricular septal defects

◆ Additional VSDs

◆ Abnormal coronary arterial anatomy

**Adult tetralogy palliated patients**

Palliated patients may have pulmonary hypertension, biventricular dysfunction, and sudden cardiac death

**The majority of patients seen as adults are repaired and the focus of this chapter is therefore on echocardiography aspects in the repaired Fallot population**

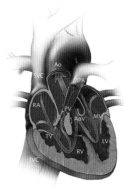

| RA. Right Atrium | SVC. Superior Vena Cava | TV. Tricuspid Valve |
| RV. Right Ventricle | IVC. Inferior Vena Cava | MV. Mitral Valve |
| LA. Left Atrium | MPA. Main Pulmonary Artery | PV. Pulmonary Valve |
| LV. Left Ventricle | Ao. Aorta | AoV. Aortic Valve |

**Fig. 13.3.6** Schematic representation of TOF

**Box 13.3.1B** Role of echo in repaired Fallot (Figs. 13.3.7–13.3.10)

- RV size and function and assessment for volume and pressure overload
- Assess RVOT for residual outflow stenosis and the level at which it occurs (infundibulum, valvar, main or branch pulmonary artery)
- Assessment of PR
- Review TV function and quantify TR (as well as estimate RV pressure)
- Exclude residual shunt (atrial or ventricular level)
- Assess LV size and function
- Review atrial size
- Assess aortic root size and AV function

**TTE best views**

- **RV size:** apical 4CV, parasternal views
- **RVOT:** PTLAX and PTSAX
- **PR:** PTLAX and PTSAX
- **TV:** apical 4CV, PTSAX
- **Residual ventricular shunt:** apical 5CV colour box subaortic, PTSAX with colour box over entire septum moving from basal to apical
- **Aortic root**—PTLAX (see sections on LV and RV function assessment)

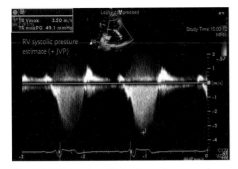

**Fig. 13.3.7** Estimation of RV end-systolic pressure from the TR jet – use the most aligned Doppler

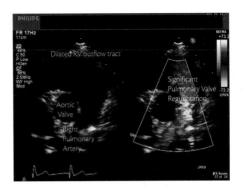

**Fig. 13.3.8** Parasternal short-axis showing reversal of flow extending from branch pulmonary arteries in diastole via the pulmonary valve

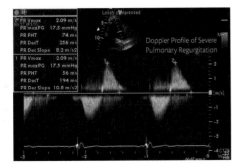

**Fig. 13.3.9** Assessment of PR severity from pressure half time

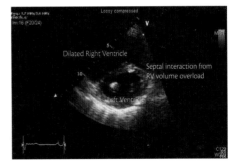

**Fig. 13.3.10** Parasternal SAX view of ventricles in patient with RV dilatation

**Box 13.3.2A  Role of TOE**

- If TTE views poor, or there is a specific question, e.g. TR or residual shunts
- Branch pulmonary arteries are generally poorly assessed with this
- **0°** Mid-oesophageal 4CV (RV and TV anatomy)
- **0°** High-oesophageal right pulmonary artery seen
- **30°–60°** Mid-oesophageal RV inflow and outflow
- **90°–130°** to assess the long axis of the PV and pulmonary artery bifurcation
- Transgastric **0°** clockwise for the RVOT

**Box 13.3.2B  Specific echo considerations in tetralogy**

**Aneurysmal and akinetic RVOT**

- Common following tetralogy repair
- It can impact significantly the RV size and global function assessment

**Features of severe PR**

- Broad laminar colour Doppler retrograde jet seen at or beyond the PV
- Dense CW Doppler signal
- Early PW spectral Doppler termination
- Paradoxical septal motion

**'Restrictive RV physiology'**

- Diastolic dysfunction may offer some protection from RV dilatation in tetralogy patients
- Antegrade flow on PV PW Doppler in late diastole throughout the respiratory cycle

# Ebstein's anomaly of the tricuspid valve (Boxes 13.3.3A, 13.3.3B, 13.3.4A, 13.3.4B)

**Box 13.3.3A** Findings (Fig. 13.3.11)

- Adherence of TV leaflets to underlying myocardium
- Downward or apical displacement of the functional annulus (septal the most, anterosuperior the least)
- Dilation of the 'atrialized' portion of the RV with variable wall hypertrophy and thinning
- Redundancy, fenestrations, and tethering of the anterosuperior leaflet
- Dilation of the right atrioventricular junction (the true annulus)

**Box 13.3.3B** Role of echo

- Assessment of TV morphology
- Does it fulfil the criteria for Ebstein's anomaly? (> 20 mm or > 8 mm/m$^2$ apically displaced functional annulus)
- Degree of valve dysfunction (stenosis/regurgitation)
- RA and RV size and function
- RV pressure
- Pulmonary valve and branch arterial anatomy and function
- Associated congenital cardiac abnormalities (majority have an ASD)
- Effect on left heart valves and function

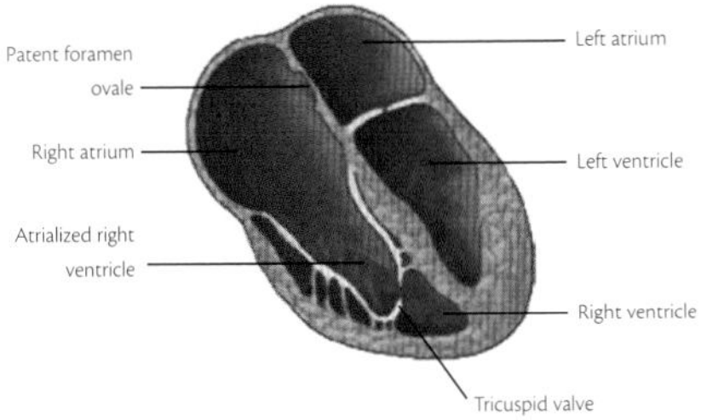

**Fig. 13.3.11** Schematic representation of Ebstein's anomaly

Patent foramen ovale
Right atrium
Atrialized right ventricle
Left atrium
Left ventricle
Right ventricle
Tricuspid valve

**Box 13.3.4A** Role of TTE and TOE

**Role of TTE** (Figs. 13.3.12 and 13.3.13)

- **Best views:** Apical 4CV for valve function and assessment of RV degree of atrialization and size compared to the left side, + LV outflow assessment

- Parasternal SAX—review of displacement of valve towards the RVOT, TV function, and PV and branch pulmonary artery flow and size (subcostal sagittal view where available, is also good for this)

- Parasternal LAX assessment of LVOT and of MV function

**Role of TOE** (Fig. 13.3.14)

- **Mid oesophagus 0°** 4CV for apical displacement and relative size of the RA and RV compared to the left

- **~30°–60°** SAX, keep rotating for a LAX from RA, to the RV outflow showing the morphology of the valve and distal attachments of the anterosuperior leaflet

- **~90°–130°** shows the PV and artery in long axis

- **N.B.** the TV should be assessed **0°–180°** to fully delineate the mechanism of dysfunction and severity

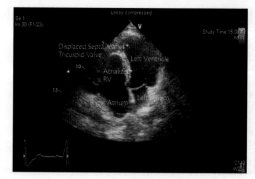

**Fig. 13.3.12** Apical 4CV of the AV valves showing displacement of TV septal leaflet attachment

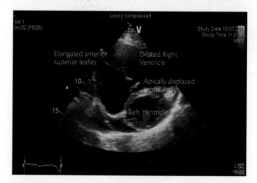

**Fig. 13.3.13** TTE parasternal SAX of the AV valves showing Ebstein's valve and right heart dilatation

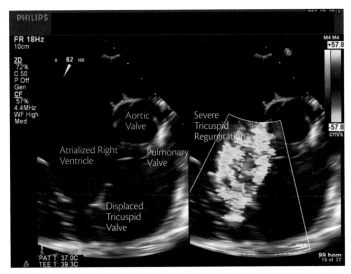

**Fig. 13.3.14** TOE view 60° of an Ebstein's TV

**Box 13.3.4B** Echo assessment post surgical intervention

Assessment for TV stenosis or regurgitation
LV and RV function
Assessment for elevated RV pressure
Residual RA and RV size over time
Other residual congenital defects and shunts

# CHAPTER 14

# Cardiac Source of Embolism (SOE) and Cardiac Masses

# Introduction

## Aetiology of SOE (Fig. 14.1)

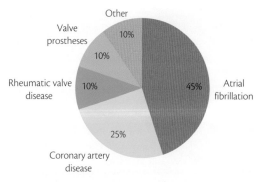

**Fig. 14.1** Principal causes of SOE

# 14.1 Atrial fibrillation (AF)

## TTE is clinically indicated in patients with AF

- To detect an underlying pathology affecting management or therapeutic decision (ischaemic heart disease, valvulopathy, cardiomyopathy or reduced ventricular function)
- Before cardioversion of atrial flutter (since this arrhythmia is often a marker of severe cardiac pathologies)
- To indicate, guide, and follow up invasive surgical procedures, such as substrate AF ablation (RF or surgical) or LAA closure

## The addition of TOE in patients with AF is indicated

- In guiding cardioversion in short-term anticoagulated patients
- In clinically selected cases (pre-ablation and closure LAA, suspect aortic arch atherosclerosis, repetitive embolism during correct anticoagulation)
- In determining the risk for future embolism (study of LAA function)

### TOE to guide cardioversion

**Abolishes the three weeks of pre-cardioversion anticoagulation in patients with no evidence of thrombi in the LA or in the LAA at TOE. This 'TOE-guided approach' is equally safe to the 'conventional approach' (oral anticoagulation for at least three weeks pre-cardioversion)**

◆ Echo findings

◆ **No thrombus at TOE** (Fig. 14.1.1): cardioversion is performed after few hours of anticoagulation and soon after TOE

◆ **Thrombus identified at TOE** (Fig. 14.1.2): oral anticoagulation is usually performed lifelong, cancelling the cardioversion because of the high thromboembolic risk (most often the TOE is repeated after at least three weeks of anticoagulation, before attempting the cardioversion)

## TOE to stratify the risk of embolism

◆ Left ventricular systolic dysfunction (EF < 35%)

◆ Complex aortic plaques

◆ LAA thrombi or SEC (spontaneous echo contrast) (Fig. 14.1.3)

◆ LAA dysfunction (emptying velocities < 25 cm/s) (Fig. 14.1.4)

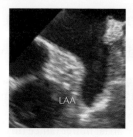

**Fig. 14.1.1** No thrombus at TOE

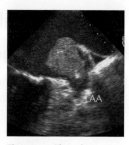

**Fig. 14.1.2** Thrombus identified at TOE

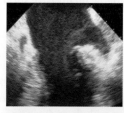

**Fig. 14.1.3** LAA thrombi or SEC

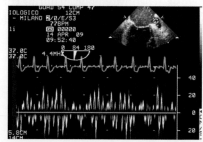

**Fig. 14.1.4** LAA dysfunction

# 14.2 Cardiac masses

## Cardiac tumours

### Secondary

6% of malignancies of various aetiologies (Fig. 14.2.1AB)

### Primary

(< 0.1% in adults) (Figs. 14.2.2–14.2.9)

- Benign (75% ) (Figs. 14.2.2–14.2.6, Box 14.2.1)
- Malignant (25%) (Figs. 14.2.7–14.2.9)

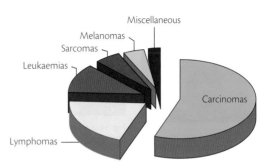

**Fig. 14.2.1A** Main aetiologies of metastasis to the heart

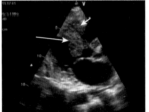

**Fig. 14.2.1B** PTLAX view illustrating multiple metastasis (arrows) from a melanoma

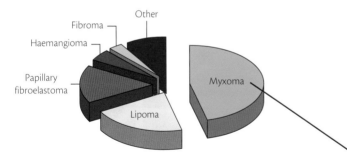

**Fig. 14.2.2** Main aetiologies of benign tumours

---

**Box 14.2.1  Cardiac tumours**

- Intracavitary
- Attachment site at the left side of atrial septum (80–85%)
- Rarely: RA > LV, RV, AV

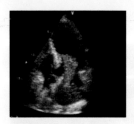

**Fig. 14.2.3** LA myxoma producing a functional mitral stenosis

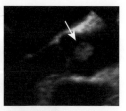

**Fig. 14.2.4** Ao valve fibroelastoma

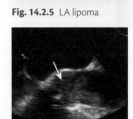

**Fig. 14.2.5** LA lipoma

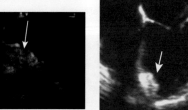

**Fig. 14.2.6** LV fibroma

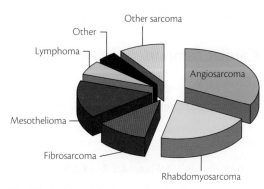

**Fig. 14.2.7** Main aetiologies of malignant tumours

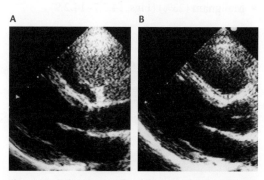

**Fig. 14.2.8** RV lymphoma before (A) and after (B) chemotherapy

**Fig. 14.2.9** Aortic synoviosarcoma

# Thrombus

## Atrial

- Left, usually at the level of LAA (contrast may be useful)
- Right, body of the RA (rarely) or in the RA appendage (generally as a consequence of AF). Distinguishing thrombi in the RA appendage from trabeculations is challenging (Fig. 14.2.10)
- Masses in transit arising from the lower limbs or pelvic veins are generally multilobulated, and freely mobile with a worm-like shape in the RA (Fig. 14.2.11)

## Ventricular

- Flat (mural) (Fig. 14.2.12), lying along the LV wall or protruding within the cavity (Fig. 14.2.13)
- Homogeneously echogenic, or present a heterogeneous texture often with central lucency
- The risk of peripheral emboli is higher in patients with larger thrombus size, protruding and mobile LV thrombi, and thrombi found in the older patients

## Paradoxical embolism

- Thrombus crossing the patent foramen ovale
- IV agitated saline serum to detect passage (TOE > TTE) + Valsalva (role as SOE debatable)

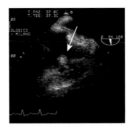

**Fig. 14.2.10** Thrombi in the RA appendage

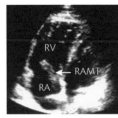

**Fig. 14.2.11** Masses in transit

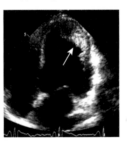

**Fig. 14.2.12** Ventricular flat

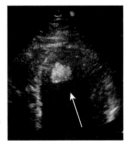

**Fig. 14.2.13** Ventricular protruding within the cavity

# Vegetation

## Endocarditis (Fig. 14.2.14)

Risk of embolism

- Related to vegetation size, and mobility
- High risk: large (> 10 mm) vegetations
- Particularly high with very mobile and large (> 15 mm) vegetations

## Strands or Lambl's excrescence (Fig. 14.2.15)

Role in embolism debatable

# Iatrogenic material

- Sewing stitches (Fig. 14.2.16)
- Catheter (+ thrombus) (Fig. 14.2.17AB)

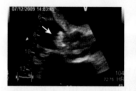

**Fig. 14.2.14** Aortic valve endocarditis

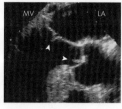

**Fig. 14.2.15** Aortic and mitral valve strands

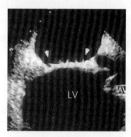

**Fig. 14.2.16** Iatrogenic material

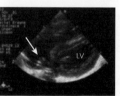

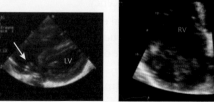

A  B

**Fig. 14.2.17** Catheter

# Extracardiac structure

♦ Hernia hiatalis (ingestion of sparkling water helpful) (Fig. 4.2.18AB)

# Normal variants (Figs. 14.2.19–14.2.26)

**A** 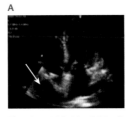 **B**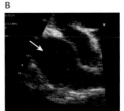

**Fig. 14.2.18AB** Hernia hiatalis

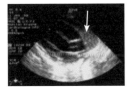

**Fig. 14.2.19** Thymus

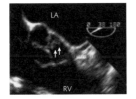

**Fig. 14.2.20** Tangential view of the aortic valve

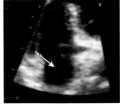

**Fig. 14.2.23** Chiari network

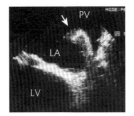

**Fig. 14.2.24** Junction left upper pulmonary vein—LAA

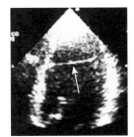

**Fig. 14.2.21** False tendon

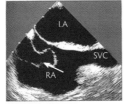

**Fig. 14.2.22** Eustachian valve

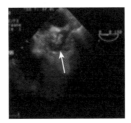

**Fig. 14.2.25** Transverse sinus

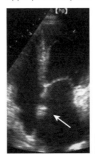

**Fig. 14.2.26** Stitching heart transplant

# Artefacts (Fig. 14.2.27)

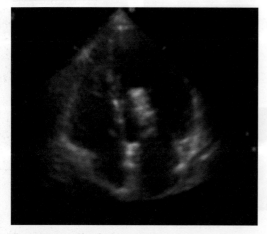

**Fig. 14.2.27** Artefact (motion parallel to other structure)

# 14.3 Differential diagnosis of LV/RV masses (Box 14.3.1)

---

**Box 14.3.1** Differential diagnosis of LV/RV masses

- ◆ Benign tumours
  - ◆ myxoma, lipoma
- ◆ Malignant tumours
  - ◆ vena caval extension of hypernephroma, hepatoma, sarcoma
- ◆ Thrombi
  - ◆ in situ or extension through vena cava
- ◆ Normal variants
- ◆ Iatrogenic masses
  - ◆ indwelling catheter, PM wires, embolized vena caval umbrella
- ◆ Others
  - ◆ artefacts, reverberations from mechanical TV prosthesis

---

# 14.4 Differential diagnosis of valvular masses (Box 14.3.2)

---

**Box 14.3.2** Differential diagnosis of valvular masses

- Benign tumours
  - myxoma
- Malignant tumours
  - sarcoma, pulmonary venous extension, bronchogenic and mediastinal tumours
- Thrombi
  - in situ or paradoxical (ASD or PFO)
- Normal variants
- Iatrogenic masses
- Others
  - artefacts, reverberations from mechanical MV prosthesis

---

# Suggested reading

1. Sherman DG. Cardiac embolism: the neurologist's perpective. *Am J Cardiol* 1990;65:32C–37C.

2. Yuan SM, Shinfeld A, Lavee J, et al. Imaging morphology of cardiac tumours. *Cardiol J* 2009;16:26–35.

3. Wann LS, Sampson C, Liu Y. Cardiac and paracardiac masses: Complementary role of echocardiography and magnetic resonance imaging. *Echocardiography* 1998;15:139–46.

# CHAPTER 15

# Diseases of the Aorta

# Introduction

- Evaluation of the aorta is a routine part of the standard echocardiographic examination. The major advantages include its portability, rapid imaging time, and lack of radiation

- TTE is an excellent modality for imaging the aortic root and is important in the serial measurement of maximum aortic root diameters, aortic regurgitation evaluation, and timing of elective surgery for several entities such as annuloaortic ectasia, Marfan syndrome, and bicuspid aortic valve

- TOE provides a good visualization of the entire thoracic aorta, with the exception of the distal part of the ascending aorta. The descending aorta is easily visualized in short-axis and long-axis views from the coeliac trunk to the left subclavian artery. Further withdrawal of the probe shows the aortic arch. TOE is safe and can be performed at the bedside, with a low risk of complications

- Intra-operative TOE is essential for planning the surgical treatment of acute aortic syndromes (AAS), in deciding whether to replace the aortic valve and for guiding thoracic endovascular therapy

# 15.1 Acute aortic syndromes (AAS)

**AAS is an acute process of the aortic wall that implies its weakening, leading to an increased risk of aortic rupture or other complications**

## Classification (entities) (Table 15.1.1, Box 15.1.1)

**Classical aortic dissection (AD):** separation of the aorta media with presence of extraluminal blood within the layers of the aortic wall. The intimal flap divides the aorta into two lumina, the true and the false (Fig. 15.1.1)

**Intramural haematoma (IMH):** aortic wall haematoma with no entry tear and no two-lumen flow

**Penetrating aortic ulcer (PAU):** atherosclerotic lesion penetrates the internal elastic lamina of the aorta wall

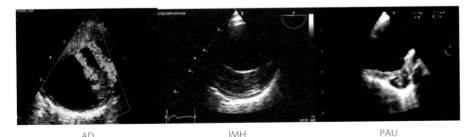

AD                          IMH                          PAU

**Fig. 15.1.1** Aortic dissection (AD), intramural haematoma (IMH), and penetrating aortic ulcer (PAU) by transoesophageal echocardiography (TOE)

**Table 15.1.1** Classification: extension of involvement (Fig. 15.1.2)

| | DeBakey | Stanford |
|---|---|---|
| Involving ascending aorta (AA) | I: originates in the AA and includes at least the aortic arch and typically the descending aorta (60%) | |
| | II: originates in and is confined to the AA (10%) | A |
| Involving descending aorta (DA) | III: originates in and is confined to the DA | B |

---

**Box 15.1.1  Classification**

Time course from presentation

◆ Acute: ≤ 14 days

◆ Sub acute: 15–90 days

◆ Chronic: > 90 days

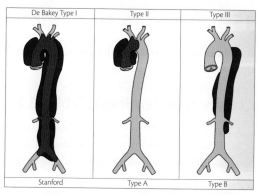

**Fig. 15.1.2**  The most common classification systems of thoracic aortic dissection: Stanford and DeBakey, Nienaber CA, and Eagle (Table 15.1.1)

# Diagnostic findings (Table 15.1.2)

**Table 15.1.2** Diagnostic findings

| Diagnosis | Secondary findings | Complications |
|---|---|---|
| AD: presence of intimal flap dividing aorta into true and false lumina* | ◆ Entry tear site/re-entry site<br>◆ Secondary communications | ◆ Acute aortic regurgitation<br>◆ Arterial vessel involvement/visceral ischaemia<br>  ◆ coronary arteries<br>  ◆ major branches<br>◆ Pericardial effusion<br>◆ Aortic rupture (pericardial/pleural effusion, mediastinal haematoma) |
| IMH: thickening of the aortic wall >5 mm in a crescentic or concentric pattern | ◆ Curvilinear and smooth luminal wall, as opposed to a rough, irregular border in atherosclerosis and PAU<br>◆ Central displacement of intimal calcium<br>◆ Echo-lucent regions may be present | ◆ Fusiform or saccular dilation<br>◆ Localized dissection (ulcer-like projections)<br>◆ Classical dissection<br>◆ Aortic rupture (pericardial/pleural effusion, mediastinal haematoma) |
| PAU: atherosclerotic lesion outpouching in the aortic wall | PAUs can only be detected when they protrude outside the contour of the aortic lumen | ◆ Intramural haemorrhage surrounding PAU<br>◆ Aortic rupture (pericardial/pleural effusion, mediastinal haematoma) |

* The echocardiographic diagnosis of classical aortic dissection is based on the demonstration of the presence of an **intimal flap** that divides the aorta into two, **true and false**, lumina. In most cases, false lumen flow is detectable by colour Doppler but may be absent in totally thrombosed and retrograde dissections

# Role of transthoracic echocardiography (TTE)

◆ Good initial imaging modality for diagnosing **proximal AD** (mainly aortic root)

◆ **Harmonic imaging** and **contrast agents** improve diagnostic sensitivity and specificity mainly in AA, arch, proximal descending aorta and abdominal aorta. Although TTE has intermediate sensitivity for AD (> 80%) and high specificity (> 90%), AAS cannot be completely ruled out

## Advantages

◆ Superior to CT and MRI in
  ◆ acute aortic regurgitation
  ◆ pericardial tamponade
  ◆ LV function/abnormal segmental wall contractility

## Disadvantages

◆ Poor ultrasonic window
◆ Limited visualization of several aortic segments
◆ Limited in IMH and PAU diagnosis

## TTE examination for AD includes the evaluation of: (Figs. 15.1.3 and 15.1.4AB)

◆ AA from the standard and high parasternal windows

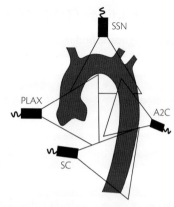

**Fig. 15.1.3** TTE approach for the evaluation of aorta: various TTE projections should be used in order to visualize the different aortic segments. SSN: suprasternal notch; PTLAX: parasternal long-axis; A2C: apical two-chambers; SC: subcostal

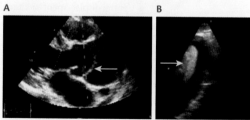

**Fig. 15.1.4** A: Parasternal long-axis TTE visualizing the intimal flap (arrow) in a type A of aortic dissection (AD) B: Contrast TTE by suprasternal view diagnoses a type B AD. Early contrast filling of the true lumen (arrow)

- Aortic arch and proximal descending aorta from the suprasternal window
- Distal descending thoracic aorta from parasternal and apical windows
- Proximal abdominal aorta from a subcostal approach

## Role of transoesophageal echocardiography (TOE)

- **AA, aortic root and aortic valve, best visualized at high TOE long-axis (120–150°) and short-axis (30–60°) views**
- **Descending aorta: best visualized in short-axis (0°) and long-axis (90°) views from the coeliac trunk to the left subclavian artery**

### Pitfalls

- 'Blind spot': short segment of distal AA, just before innominate artery (interposition of the right bronchus and trachea)
- Reverberations from the aortic or right pulmonary artery walls in the aortic root and AA. Location and movement assessment by M-mode permits correct identification. Other reverberations or artefacts: catheters, atherosclerotic plaques, or calcium shadow
- Total FL thrombosis vs IMH vs aneurysm with mural thrombus

### Features of AD on TOE

- A dissection flap that appears as a bright, linear echogenic structure in the aortic lumen with erratic motion compared with normal systolic pulsations (Fig. 15.1.5)

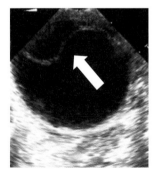

**Fig. 15.1.5** TOE illustration of AD with the dissection flap (arrow)

◆ Colour Doppler evidence of blood flow in both the true (bounded by endothelium) and false (bounded by media) lumen (Tables 15.1.3, 15.1.4)

**Table 15.1.3** Communications between true and false lumina

| Type of communication | Blood flow pattern |
|---|---|
| Entry site | From the true towards the false channel TL → FL |
| Re-entry site | Flow re-enters the true from the false lumen. May occur alone or at multiple sites TL ← FL |
| Secondary communications | Communication between true and false lumina with bidirectional flow. Mainly TL to FL in systole and FL to TL in diastole. Several TL ↔ FL patterns |

**Table 15.1.4** Differentiation between true and false lumina

| | True lumen | False lumen |
|---|---|---|
| **Size** | Most often: true < false | Most often: false > true |
| **Pulsation** | Systolic expansion | Systolic compression |
| **Flow direction** | Systolic anterograde flow | Systolic anterograde flow: <br> ◆ reduced or absent, or <br> ◆ retrograde flow |
| **Communication flow** | From true to false lumen | – |
| **Contrast echo flow** | Early and fast | Delayed and slow (even spontaneous echo contrast or partial thrombosis) |

**Colour Doppler** can reveal the presence of multiple small communications between the two lumina

- The entry site into the false lumen
- Secondary communications between the two lumina
- Thrombosis of the false lumen

## Complications of AD (Fig. 15.1.6AB)

- **Acute aortic regurgitation (AR)** mechanisms and severity (Table 15.1.5)
- **Pericardial effusion/tamponade**
- **Aortic rupture:** other indirect signs are better defined by CT: pleural effusion, pseudoaneurysm, mediastinal haematoma
- **Arterial branch involvement:** dissection vs compression
  - coronary arteries: direct flap visualization (TOE)/regional wall-motion abnormalities (TTE/TOE)
  - other major branch involvement: direct flap visualization, assessment of blood flow pattern of left subclavian artery and coeliac trunk by TOE, and brachiocephalic trunk and left carotid artery by TTE

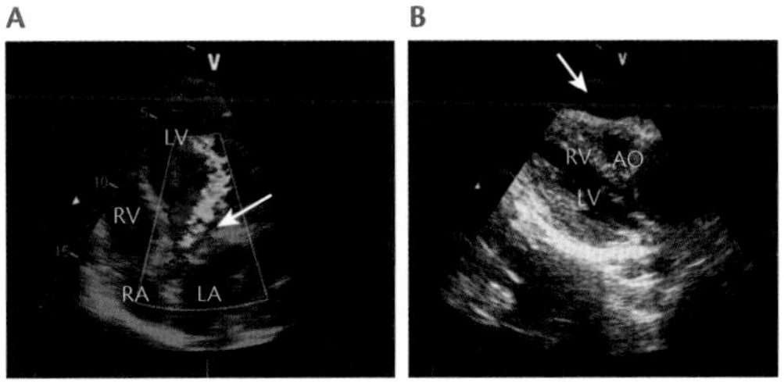

**Fig. 15.1.6** AD complications diagnosed by TTE:
A: Apical 5CV with colour-flow Doppler that shows a diastolic jet (arrow) reaching the left ventricular apex due to an acute and severe aortic regurgitation
B: Parasternal long-axis view showing a severe pericardial effusion (arrow) that compresses right ventricle. Dilated aortic root is also evident in this projection
LV: left ventricle; RV: right ventricle; RA: right atrium; LA: left atrium; Ao: aorta

**Table 15.1.5** Related to dissection

| | Annulus dilation secondary to AA dilation (incomplete leaflet closure) |
|---|---|
| **Previous valvular abnormalities** | Leaflet prolapse secondary to extending dissection into the aortic root |
| | Prolapse of dissected intima through structurally normal leaflets |
| | Aortic valve sclerosis/calcification, bicuspid aortic valve |

## Imaging approach when acute AD is suspected (Fig. 15.1.7)

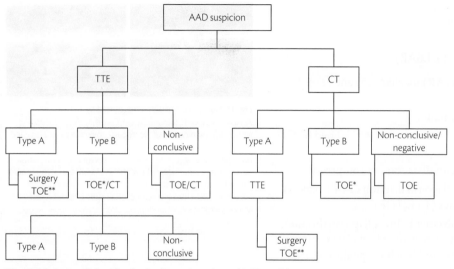

**Fig. 15.1.7** Proposed algorithm for the diagnostic work-up of AAD suspicion

♦ *Definitive diagnosis of type A AD by TTE to indicate surgical treatment whenever intra-operative TOE is performed in the operating theatre

♦ **Definitive diagnosis of type A dissection by TTE permits the patient to be sent directly to surgery. Intra-operative TOE will be performed before surgery

TTE: transthoracic echocardiogram; TOE: transoesophageal echocardiogram; CT: computed tomography

## Intramural haematoma

Considered to be a variant of aortic dissection, accounts for 10–15% of AAS

**Pathogenesis:** from vasa vasorum rupture, small intimal tears, PAU, or trauma

**Echo findings** (Fig. 15.1.8)

- Eccentric, crescent-shaped or circular thickening of the aortic wall (≥ 5 mm) extending longitudinally
- Absence of dissection flap
- Preserved aortic lumen without evidence of flow in the thickened aortic wall

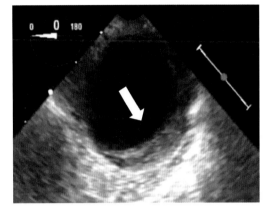

**Fig. 15.1.8** TOE illustration of intramural haematoma (arrow)

### Differential diagnosis

- Classical aortic dissection with thrombosed false lumen
- Atherosclerosis, aortitis
- Aortic aneurysm with mural thrombus
- Hemiazygos sheath (fat-pad)
- Ulcer-like projection (ULP) secondary to focal intimal disruption during IMH evolution vs PAU. Generally, PAU is defined by an atherosclerotic plaque with jagged edges, multiple irregularities in the intimal layer, and may be accompanied by localized IMH

# Follow-up of AAS echo findings

◆ Patent false lumen with persisting intimal flap (entry site dimension) and false lumen features (flow/thrombosis)

◆ Progression of the disease: false lumen enlargement, dilatation/dissection non-contiguous/non-operated aortic segments

◆ Post-operative complications
  ◆ residual aortic regurgitation
  ◆ pseudoaneurysm formation (graft tube dehiscence or at coronary artery reimplantation level after Bentall procedure) (Fig. 15.1.9)

◆ IMH evolution to reabsorption, fusiform or saccular aneurysm, localized dissection (ULP) or classical dissection

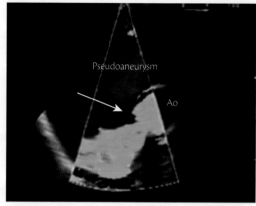

**Fig. 15.1.9** Large pseudoaneurysm formation at the suture-site after right-coronary reimplantation using the coronary button technique in a Bentall´s procedure diagnosed by TOE in short-axis (0°) view. The turbulent jet by colour Doppler represents the flow from the endograft tube implanted in ascending aorta to the large pseudoaneurysm through the ruptured coronary button

# 15.2  Thoracic aortic aneurysm (AA)

Significant aortic dilatation which contains all three aortic wall layers with an enlargement exceeding 1.5 times the expected aortic diameter according to the individual's age and body surface area

## Aetiology and most frequent AA morphology

- **Degenerative**: related to the ageing process (high blood pressure and atherosclerosis favour medial degeneration). Enlargement in tubular AA
- **Marfan syndrome, other inherited connective tissue disorders** (Loeys–Dietz, Ehler–Danlos), **idiopathic** (annuloaortic ectasia). Pyriform appearance of aortic root
- **Other inherited disorders**: Turner syndrome, Noonan syndrome, osteogenesis imperfecta
- **Bicuspid aortic valve**: Tubular AA with/without aortic root dilatation
- **Syphilis** (tertiary stage): characteristic calcification pattern
- **Non-infectious aortitis** (giant-cell, Takayasu's syndrome)

## Location and morphology

- Thoracic aneurysms are six times less frequent than abdominal aneurysms
- Thoracic aneurysms are classified according to their location: AA (50%), aortic arch (10%) and descending aorta (40%)
- One or more aortic segments can be affected (15% multiple)
- Morphology: tubular/saccular, symmetric/asymmetric

# Echo assessment

- TTE aortic measurements are taken on 2D (leading-edge-to-leading edge) in end-diastolic frame
- Absolute values/normograms/indexed measurements per body surface area (Table 15.2.1, Fig. 15.2.1)

**Table 15.2.1** Upper-limit of normality for aortic root dimensions in adults (20–74 y)

| Aortic level | MEN | | WOMEN | |
|---|---|---|---|---|
| | Absolute (mm) | Indexed (mm/m²) | Absolute (mm) | Indexed (mm/m²) |
| Aortic annulus | 31 | 16 | 26 | 16 |
| Sinus of Valsalva | 40 | 21 | 36 | 21 |
| Sinotubular junction | 36 | 19 | 32 | 19 |

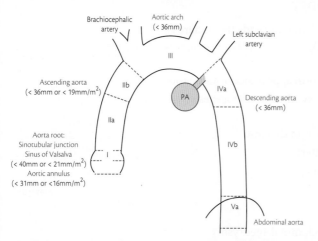

**Fig. 15.2.1** Schematic representation of thoracic aorta illustrating its segmentation. Upper limits of normal dimensions for the different segments are given. PA: pulmonary artery

# Different types and localization of aortic aneurysms (Fig. 15.2.2ABC, Box 15.2.1)

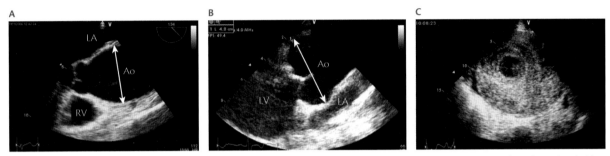

A                                    B                                    C

**Fig. 15.2.2** A: TOE long-axis view (120°) of the aortic root and tubular ascending aorta in a patient with ascending aorta aneurysm (arrow) associated with a bicuspid aortic valve. B: TTE parasternal long-axis view in a patient with Marfan syndrome and aortic root aneurysm (arrow). C: Abdominal view that shows a large, partially thrombosed atherosclerotic abdominal aneurysm. LA: left atrium; Ao: aorta; RV: right ventricle; LV: left ventricle

**Box 15.2.1** Assessment

Post-operative assessment (risk of dilation of the remaining aorta) is mandatory during follow-up (Table 15.2.2)

**Table 15.2.2**  AA follow-up and surgical timing

| Diameter | Ascending aorta | Aortic arch and descending aorta | Abdominal aorta |
|---|---|---|---|
| > 60 mm | | General indication | |
| > 55 mm | ◆ General indication<br>◆ BAV without risk factors | ◆ Aneurysms suitable for TEVAR<br>◆ Aortic expansion rate ≥ 5 mm/year | General indication |
| > 50 mm | ◆ Marfan syndrome and other genetic disorders<br>◆ BAV with risk factors*<br>◆ TAV with more than mild AR<br>◆ Aortic expansion rate ≥ 5 mm/year | | |
| > 45 mm | ◆ Marfan syndrome with risk factors**<br>◆ Aortic valve surgery indicated (BAV)<br>◆ Pregnancy desire | | |
| > 40 mm | ◆ Loeys–Dietz syndrome with family history of aortic dissection (lower level of evidence) | | |

BAV: bicuspid aortic valve; TEVAR: thoracic endovascular aortic repair; TAV: tricuspid aortic valve

* Aortic dissection/rupture in first-degree relatives; aortic coarctation; aortic expansion rate ≥ 5 mm/year; high blood pressure

**Aortic dissection/rupture in first-degree relatives; ratio aortic diameter: body surface area > 27.5 mm/m$^2$; aortic expansion rate ≥ 5 mm/year

# 15.3 Traumatic injury of the aorta

## Aetiology

- **Blunt chest trauma** (aortic rupture, complete transection—may be contained by surrounding tissues, pseudoaneurysm, aortic dissection, intramural haematoma)
- **Laceration of the aortic wall** (usually horizontal, small (limited)/large (circumferential), extend outward from the intima)
- **Iatrogenic trauma** (cardiac catheterization, angioplasty of aortic coarctation, cardiac surgery—cross-clamping of the aorta, intra-aortic balloon pump)

## Location

- Usually just distal to left subclavian artery origin at ligamentum arteriosum (50–70%)
- Other vulnerable sites: origin of the right brachiocephalic artery (particularly with vertical forces from falls), ascending aorta above SV
- Frequently, proximal thoracic aorta (18%)

## Diagnosis (echo findings)

- Localized AD often limited to a few centimetres
- IMH (without apparent intimal discontinuity)
- False aneurysm with/without mediastinal haematoma

# Role of TOE

- Safe and highly sensitive
- Contraindicated with unstable injuries of the cervical spine or in the setting of suspected oesophageal injury
- Mainly applied in the operating room and during the intensive care unit course, where it can be performed serially if necessary

# 15.4 Aortic atherosclerosis

- TTE from a suprasternal view is not adequate for reliable detection or characterization of plaque
- Risk of embolization
- Marker of atherosclerotic disease (**TOE findings:** Table 15.4.1, Fig. 15.4.1ABCD)

**Table 15.4.1** Grading based on thickness, mobile components, and ulceration

| Grade | Severity | Description |
|-------|----------|-------------|
| I | Normal | No or minimal intimal thickening |
| II | Mild | Intimal thickening 1–3.9 mm without atheroma |
| III | Moderate | Sessile atheroma < 4 mm |
| IV | Severe | Intimal thickening or atheroma > 4 mm |
| V | Severe | Ulcerated or mobile atheroma |

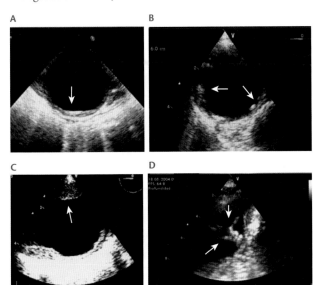

**Fig. 15.4.1** TOE visualization aorta with different grades of atheromas (arrows). A: Mild atheroma (grade II); B: Moderate atheroma (grade III); C: Severe atheroma (grade IV); D: Severe atheroma (> 4 mm) with mobile component (grade V)

## 15.5 Sinus of Valsalva aneurysm

### Aetiology

**Congenital or iatrogenic (during procedures, i.e. ablation or aortic valve replacement)**

### Echo findings

- Dilation located in one sinus of Valsalva: round or finger-like (windsock) aneurysm
- Size: measurement from one to contralateral cusp in end-diastole

### Complication

Rupture, secondary aortic regurgitation

- Right coronary cusp rupture—communication with right ventricle or right atrium
- Non-coronary cusp rupture—communication with left atrium
- Echo findings of ruptured sinus of Valsalva (Fig. 15.5.1ABC)
  - Colour Doppler: jet flow through pathological communication
  - Continuous-wave Doppler with continuous systo-diastolic flow
  - Right ventricular dilation volume overload

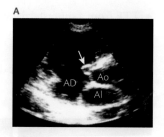

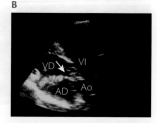

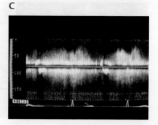

**Fig. 15.5.1** A: SAX view showing aneurysm or right-coronary sinus of Valsalva aneurysm (arrow); B: apical 5CV with colour-flow Doppler. The turbulent jet (arrow) represents left to right shunt from a ruptured right coronary sinus of Valsalva aneurysm to RV; C: continous-wave Doppler spectral signal that shows a continuous systo-diastolic flow from ascending aorta to the RV through a ruptured sinus of Valsalva aneurysm

# Suggested reading

1. Evangelista A, Flachskampf FA, Erbel R, et al. Echocardiography in aortic diseases: EAE recommendations for clinical practice. *Eur J Echocardiogr* 2010;11:645–58.

2. Pepi M, Campodonico J, Galli C, et al. Rapid diagnosis and management of thoracic aortic dissection and intramural haematoma: a prospective study of advantages of multiplane vs. biplane transoesophageal echocardiography. *Eur J Echocardiogr* 2000;1:72–9.

3. Evangelista A, Avegliano G, Aguilar R, et al. Impact of contrast-enhanced echocardiography on the diagnostic algorithm of acute aortic dissection. *Eur Heart J* 2010;31:472–79.

# CHAPTER 16

# Stress Echocardiography

# 16.1 Stress echocardiography

## Indications

Indications for stress echocardiography—grouped in very broad categories to encompass the overwhelming majority of patients:

* Coronary artery disease diagnosis
* Prognosis and risk stratification in patients with established diagnosis (for example, after myocardial infarction)
* Pre-operative risk assessment
* Evaluation for cardiac aetiology of exertional dyspnoea
* Evaluation after revascularization
* Ischaemia location
* Evaluation of heart valve stenosis severity

<u>As a rule</u>, the less informative the exercise ECG test is, the stricter the indication for stress echocardiography will be

## The main specific indications for stress echocardiography

* Patients in whom the exercise stress test is contraindicated (i.e. patients with severe arterial hypertension)
* Patients in whom the exercise stress test is not feasible (i.e. those with intermittent claudication)
* Patients in whom the exercise stress test was non-diagnostic or yielded ambiguous results

- ◆ LBBB or significant resting ECG changes that makes any ECG interpretation during stress difficult
- ◆ Sub-maximal stress ECG
- ◆ Pharmacological stress echocardiography is the choice for patients in whom exercise is unfeasible or contraindicated

## Contraindications

A poor acoustic window makes any form of stress echocardiography unfeasible to perform. This limitation of stress echocardiography today should not exceed 5% of all referrals (harmonic imaging, intravenous left ventricular opacification)

### Exercise

- ◆ Unstable haemodynamic conditions
- ◆ Uncontrolled hypertension
- ◆ Inability to exercise adequately
- ◆ Difficult resting echocardiogram

### Dobutamine

- ◆ A history of complex atrial (paroxysmal AF, paroxysmal supraventricular tachycardia) or ventricular arrhythmias (sustained ventricular tachycardia or ventricular fibrillation)
- ◆ Moderate to severe hypertension (should be referred for safer vasodilator stress)

## Dipyridamole

- ◆ Patients with second- or third-degree atrioventricular block, sick sinus syndrome, bronchial asthma or a tendency to bronchospasm should not receive dipyridamole
- ◆ Patients using dipyridamole chronically should not undergo adenosine testing for at least 24 h after withdrawal of therapy, since their blood levels of adenosine could be unpredictably high

# Echo views for LV wall motion assessment

Analysis and scoring of the study are usually performed using a 16- or 17- segment model of the left ventricle and a four-grade scale of regional wall motion analysis (Fig. 16.1.1)

Regional wall motion is semi-quantitatively graded from 1 to 4 as follows

- ◆ 1 = normal; 2 = hypokinetic; 3 = akinetic; 4 = dyskinetic
- ◆ WMSI is the sum of individual segment scores divided by the number of interpretable segments

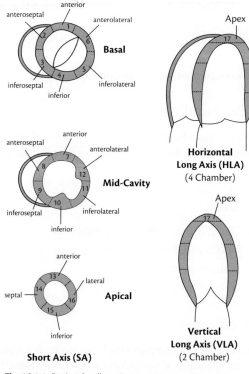

**Fig. 16.1.1** Regional wall motion assessment

# Left ventricular segmentation (Fig. 16.1.2)

A circumferential polar plot display of the 16, 17, or 18 myocardial segments and the recommended nomenclature for tomographic imaging of the heart

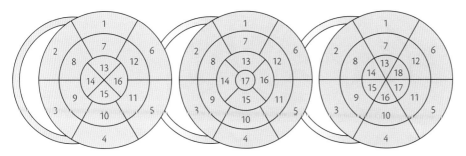

**all models**
1. basal anterior
2. basal anteroseptal
3. basal inferoseptal
4. basal inferior
5. basal inferolateral
6. basal anterolateral
7. mid anterior
8. mid anteroseptal
9. mid inferoseptal
10. mid inferior
11. mid inferolateral
12. mid anterolateral

**16 and 17 segment model**
13. apical anterior
14. apical septal
15. apical inferior
16. apical lateral

**17 segment model only**
17. apex

**18 segment model only**
13. apical anterior
14. apical anteroseptal
15. apical inferoseptal
16. apical inferior
17. apical inferolateral
18. apical anterolateral

**alternatively, walls are commonly labelled as:**
3. , 9. , 15(18-seg). : septal;    5. , 11. , 17(18-seg). : posterior;    6. ,12. ,18(18-seg). : lateral

**Fig. 16.1.2**  Polar plot display: schematic diagram of the different LV segmentation models

# Coronary artery territories and myocardial segmentation (Fig. 16.1.3)

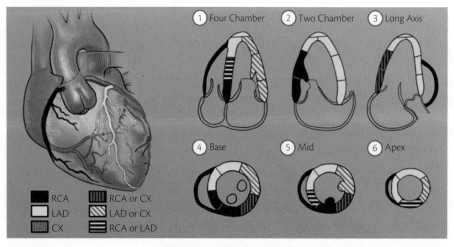

**Fig. 16.1.3** A schematic representation of the perfusion territories of the three major coronary arteries

♦ Assignment of the myocardial segments to the territories of the left anterior descending (LAD), right coronary artery (RCA), and the left circumflex coronary artery (LCX)

## Stress types (general test protocol: 1)

- A 12-lead ECG is recorded in resting condition and each minute throughout the examination. An ECG lead is also continuously displayed on the echo monitor to provide the operator with a reference for ST segment changes and arrhythmias
- Cuff blood pressure is measured in resting condition and each stage thereafter
- Echocardiographic imaging is typically performed from the parasternal long- and short-axis, apical long-axis, and apical four- and two-chamber views. In some cases the sub-xyphoidal and apical long-axis views are used
- Images are recorded in resting condition from all views and captured digitally. A quad-screen format is used for comparative analysis
- Echocardiography is then continuously monitored and intermittently stored
- In the presence of obvious or suspected dyssynergy, a complete echo examination is performed and recorded from all employed approaches to allow optimal documentation of the presence and extent of myocardial ischaemia

## Stress types (general test protocol: 2)

- It is critical to obtain the same views at each stage of the test
- These same projections are obtained and recorded during the recovery phase, after cessation of stress (exercise or pacing), or administration of the antidote (aminophylline for dipyridamole, beta-blocker for dobutamine, nitroglycerine for ergometrine) an ischaemic response may occasionally occur late, after cessation of drug infusion

- The transiently dyssynergic area during stress can be evaluated by a triple comparison: stress versus resting state; stress versus recovery phase; at peak stress
- Pharmacological stress tests should always be performed with an attending physician. Every test carries a definite, albeit minor risk
- Contrast for endocardial border enhancement, which should be used whenever there are suboptimal resting or peak stress images. Intravenous contrast for LV opacification improves endocardial border definition and may salvage an otherwise suboptimal study

## Exercise vs pharmacological stress echo (Table 16.1.1)

**Table 16.1.1** Instructions for use

| Parameter | Exercise | Pharmacological |
|---|---|---|
| Intravenous line required | | ✓ |
| Diagnostic utility of heart rate and blood pressure response | ✓ | |
| Use in deconditioned patients | | ✓ |
| Use in physically limited patients | | ✓ |
| Level of echocardiography imaging difficulty | High | Low |
| Safety profile | High | Moderate |
| Clinical role in valvular heart disease | ✓ | |
| Clinical role in pulmonary hypertension | ✓ | |
| Fatigue and dyspnoea evaluation | ✓ | |

# Reasons for test termination

1. **Submaximal non-diagnostic end points**

   - Non-tolerable symptoms (severe chest pain)
   - Hypertension, with systolic blood pressure >220 mmHg or diastolic blood pressure >120 mmHg
   - Symptomatic hypotension, with >40 mmHg drop in blood pressure
   - Supraventricular arrhythmias, such as supraventricular tachycardia or atrial fibrillations
   - Complex ventricular arrhythmias, such as ventricular tachycardia or frequent, polymorphic premature ventricular beats
   - Electrocardiographic positivity (>2 mV ST-segment shift) not associated with wall motion abnormalities

2. **Diagnostic end points**

   - Maximum workload (for exercise testing)
   - Maximum dose (for pharmacological)
   - Achievement of target heart rate for dobutamine and exercise
   - Echocardiographic positivity (dyssynergy ≥ 2 LV segments)

# Types of stress echocardiography responses
## (Fig. 16.1.4, Tables 16.1.2, 16.1.3)

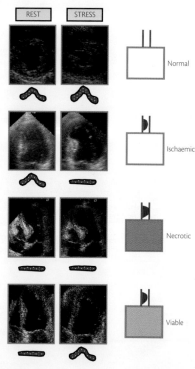

**Fig. 16.1.4** Echocardiographic examples of normal (upper row), ischaemic (second row), necrotic (third row), and viable (fourth row) response

**Normal response:** A segment is normokinetic at rest and normal or hyperkinetic during stress

**Ischaemic response**: The function of a segment worsens during stress from normokinesia to hypokinesia (decrease of endocardial movement and systolic thickening), akinesia (absence of endocardial movement and systolic thickening), or dyskinesia (paradoxical outward movement and possible systolic thinning). However, a resting akinesia becoming dyskinesia during stress reflects purely passive phenomenon of increased intraventricular pressure developed by normally contracting walls and should not be considered a true active ischaemia

**Necrotic response**: A segment with resting dysfunction remains fixed during stress

**Viability response**: A segment with resting dysfunction may show either a sustained improvement during stress indicating a nonjeopardized myocardium (stunned), or improve during early stress with subsequent deterioration at peak (biphasic response). The biphasic response is suggestive of viability and ischaemia, with jeopardized myocardium fed by a critically coronary stenosis

**Table 16.1.2** Stress echocardiography in four equations

| Rest | + | Stress | = | Diagnosis |
|------|---|--------|---|-----------|
| Normokinesis | + | Normohyperkinesis | = | Normal |
| Normokinesis | + | Hypo, A-, dyskinesis | = | Ischaemia |
| Akinesis | + | Hypo, normokinesis | = | Viable |
| A-, dyskinesis | + | A-, dyskinaesis | = | Necrosis |

**Table 16.1.3** Stress echo protocols

| Test | Equipment | Protocols |
|------|-----------|-----------|
| Exercise | Semi-supine bicycle ergometer | 25 W × 2′ with incremental loading |
| Dobutamine | Infusion pump | 5 mcg/kg/min 10−20−30−40 + atropine (0.25 × 4) up to 1mg |
| Dipyridamole | Syringe | 0.84 mg/Kg in 6′ or 0.84 mg/kg in 10′ + atropine (0.25 × 4) up to 1mg |
| Adenosine | Syringe | 140 mcg/Kg/min in 6′ |
| Pacing | External pacing | From 100 bpm with increments of 10 beats/min up to target heart rate |

# Complications

◆ Minor, but limiting, side effects preclude the achievement of maximal pharmacological stress in less than 10% of patients with dobutamine and less than 5% in patients with dipyridamole stress

◆ Not all stress tests carry the same risk of major adverse reactions and dobutamine stress testing may be more dangerous than other forms of pharmacological stress, such as those produced by dipyridamole or adenosine

◆ Both the doctor and the patient should be aware of the rate of complications, and the rate of complications (derived from literature and from the lab experience) should be spelled out in the informed consent

# Exercise stress echo

## Contraindications

◆ Unstable haemodynamic conditions

◆ Severe, uncontrolled hypertension

◆ Additional relative contraindications are inability to exercise adequately and a difficult resting echocardiogram

## Patient preparation

◆ No particular indications are to be given to patients

## Protocol

◆ Exercise echocardiography can be performed using either a **treadmill** or semi-supine **bicycle** protocol

◆ When a **treadmill** test is performed, scanning during exercise is not feasible, so most protocols rely on immediate post-exercise imaging

◆ It is imperative to accomplish post-exercise imaging as soon as possible (<1 min from cessation of exercise)

◆ The advantages of treadmill exercise echocardiography are the widespread availability of the treadmill system and a greater feasibility (a number of patients are unable to cycle)

◆ **Bicycle** exercise echocardiography is performed during either an upright or recumbent posture.

◆ The workload is escalated in a stepwise fashion while imaging is performed

◆ The most important advantage of semi-supine bicycle exercise is the chance to obtain images during the various levels of exercise (rather than relying on post-exercise imaging)

## Limiting side effects

◆ The safety of exercise stress is witnessed by decades of experience with electrocardiographic testing and stress imaging

◆ Death occurs at an average in 1 in 10 000 tests

◆ Major life-threatening effects, including myocardial infarction, ventricular fibrillation, sustained ventricular tachycardia, and stroke, were reported in about 1 in 6000 patients with exercise in the international stress echocardiography registry

# Dipyridamole stress echo

## Contraindications

Patients with the following should not receive dipyridamole

◆ Second- or third-degree atrioventricular block
◆ Sick sinus syndrome
◆ Bronchial asthma or a tendency to bronchospasm

## Patient preparation

◆ Patients should abstain from the assumption of caffeine-containing drinks (tea, coffee, cola) for 24 h prior to test
◆ Patients on chronic xanthine medication should not undergo dipyridamole stress echo

## Infusion protocol

◆ The standard dipyridamole protocol: intravenous infusion of 0.84 mg/kg over 10 min, in two separate infusions: 0.56 mg/kg over 4 min ('standard dose'), followed by 4 min of no dose and, if still negative, an additional 0.28 mg/kg over 2 min
◆ If no end point is reached, atropine (doses of 0.25 mg up to a maximum of 1 mg) is added
◆ The 'accelerated protocol': the same overall dose of 0.84 mg/kg can be given over 6 min—the shorter the infusion time, the higher the sensitivity. No need for atropine
◆ Coronary flow reserve can be assessed at peak hyperaemic dose

- Aminophylline (240 mg IV) should be available for immediate use in case of an adverse dipyridamole-related event
- Aminophylline is routinely infused at the end of the test regardless of test result

## Limiting side effects

- Limiting side effects occur in 3% of patients tested with dipyridamole. In order of frequency: hypotension, supraventricular tachycardia, general malaise, headache, dyspnoea, atrial fibrillation
- Major life-threatening complications, such as myocardial infarction, third-degree atrioventricular block, cardiac asystole, sustained ventricular tachycardia or pulmonary oedema, occur in about 1 in 1000 cases with high-dose dipyridamole stress

# Adenosine stress echo

## Patient preparation

- Similar to dipyridamole
- Patients using dipyridamole chronically should not undergo adenosine testing for at least 24 h after withdrawal of therapy, because their blood levels of adenosine could be unpredictably high

## Infusion protocol

- It is infused at a maximum dose of 140 ug/kg/min over 6 min
- Imaging is performed prior to and after starting adenosine infusion

- Dual imaging (wall motion and coronary flow reserve) is not possible due to the very short half-life

## Limiting side effects

- Side effects are very frequent and are limiting in up to 20% of patients investigated with adenosine stress echocardiography
- They include: high-degree atrioventricular block, hypotension, intolerable chest pain (possibly induced for direct stimulation of myocardial A1 adenosine receptors), shortness of breath, flushing, headache
- Although side effects are frequent, the incidence of life-threatening complications, such as myocardial infarction, ventricular tachycardia, and shock, has been shown to be very low, with only one fatal myocardial infarction in approximately 10 000 cases

# Dobutamine stress echo

## Contraindications

- History of complex atrial (paroxysmal atrial fibrillation, paroxysmal supraventricular tachycardia)
- Ventricular arrhythmias (sustained ventricular tachycardia or ventricular fibrillation)
- Moderate to severe hypertension should not undergo dobutamine stress echocardiography and be referred for safer vasodilator stress

## Patient preparation

◆ No particular preparation to be given to patients

## Infusion protocol

◆ The standard dobutamine stress protocol usually adopted consists of continuous intravenous infusion of dobutamine in 3-min increments, starting with 5 µg/kg/min and increasing to 10, 20, 30, and 40 µg/kg/min

◆ If no end point is reached, atropine (in doses 0.25 mg up to a maximum of 1 mg) is added to the 40 µg/kg/min dobutamine infusion

◆ Other more conservative protocols—with longer duration of steps and peak dobutamine dosage of 20 to 30 µg/kg/min—have been proposed but are limited by unsatisfactory sensitivity

◆ More aggressive protocols—with higher peak dosage of dobutamine up to 50–60 µg/kg/min and atropine sulphate up to 2 mg—have also been proposed, but safety concern remains and to date no advantages have been shown in larger studies

◆ The assessment of myocardial viability is obtained at low doses (5–10 µg/kg/min)

## Limiting side effects

◆ In order of frequency, limiting side effects during dobutamine stress include: complex ventricular tachyarrhythmias (the most frequent complications, which are independent of ischaemia in many cases and can also develop at low-dose dobutamine regimen), hypotension, atrial fibrillation, hypertension (in some cases due to dynamic intraventricular obstruction provoked by inotropic action of dobutamine, especially in hypertrophic hearts). A vasodepressor reflex triggered by left ventricular mechanoreceptors stimulation (Bezold–Jarisch reflex) due to excessive inotropic stimulation may be an alternative mechanism, bradyarrhythmias, coronary vasospasm (through α-receptor stimulation)

◆ The rate of major complications may occur in 1 of 300 cases during dobutamine stress

## Stressor choice and appropriateness criteria (Table 16.1.4)

◆ Pharmacological stress echocardiography is the choice for patients in whom exercise is unfeasible or contraindicated

◆ The choice of dobutamine or dipyridamole should depend on specific contraindications of either drugs, patient characteristics, local drug cost, and the physician's preference

**Table 16.1.4.** Appropriateness criteria

| Patients with | Appropriate | Uncertain | Inappropriate | Class |
|---|:---:|:---:|:---:|:---:|
| Uninterpretable ECG, inability to cycle, or submaximal uncertain exercise ECG | ✓ | | | I |
| Uncertain coronary stenosis significance | ✓ | | | I |
| Post-revascularization with symptom changes | ✓ | | | I |
| Before surgery, at high risk, with low exercise tolerance | ✓ | | | I |
| Viability in ischaemic cardiomyopathy | ✓ | | | I |
| Asymptomatic > 5 years after CABG or > 2 after PCI | | ✓ | | IIb |
| Asymptomatic, low risk | | | ✓ | III |
| Pre-op, intermediate risk surgery, good exercise tolerance | | | ✓ | III |
| Low pre-test probability, interpretable ECG, ability to exercise | | | ✓ | III |
| Asymptomatic < 5 years after CABG or < 2 after PCI | | | ✓ | III |

# Suggested reading

1. Sicari R, Nihoyannopoulos P, Evangelista A, et al. European Association of Echocardiography. Stress echocardiography expert consensus statement: European Association of Echocardiography (EAE) (a registered branch of the ESC). *Eur J Echocardiogr* 2008;9:415–37.
2. Nedeljkovic I, Ostojic M, Beleslin B, et al. Comparison of exercise, dobutamine-atropine and dipyridamole-atropine stress echocardiography in detecting coronary artery disease. *Cardiovasc Ultrasound* 2006;4:22.

# CHAPTER 17

# Systemic Disease and Other Conditions

# 17.1 Athlete's heart

## Introduction

**Physiological morphological adaptations of the heart to physical activity is shown in** Fig. 17.1.1

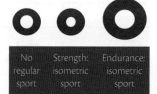

**Fig. 17.1.1** Morganroth hypothesis. The morphologic adaptations result from the type of the haemodynamic overload during exercise

- **Endurance training, dynamic isotonic exercise** (running, walking, cycling, swimming, rowing, skiing) ➜ volume overload and increased diastolic wall stress ➜ LV eccentric hypertrophy (increased LV cavity dimension/volume, and thus LV mass; mildly increased wall thickness)

- **Resistance training, static isometric exercise** (wrestling, weightlifting) ➜ pressure overload and increased systolic wall stress ➜ LV concentric hypertrophy (increased wall thickness with no increase in cavity size/volume)

- **Mixed training disciplines** (soccer, rugby, hockey) ➜ combined effects of both volume and pressure overload

## Echocardiographic findings

### Morphology (Fig. 17.1.2ABCD, Box 17.1.1)

- **LV:** normal or mildly increased LV wall thickness (< 15 mm); normal or mildly increased LV end-diastolic diameter/volume (a small LV plays against athlete's heart)

- **LA:** normal or mild dilation, indexed LA volume usually above the normal range

- **RV:** larger RV wall thickness and larger RV diameters at both the RV inflow and outflow (endurance athletes), as well as inferior vena cava, when compared to published normal ranges

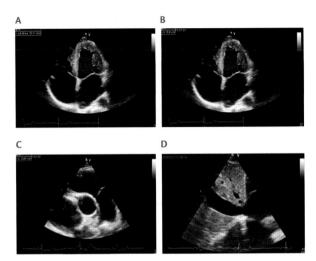

**Fig. 17.1.2** Top-level basketball player with increased non indexed LA volume (A) and longitudinal diameter (B); increased RV outflow diameter (C) and inferior vena cava (D). Courtesy of A. D'Andrea

> **Box 17.1.1  Key points regarding LV morphology in athlete's heart**
>
> ◆ Only a minority of athletes (about 3% in Caucasians, about 10% in blacks) show 'grey zone LV hypertrophy' (mild to moderate increased wall thickness: 12–15 mm)
>
> ◆ Racial and gender differences **MUST BE** taken into account (black athletes ➜ more hypertrophy, female athletes ➜ less hypertrophy)
>
> ◆ Endurance training, dynamic isotonic exercise ➜ LV eccentric hypertrophy pattern, mildly increased LV end-diastolic diameter/volume, normal/mildly increased relative wall thickness, increased LV mass
>
> ◆ Resistance training, static isometric exercise ➜ LV concentric hypertrophy pattern, mildly to moderate increased wall thickness (< 15 mm), no change in LV end-diastolic diameter/volume, increased LV mass
>
> ◆ 'Pure' types of training are rare in the real world ➜ mixed training programs are the rule and that 'resistance–static–strength–isometric' exercise often does not show remodelling

## LV systolic function (Fig. 17.1.3)

- ◆ Normal/supernormal myocardial function, more evident in endurance and combination sports (volume overload)
- ◆ Causes: loading conditions (Frank–Starling law) + lower heart rate + better myofibril properties (high ATPase content myosin)
- ◆ **Conventional assessment** (volumetric and blood flow Doppler methods): normal ejection fraction and normal/increased stroke volume and cardiac output
- ◆ **Doppler myocardial imaging (DMI) and deformation imaging**: normal or supernormal systolic function: normal/increased s' (pulsed DMI) and increased regional longitudinal systolic strain and strain rate (pulsed DMI–derived and STE)

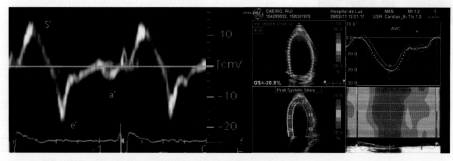

**Fig. 17.1.3** Left: DMI typical pattern of athlete's heart, normal/supernormal systolic and diastolic function: normal/increased s' and e' velocities, normal/increased e'/a'. Right: 2D speckle tracking echocardiography typical pattern, normal/supernormal global and regional longitudinal strain, with global and regional longitudinal systolic strain

## LV diastolic function

◆ Conventional assessment (PW Doppler trans-mitral inflow and pulmonary venous flow): usually normal

◆ DMI: increased e' leading to reduced E/e' and increased e'/a'

## RV functional adaptation (Fig. 17.1.4)

◆ Classically normal/supernormal systolic and diastolic function

◆ In well-trained ultra-endurance endurance athletes, RV global and regional (basal segments) dysfunction may be seen after exercise, usually reversible in one to two weeks

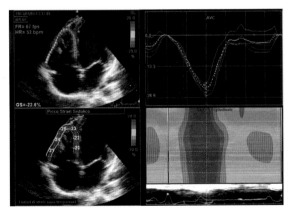

**Fig. 17.1.4** 2D STE echocardiography of the RV of a top-level basketball player. Normal/high negative regional systolic strain in all RV segments in this view. Courtesy of A. D' Andrea

# Differential diagnosis

## HCM versus athlete's heart (Table 17.1.1 and Fig. 17.1.5AB)

**Table 17.1.1** EACVIs updated Maron's criteria to distinguish hypertrophic cardiomyopathy from athlete's heart

| HCM | Echo criteria | Athlete's heart |
|---|---|---|
| + | Atypical patterns of LVH | – |
| – | LVH regression after deconditioning | ++ |
| + | Small LV cavity (< 45 mm) | – |
| – | Big LV cavity (> 55 mm) | + |
| + | RV hypertrophy (right ventricular subcostal thickness > 5 mm) | – |
| + | LA dilatation (> 45 mm or ≥ 34 ml/m²) | ± |
| + | MV apparatus abnormalities | – |
| + | Dynamic obstruction (> 30 mmHg) | – |
| + | MR > mild | – |
| + | LV subendocardial systolic dysfunction<br>Pulsed DMI: mitral annulus velocities (average four sites):<br>s'< 9 cm/s; 2D-STE peak regional strain ≤ -15% | – |
| + | Abnormal global diastolic function<br>Impaired LV relaxation | – |
| + | LV subendocardial diastolic dysfunction<br>Pulsed DMI: mitral annulus velocities (average four sites):<br>e'< 7 cm/s; e'/a'< 1 in any site | – |
| + | Delayed LV untwist (LV untwist extending beyond 25% of diastole) | – |

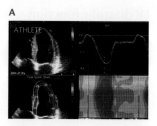

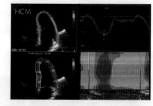

**Fig. 17.1.5** 2D speckle tracking: two athletes with mild LVH in the 'grey zone' range: in opposition to the healthy athlete (A), the HCM patient (B) shows mildly reduced regional longitudinal strain in several LV segments

## Athlete's heart vs idiopathic dilated cardiomyopathy (IDCM) (Table 17.1.2, Fig. 17.1.6)

- ◆ LV dilation (LV internal diastolic diameter > 60 mm) with reduced EF and abnormal LV diastolic function ➜ suspicion of IDCM ➜ LGE cardiac MRI (mid-myocardial streaks in about one-third of subjects)

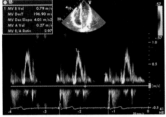
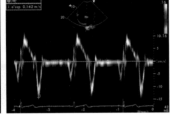
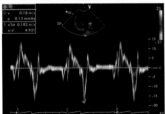

**Fig. 17.1.6** Standard trans-mitral Doppler and pulsed DMI of septal and lateral mitral annulus in a competitive runner. Trans-mitral E/A ratio (top panel) is 2.97 but E/e' ratio (pulsed DMI in the lower panel) is 4.9, consistent with normal degree of LV filling pressure. In IDCM, LV filling pressures are often increased

**Table 17.1.2** Differential diagnosis criteria between IDCM and athlete's heart

| IDCM | Echocardiographic data | Athlete's heart |
|:---:|---|:---:|
| + | LV dilatation | + |
| + | Increased sphericity index | − |
| + | LV systolic dysfunction | − |
| + | LV diastolic dysfunction | − |
| ± | Increased LV filling pressures | − |
| + | Left atrial dilation | − |
| + | RV dilatation | ± |
| ± | RV systolic dysfunction | − |
| ± | Increased pulmonary artery systolic pressure | + at exercise |
| + | Vena cava dilation | + |
| − | Vena cava respiratory reactivity | + |

## Athlete's heart vs arrhythmogenic right ventricular cardiomyopathy (ARVC) (Table 17.1.3, Fig. 17.1.7)

- RV dilation in an athlete with palpitations/arrhythmias → suspicion of ARVC → cardiac MRI (abnormalities of RV wall motion, RV dimensions and function)
- However, neither cardiac imaging can confirm or exclude ARVC which remains a clinical diagnosis

**Table 17.1.3** Differential diagnosis criteria between IDCM and ARVC

| ARVC | Echocardiographic data | Athlete's heart |
|------|------------------------|-----------------|
| − | LV dilation | + |
| − | LV hypertrophy | + |
| + | RV dilation | ± |
| + | RV systolic dysfunction | − |
| ± | Dilation of RV outflow | − |
| ± | Thickened moderator band | ± |
| + | RV wall bulging | − |

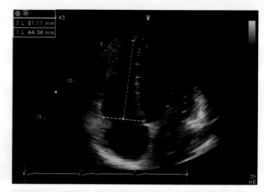

**Fig. 17.1.7** RV enlargement in an endurance athlete. The apical 4CV shows an increase of both RV basal diameter (1 = 44 mm) and of RV base-to-apex length diameter (2 = 81 mm). References normal values (RV basal diameter = 20–28 mm, RV base-to-apex length diameter = 71–79 mm). In ARVC, RV dilation is combined with RV segmental morphological (thinning, bulging, aneurysm) and functional (regional wall motion) abnormalities

# Suggested reading

1. Morganroth J, Maron BJ, Henry WL, et al. Comparative left ventricular dimensions in trained athletes. *Ann Intern Med* 1975;82:521–24.

2. George K, Whyte GP, Green DJ, et al. The endurance athlete's heart: acute stress and chronic adaptation. *Br J Sports* Med 2012;46:i29–i36.

3. D'Andrea A, Riegler L, Golia E, et al. Range of right heart measurements in top-level athletes: the training impact. *Int J Cardiol* 2013;164:48–57.

4. La Gerche A, Burns AT, Mooney DJ, et al. Exercise-induced right ventricular dysfunction and structural remodelling in endurance athletes. *Eur Heart J* 2012;33:998–1006.

5. Maron BJ, Pelliccia A, Spirito P. Cardiac disease in young trained athletes. Insights into methods for distinguishing athlete's heart from structural heart disease, with particular emphasis on hypertrophic cardiomyopathy. *Circulation* 1995;91:1596–1601.

6. Cardim N, Oliveira AG, Longo S, et al. Doppler tissue imaging: regional myocardial function in hypertrophic cardiomyopathy and in athlete's heart. *J Am Soc Echocardiogr* 2003;16:223–32.

7. Galderisi M, Lomoriello VS, Santoro A, et al. Differences of myocardial systolic deformation and correlates of diastolic function in competitive rowers and young hypertensives: a Speckle Tracking echocardiographic study. *J Am Soc Echocardiogr* 2010;23:1190–8.

8. D'Andrea A, Caso P, Sarubbi B, et al. Right ventricular myocardial adaptation to different training protocols in top-level athletes. *Echocardiography* 2003;20:329–36.

9. Elliott P, Andersson B, Arbustini E, et al. Classification of the cardiomyopathies: a position statement of the European Society Working Group on myocardial and pericardial diseases. *Eur Heart J* 2008;29:270–6.

10. Galderisi M, Caso P, Severino S, et al. Myocardial diastolic impairment caused by left ventricular hypertrophy involves basal septum more than other walls: analysis by pulsed Doppler tissue imaging. *J Hypertens* 1999;17:685–93.

# 17.2  Heart during pregnancy

## Haemodynamic changes during pregnancy (Table 17.2.1)

- Changes start during first trimester and are maximum between five and eight months
- Other changes: hypercoagulability, increased platelets activity, increased coagulation factors, and decrease in fibrinolysis
- Cardiac output and blood pressure increase with uterine contraction during labour up to 20%. Pain, anaesthesia-related change, and mode of delivery may influence haemodynamic changes during delivery
- Haemodynamic values are back to normal within six weeks following delivery

## Echocardiographic findings during normal pregnancy (Table 17.2.2)

- Changes are maximal during third trimester of pregnancy compared to baseline or post-partum values
- Small pericardial effusion could be seen close to term in normal pregnancy

**Table 17.2.1**  Haemodynamic changes during pregnancy

|  | Change |
|---|---|
| Blood volume | Up to 50% |
| Heart rate | ↑ 25–30% |
| Stroke volume | ↑ |
| Cardiac output | ↑ ± 50% |
| Systolic blood pressure | Unchanged or slightly ↓ |
| Systemic vascular resistance | ↓ |
| Pulmonary arterial resistance | Unchanged |

# Role of echo in pregnancy

**Echo should be performed in all pregnant women with unexplained or new cardiovascular signs or symptoms**

## Evaluation of cardiac murmur

- Frequent in pregnant woman, most of the time = flow murmur (soft, mid systolic) due to increase in cardiac output

### Indication for echo

- History of cardiac disease
- Murmur with cardiac symptoms (at least grade 3/6 murmur or diastolic murmur)
- Any doubt regarding underlying cardiac disease

### Other echo findings

- Unknown or neglected cardiovascular disease (may change with ethnicity of the patient)
- Valvular heart disease
- Congenital heart disease: ASD, VSD, etc.
- Hypertrophic cardiomyopathy, etc.

**Table 17.2.2** Echocardiographic findings during normal pregnancy

| | Change |
|---|---|
| LV end diastolic dimension | ↑ |
| LV end systolic dimension | Unchanged |
| Fractional shortening | Unchanged or slightly ↑ |
| LV end diastolic volume | ↑ |
| LV ejection fraction (EF) | Unchanged or slightly ↑ (recent 3D echo studies, not change in EF) |
| LV shape | ↑ Sphericity index |
| LV mass | ↑ (5–10%) |
| LA size | ↑ |
| VCF | Unchanged or slightly ↑ |
| E/A | ↓ (Due to enhanced atrial contractility) |
| E/e' | Unchanged or slightly ↓ |
| Transvalvular flow | ↑ |

## Evaluation of cardiac symptoms or signs

**Many cardiac symptoms could already be present in a normal pregnancy (dyspnoea, palpitation, elevated venous pressure, legs oedema…)**

### Dyspnoea

◆ Indication for echo: differentiate non-cardiac (pulmonary embolism, pneumonia, etc.) from cardiac cause

### Echo findings

◆ Depressed LV function: suggest peri-partum cardiomyopathy in absence of other cause to explain depressed LV function (known cardiomyopathy, congenital disease, etc.)

◆ Valvular disease and especially stenotic disease (aortic or mitral)

◆ Diastolic dysfunction: hypertension, etc.

◆ Congenital heart disease: ASD, VSD, etc.

◆ Other structural heart disease: hypertrophic cardiomyopathy, etc.

### Palpitations

◆ Presence of significant arrhythmia warrants echographic evaluation to search structural cardiac disease

## Evaluation of pre-existing cardiac disease

**All woman with cardiac condition should have complete cardiac evaluation (comprising complete echocardiography) before pregnancy to assess and discuss the**

risk related to pregnancy in their situation. This also permits a baseline echo value to be taken

## Specific cardiac disease

### Valvular stenosis

◆ Asymptomatic patients with valvular stenosis may become symptomatic during pregnancy because of the increase in cardiac output
◆ Aortic stenosis: echocardiography useful for monitoring
  ◆ increase in pressure gradient measured by Doppler, continuity equation can still be used for valve area
  ◆ worsening of severity of stenosis in some patients (hormonal changes?)
◆ Mitral stenosis: echocardiography useful for monitoring
  ◆ increase in trans-mitral flow, heart rate (shortening filling time), increase in LA pressure
  ◆ echo measurement (2D, Doppler, etc.) remain valid during pregnancy
  ◆ role if percutaneous dilatation is proposed

### Valvular regurgitation

Regurgitant lesions are usually well tolerated during pregnancy

Assessment could be performed by the same echo method than in the non-pregnant patient but evaluation could be misinterpreted during pregnancy

◆ Severity may apparently decrease due to decrease in systemic vascular resistance and thus LV function may appear to be improved

- LV dimension change due to pregnancy could lead to a misdiagnosis in a patient with only moderate lesion
- Severity of regurgitant lesion and ventricular function must be assessed in the post-partum period before taking any treatment decision

**Valvular prosthesis**

- Echocardiography plays a critical role for monitoring during pregnancy
- Mechanical valve: increased risk of thrombosis
- Bioprosthesis: increased risk of structural deterioration (controversial!)
- Increased heart rate and stroke volume influence Doppler evaluation of gradient and velocities across the valve
- Alteration on loading conditions may affect pressure half-time measurement
- It is important to have baseline value and to interpret the result according to haemodynamic status

**Marfan syndrome**

- Risk during pregnancy or post partum: aortic dissection
- Important to have a pre-pregnancy assessment of the dimension of the aortic root to estimate the risk related to pregnancy
- Echo will be used to monitor change in aortic root dimension during pregnancy and to advise mode of delivery
  - **aortic root < 40 mm ➜ vaginal delivery**
  - **aortic root > 45 mm ➜ caesarean delivery**
- Echo should also be performed in early post-partum period: assessment of aortic root

## Aortic dissection

◆ Rare!

◆ Echo should be performed as first-stage diagnosis of symptoms are suspect and especially in patients with connective tissue disease such as Ehlers–Danlos, bicuspid aortic valve and root dilatation, Turner syndrome, severe hypertension

## Ischaemic heart disease

◆ Rare!

◆ More frequent in older woman and women with at least one risk factor for myocardial infarction

◆ Segmental abnormalities with or without depressed LV function on echo should lead to considering this diagnosis

## Congenital heart disease

### Atrial septal defect

◆ The most frequently newly diagnosed congenital heart disease during pregnancy (murmur)

◆ Contrast injection to confirm diagnosis should be avoided to minimize embolic risk

◆ Shunt calculation may be difficult due to increase in cardiac output, ventricular volume, and decrease in systemic vascular resistance

◆ Well tolerated during pregnancy if there is no pulmonary hypertension

◆ After surgical repair, echo examination is normal (check for pulmonary hypertension). Outcome of pregnancy is similar to normal patient

### Ventricular septal defect

◆ Pregnancy: well tolerated in patient with small defect, left to right shunt in the absence of pulmonary hypertension

◆ Echo assessment before pregnancy: severity of the shunt, haemodynamic repercussion of the shunt, pulmonary hypertension, RV function

◆ Echo assessment during pregnancy: not mandatory if no haemodynamic repercussion and small shunt

◆ RV function, pulmonary hypertension

### Coarctation of the aorta

◆ Pregnancy: well tolerated if repair and residual gradient < 20 mmHg or unrepaired with moderate severity. Increased risk of hypertension and complication related to hypertension

◆ Echo assessment before pregnancy: residual gradient, LV function, search for aneurysm at the site of repair (may need assessment by MRI or MDCT)

◆ Echo assessment during pregnancy: LV function, residual gradient (increased cardiac output), aneurysm, diastolic dysfunction related to hypertension

### Tetralogy of Fallot

◆ Pregnancy: well tolerated in repaired patients if no RV/LV dysfunction or RVOT obstruction. Potential risk of further deterioration of RV/LV dysfunction if pre-existent or pre-existent RV dilatation

◆ Echo assessment before pregnancy: RV function and dilatation, RVOT obstruction, pulmonary regurgitation, pulmonary hypertension, LV function

- Echo assessment during pregnancy: RV function and dilatation, pulmonary hypertension, LV function

## Congenitally corrected transposition of the great arteries (CCTGA)

- Pregnancy: well tolerated in the absence of RV dysfunction, depending on the associated lesion (shunt, etc.). Risks related to pregnancy are: heart failure, cyanosis (shunt), stroke (shunt)
- Echo assessment before pregnancy: RV function, presence of associated lesion (VSD, pulmonary stenosis, etc.)
- Echo assessment during pregnancy: RV function, associated lesions

## Transposition of the great arteries (TGA)

### Atrial correction

- Pregnancy: tolerance is related to RV function, risk associated with permanent decline of RV function
- Echo assessment before pregnancy: RV function, systemic atrioventricular valve regurgitation, baffle leakage, or stenosis
- Echo assessment during pregnancy: RV function, systemic atrioventricular valve regurgitation

### Arterial correction

- Pregnancy: less experience, depend on associated lesions and repair (i.e. mechanical valve)
- Echo assessment before pregnancy: aortic or pulmonary stenosis of regurgitation, associated lesion, LV function

◆ Echo assessment during pregnancy: aortic or pulmonary stenosis of regurgitation, associated lesion, LV function

### Ebstein's valve abnormality

◆ Pregnancy: well tolerated in the absence of cyanosis
◆ Echo assessment before pregnancy: RV function, tricuspid regurgitation, importance of the shunt, LV function
◆ Echo assessment during pregnancy: RV function, tricuspid regurgitation, LV function

### Fontan repair

◆ Pregnancy: high-risk pregnancy (± risk of anticoagulation), limited data, high rate of foetal loss and maternal complication (arrhythmia, heart failure)
◆ Echo assessment before pregnancy: ventricular function, functioning of the Fontan anastomosis
◆ Echo assessment during pregnancy: ventricular function, functioning of the Fontan anastomosis

### Pulmonary hypertension

◆ Pregnancy: is contraindicated in patients with pulmonary hypertension and Eisenmenger syndrome. High maternal and foetal morbidity and mortality
◆ Echo assessment before pregnancy: pulmonary hypertension (exact value may be difficult to evaluate using tricuspid regurgitation), RV function
◆ Echo assessment during pregnancy: pulmonary hypertension, RV function

# Suggested reading

1. Thorne S, et al. Risks of contraception and pregnancy in heart disease. *Heart* 2006;92:1520–25.
2. Baumgartner H, MacGregor A, Nelson-Piercy C. ESC Guidelines for the management of grown-up congenital heart disease (new version 2010). *Eur Heart J* 2010;31:2915–57.
3. Vera Regitz-Zagrosek V, Blomstrom Lundqvist C, et al. ESC Guidelines on the management of cardiovascular diseases during pregnancy: The Task Force on the Management of Cardiovascular Diseases during Pregnancy of the European Society of Cardiology (ESC). *Eur Heart J* 2011;32: 3147–97.
4. Naqvi TZ, Elkayam U. Serial echocardiographic assessment of the human heart in normal pregnancy. *Circ Cardiovasc Imaging* 2012;5:283–5.
5. Savu O, Jurcuţ R, Giuşcă S, et al. Morphological and functional adaptation of the maternal heart during pregnancy. *Circ Cardiovasc Imaging* 2012;5:289–97.
6. Naqvi, TZ, Lee MS, Aldridge M, et al. Normal cardiac adaptation during pregnancy—assessment by velocity vector imaging and three-dimensional echocardiography in healthy pregnant women. *Circulation* 2013;128:A16377.

# 17.3  Systemic diseases

## Introduction

- The heart is not the principal affected organ in systemic disease
- There is some involvement of the heart in systemic disease
- There are no pathognomonic symptoms of cardiovascular disease
- Late mortality results primarily from cardiovascular complications

## Main echo findings refer to:

- Pericardium
- Cardiac valves
- Left and right ventricular myocardium
- Arteries
- Intracardiac thrombi
- Pulmonary hypertension

## Amyloidosis

### Echo findings

- Increased LV wall thickness without left ventricular enlargement, i.e. concentric remodelling/hypertrophy (Fig. 17.3.1A)
- Increased right ventricular wall thickness (**biventricular thickening is strongly suggestive of infiltrative heart disease**) (Fig. 17.3.1B)

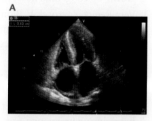

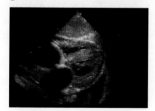

**Fig. 17.3.1** A: 4CV. Thickened LV walls with granular sparkling is apparent. Biatrial enlargement is visible. There is also small pericardial effusion; B: subcostal 4CV. Thickened RV free wall is visible

- Increased myocardial echogenicity ('granular sparkling') (Fig. 17.3.1A)
- LV ejection fraction is typically preserved until late
- Long-axis LV dysfunction (use strain, strain rate imaging) is impaired in early stage
  - depressed longitudinal myocardial velocities and mainly deformation can detect early cardiac involvement
- LV filling—progressive diastolic dysfunction
  - restrictive trans-mitral flow pattern - short E-wave deceleration time and a low-velocity A-wave are observed in advanced stages (Fig. 17.3.2)
- Biatrial dilatation—may be an isolated atrial amyloidosis
- Interatrial septum infiltration is relatively frequent
- Atrial thrombus may be observed even in sinus rhythm
- Valvular leaflet thickening resulting usually in mild regurgitation
- Usually minor pericardial effusion

## Haematochromatosis

### Echo findings

- Systolic LV function
  - usually preserved in early stages
  - significantly depressed in later stages (Fig. 17.3.3AB)

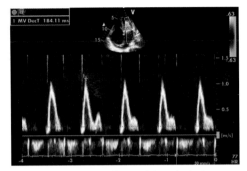

**Fig. 17.3.2** Restrictive LV filling with low velocity A-wave

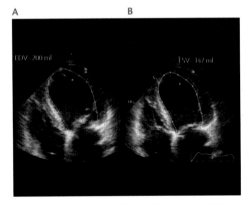

**Fig. 17.3.3** TTE. 4CV: LV in diastole (A) and systole (B) in patients with late-stage haematochromatosis

- Biatrial enlargement
- Increased LV wall thickness, increased LV mass in advanced phase
- Various degrees of mitral and tricuspid valve regurgitation
- LV diastolic dysfunction (correlates with the severity of iron overload)
- RV involvement with normal size and increased wall thickness
- Increased pulmonary pressures
- Global longitudinal systolic strain could be reduced (Fig. 17.3.4)

## Sarcoidosis

### Echo findings

- LV dilatation with thinning or thickening of the LV walls (usually the basal interventricular septum thinning and ventricular aneurysm in the inferoposterior wall)
- Increased echogenicity
- LV wall-motion abnormalities (regional or global): coexistence of dyskinetic and normokinetic segments
- LV diastolic dysfunction (from mild to severe)
- Mitral and tricuspid valve regurgitation
- RV involvement with increased wall thickness due to direct granulomatous involvement (Fig. 17.3.5)
- Increased pulmonary pressures secondary to lung implication

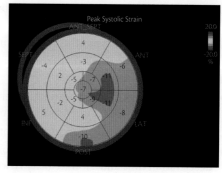

**Fig. 17.3.4** Reduced LV global longitudinal systolic strain (average GLS = - 4.6%) in patients with late-stage haematochromatosis

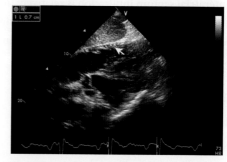

**Fig. 17.3.5** Subcostal view of RV involvement with increased wall thickness (7 mm, see arrow). Courtesy of Prof J Kasprzak.

- Global longitudinal strain: peak systolic shortening is significantly reduced (can be regional or diffuse)
- Pericardial effusion, tamponade, and constrictive pericarditis have been infrequently found

## Carcinoid syndrome

### Echo findings

- Right-sided valvular heart lesions: tricuspid regurgitation (90%) and pulmonary stenosis (50–69%)
  - tricuspid valve leaflets and subvalvular apparatus are thickened and shortened
- In advanced stages leaflets become retracted with reduced mobility (septal and anterior leaflets)
- In more advanced stages the leaflets become fixed in a semi-open position
- Enlargement of the right atrium and right ventricle, RV systolic dysfunction
- Left-sided valvular heart involvement is less frequent (7–29%) and indicates lung metastasis or shunt
- Pericardial effusion is rather small and not frequent
- Myocardial carcinoid metastases are very rare
- Usefulness of 3D and contrast echocardiography

## Connective tissue disease (CTD)

Connective tissue diseases (CTDs) are chronic inflammatory diseases characterized by a systemic and heterogeneous spectrum of clinical symptoms

# Rheumatoid arthritis (RA)

## Echo findings

- Pericarditis is the most frequent cardiac complication of RA
  - small or moderate pericardial effusion (20–25% of RA patients) (Fig. 17.3.6)
  - cardiac tamponade is very rare
  - constrictive pericarditis is also very rare
- Regional wall-motion abnormalities after myocardial infarction (premature coronary artery disease)
- Diastolic dysfunction is frequent—the impaired relaxation of left ventricle (20–30%)
- **The prevalence of subclinical amyloidosis among RA patients is about 30%**
- Valves are affected in about 30–40% of RA patients
  - mitral valve insufficiency is most prevalent (Fig. 17.3.7)— nodules and fibrosis of the leaflets (basal or mid portions), annulus, and subvalvular apparatus
  - mitral valve prolapse; aortic stenosis is rare; aortic dilatation is also rare

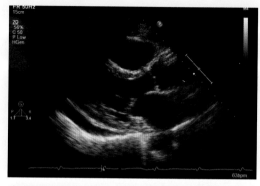

**Fig. 17.3.6** PTLAX showing a small pericardial effusion

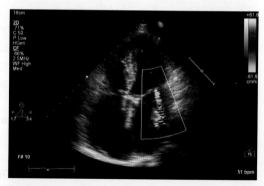

**Fig. 17.3.7** 4CV showing a mild mitral regurgitation

# Systemic lupus erythematosus (SLE)

## Echo findings

- Pericarditis—one of the most characteristic manifestations of SLE
  - pericardial effusion, usually small or moderate (11–54%)
  - cardiac tamponade and constrictive pericarditis are rare (< 1%)
- Valvular disease is the most prevalent
  - SLE Libman–Sacks vegetations (Fig. 17.3.8) appear as
    - non-infective valvular masses of varying size (≥ 2 mm)
    - shape with irregular borders and echodensity firmly attached to the valve surface without independent motion, mainly on the mitral valve but also on other valves, chordae tendinae, and endocardium surface
    - **Libman–Sacks vegetations are clinically silent in the majority but sometimes progress and cause severe valve regurgitations**
  - Abnormalities of LV regional motion after myocardial infarction, or myocarditis (8–25%)
  - LV diastolic dysfunction as relaxation abnormalities (reflect myocardial inflammation)
  - Pulmonary arterial hypertension (PAH) (0.5–17.5%)

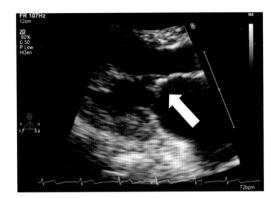

**Fig. 17.3.8** TTE. PTLAX. Libman–Sacks vegetation on anterior mitral leaflet (arrow)

# Antiphospholipid syndrome (APS)

## Echo findings

### Valvular

- Left-sided valves (especially mitral)
- Diffuse or focal leaflet thickening (40–60%)
- Vegetations, typically irregular (10–40%)—predominantly thrombotic but can be inflammatory or mixed on its atrial surface
- Aortic valve—vegetations on the ventricular or the vascular surface
- Significant valvular diseases are rare (3%)

### Cardiac thromboembolism

- Thrombus formation in all cardiac chambers—can cause pulmonary and systemic embolism
- Systemic embolization—can result from in situ mural thrombi
- Spontaneous echo contrast in LA, more often in APS than in normal subjects

### Pulmonary hypertension (PH)

**PH is one of the most important complications (1.8–3.5%)**

### Myocardial

- Regional wall-motion abnormalities and LV systolic dysfunction—small vessels thrombotic disease
- LV filling abnormalities

# Systemic sclerosis (SSc)

## Echo findings

## Pulmonary hypertension—one of the most important complications adversely influencing SSc patients' survival

- ◆ Pulmonary arterial hypertension (PAH) (7–12%)
- ◆ PAH secondary to interstitial lung disease
- ◆ Pulmonary venous hypertension (PVH) associated with LV diastolic dysfunction
- ◆ Inappropriate pulmonary pressure response to exercise (Fig. 17.3.9AB)

## Pericardial

- ◆ Pericardial involvement in 30–70% of SSc patients (symptoms occur in only 7–20%)
- ◆ Pericardial effusion—in patients with PAH and worse prognosis
- ◆ Cardiac tamponade is rare—in patients with PAH or renal crisis

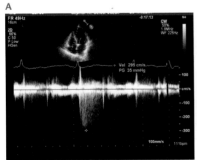
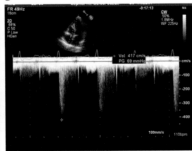

**Fig. 17.3.9** Apical 4CV. CW Doppler. Tricuspid regurgitant peak gradient (TPG) before (A) exercise in systemic sclerosis patient is 35 mmHg and after (B) exercise in systemic sclerosis patient increases to 69 mmHg

### Myocardial

◆ Myocardial fibrosis in autopsy is frequent but significant LV systolic dysfunction in echo in less than 5% SSc patients

◆ RV systolic dysfunction

◆ LV diastolic dysfunction in 20–50% of SSc patients

◆ Myocarditis usually accompanied with skeletal muscle myositis—a rare complication

## Mixed connective tissue disease (MCTD)

### Echo findings

*Pericardial (pericarditis is the most common cardiac manifestation)*

◆ An asymptomatic pericardial effusion in 25–35%, only 10% are symptomatic

◆ Cardiac tamponade is rare

*Pulmonary hypertension (main cause of death in MCTD patients)*

◆ PAH: the most severe cardiopulmonary complication (3–10%)

**Valvular:** *mitral valve prolapse in about 25% of patients* (Fig. 17.3.10)

◆ **Myocardial**

◆ Myocarditis can occur in MCTD patients—LV dilatation, hypokinesis and reduced LVEF

◆ Impaired LV diastolic function

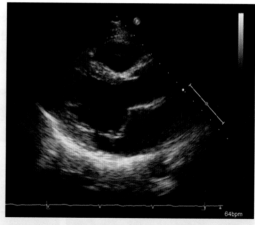

**Fig. 17.3.10** PTLAX. Mitral valve prolapse in MCTD patient

# Marfan syndrome

**An autosomal dominant connective tissue disorder caused by gene mutations**

### Role of echo

- Measure aortic root parallel to the plane of the aortic valve
  - report as an aortic root Z-score (correct for age and body size)
  - aortic root Z-score ≥ 2 or aortic dissection is diagnostic
  - < 20 years old with no ectopia lentis but with a family history of Marfan syndrome Z-score ≥ 3 is diagnostic
- Echocardiography is warranted in asymptomatic family members
- Monitor the progression of aortic aneurysm and aid the decision of aortic root replacement
- Diagnose aortic rupture/dissection
- Monitor associated pathologies—aortic and mitral regurgitation

### Echo findings

- Aortic root aneurysm—a typical annulo-aortic ectasia (Fig. 17.3.11)
- **Aortic dissection—the typical is type A, normal size of aortic root does not exclude dissection (responsible for 90% of the morbidity and mortality)** (Fig. 17.3.12)

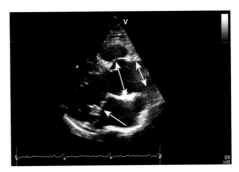

**Fig. 17.3.11** Dilated aortic annulus, sinuses of Valsalva, and ascending aorta are apparent (arrows). There is also significant mitral valve prolapse (arrow) in a patient with Marfan syndrome

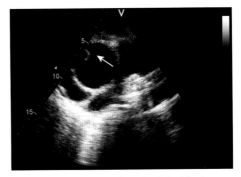

**Fig. 17.3.12** Type A aortic dissection: intimal flap in ascending aorta (short-axis slice) marked with an arrow in a patient with Marfan syndrome

- Aortic regurgitation (25%) due to aortic root dilatation (Fig. 17.3.13), acute in aortic root dissection
- Myxomatous prolapsing mitral valve—dilated annulus and mitral regurgitation are frequent
- Aortic arch, descending aorta (fusiform aneurysm), and abdominal aorta are affected in a descending order of frequency

### Follow-up echo

- Repeat echocardiogram at minimum yearly, more frequently if aortic root diameter approaches 45 mm, or there is a rapid increase in diameter > 5 mm/year
- In adults if aortic root measurements are repeatedly normal, echo performed every two to three years
- Even in the absence of aortic root dilatation, imaging of the descending thoracic aorta is indicated (Fig. 17.3.14)

## Vasculitis

### Giant cell arteritis (GCA)

#### Echo findings

- **Ascending aorta dilatation** (18% cases of GCA) → predominantly aortic aneurysm but also aortic dissection, aortic rupture, aortic arch syndrome, aortic wall haematoma, and aortopulmonary or aortodigestive fistula

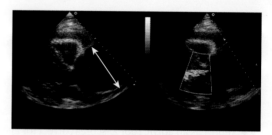

**Fig. 17.3.13** TTE PTLAX: a massively dilated (90 mm) aortic aneurysm and severe aortic valve regurgitation in a patient with Marfan syndrome

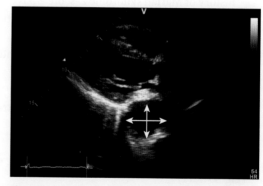

**Fig. 17.3.14** Significant dilatation of thoracic (descending) aorta is apparent in a patient with Marfan syndrome

- Aortic valve regurgitation ➜ secondary to aortic root dilatation
- Pericarditis without myocarditis in two-thirds of the cases—initial manifestation of GCA
- Acute myocarditis ➜ sometimes revealing GCA
- Pulmonary arteries ➜ occasionally affected
- Regional LV contractions abnormalities—rarely coronary arteries disease
- TOE: the presence of a clear intramural hypoechogenic halo around the lumen of the descending aorta ('**halo sign**') and circumferential thickening should suggest GCA

## Takayasu's arteritis

### Echo findings

- LV concentric hypertrophy (50%) due to arterial hypertension related to renal artery stenosis
- Aortic regurgitation (may be severe) due to both leaflet pathology and aortic root dilatation (25–40%)
- Ascending aortic aneurysm (9%); stenosis in the descending aorta (10%)
- Segmental wall motion abnormalities ➜ myocardial infarction (3–10%) or myocarditis (9–20%)
- Pulmonary hypertension (7%); pulmonary artery narrowing (right pulmonary artery more frequently)
- Pericarditis and pericardial effusion (10%); congestive heart failure (up to 10%)

### Kawasaki disease

#### *Echo findings in acute phase*

◆ myocarditis: the most common non-coronary complication (< 50% of patients with acute stage)

◆ pericarditis with pericardial effusion (about 25% of patients in the acute phase)

◆ systolic LV function should be routinely assessed (> 50% of patients develop transient LV dysfunction)

◆ mitral, tricuspid, or aortic regurgitation due to myocardial inflammation

◆ aortic root dilatation—usually mild

#### *Echo findings in subacute phase and during follow-up (Box 17.3.1)*

◆ **coronary arteries aneurysm: the most significant cardiovascular complication and occurs in 20–25% of untreated children (sometimes with thrombus) (Fig. 17.3.15)**

◆ regional wall-motion abnormalities: significant coronary artery involvement

> **Box 17.3.1** Optimize machine settings for the analysis of the coronary arteries by:
>
> ◆ using the highest possible frequency transducer
>
> ◆ reducing two-dimensional gain and compression
>
> ◆ assess coronary artery calibre from the inner edge to inner edge of the vessel wall
>
> ◆ Doppler imaging set at a low Nyquist limit for evaluating normal coronary artery flow
>
> ◆ zoom the region of interest

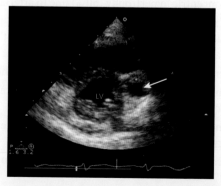

**Fig. 17.3.15** PTSAX at the mitral valve level. The arrowhead indicates the large aneurysm of the proximal part of left anterior descending branch with organized thrombus (asterisk)

- severe mitral regurgitation: papillary muscle dysfunction due to myocardial ischaemia
- TTE is highly sensitive and specific for the coronary artery involvement diagnosis, perform at the time of Kawasaki disease diagnosis or six to eight weeks after the onset of illness

## Syphilitic aortitis

### Echo findings

- **Ascending aorta aneurysm: often gigantic, above sinuses of Valsalva (most common involvement)**
- Aortic regurgitation due to annulus dilatation
- Aortic arch is involved in 91% of patients and the descending thoracic aorta in 90%
- Aortic aneurysm (occasionally multiple) is more common in syphilis than in atherosclerosis
- Rupture of the thoracic aorta is the most common cause of death—aortic dissection is less often than direct aneurysm rupture
- Aortopulmonary fistula is the rare complication of aneurysmal aortic dilatation

## Churg–Strauss

### Echo findings

- Impaired LV function in 30–50% patients
- Coronary arteries vasculitis: segmental wall motion abnormalities, intraventricular thrombus

- Myocarditis: global ventricular dysfunction
- Diastolic dysfunction (any degree) in 30–40%
- Restrictive cardiomyopathy (see Chapter 8) due to endomyocardial fibrosis
- Pericardial effusion in 20–40% of patients, cardiac tamponade, rarely pericardial constriction valvular regurgitation (any degree) in 20–70% of patients

## Hypereosinophilic syndrome (Löffler)

### Echo findings in the thrombotic phase

- Multiple intracardiac thrombi
- Thrombi can be also on the valves and could cause aortic stenosis
- Initial tethering of the chordae tendineae of atrioventricular valves causes valve insufficiency

### Echo findings in the fibrotic phase

- **Apical obliteration of one or both ventricles by an echogenic thrombotic-fibrotic material (usefulness of echo-contrast imaging )** (Fig. 17.3.16)
- Further distortion of the normal position of mitral valve structures (Fig. 17.3.17)

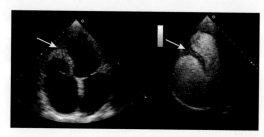

**Fig. 17.3.16** 4CV with and without contrast: apical obliteration of the right ventricle by an echogenic thrombotic-fibrotic material (arrows)

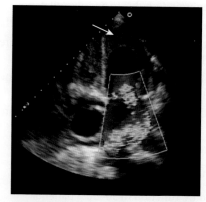

**Fig. 17.3.17** 4CV: apical obliteration of the LV by an echogenic thrombotic-fibrotic material (arrow) and severe mitral regurgitation

- Extensive left-ventricular endocardial fibrosis
- Endocardial thickening
- Hyperdynamic contraction of the spared ventricular walls
- Bilateral atrial enlargement
- Restrictive pattern in PW Doppler of AV valves

## Chronic cardiac consequences of hypereosinophilia

- Restrictive cardiomyopathy
- Dilated cardiomyopathy
- Mitral or tricuspid valves regurgitation
- Valves obstruction
- Constrictive pericarditis

# Whipple's disease

## Echo findings

- Aortic and mitral valves leaflet thickening and calcification (endocarditis, a frequent finding) ➜ mild to moderate valvular stenosis/regurgitation (Fig. 17.3.18AB)
- Endocarditis should be considered in negative blood cultures—fever, congestive heart failure, vegetations, previous valvular disease are less frequent than in patients with other endocarditis

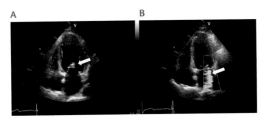

**Fig. 17.3.18** 4CV: arrow indicates thickening and fibrosis of anterior mitral valve leaflet (A); moderate mitral regurgitation (B) in patient with Whipple's disease

- Pericardial effusion, pericardial thickening, pericardial constriction
- Increased LV wall thickness, increased end-diastolic and end-systolic LV diameters
- Impaired LV function: myocardial involvement is rare
- Pulmonary hypertension is rare

# Endocrine disease

## Hyperthyroidism

### Echo findings

#### *Myocardial*

- High cardiac output, enhanced cardiac contractility ➡ the majority of hyperthyroid patients
- Sinus tachycardia or atrial fibrillation caused/related to LV systolic or diastolic dysfunction

#### *Valvular*

- Mitral or tricuspid regurgitation (hyperthyroidism can unmask valvular heart disease)
- Increased prevalence of mitral valve prolapse in autoimmune thyroid diseases (Graves disease and Hashimoto's thyroiditis)
- **Pulmonary hypertension**: PAH in 30–40% patients (usually reversible)

# Hypothyroidism

## Echo findings

### Myocardial

◆ Regional LV wall-motion abnormalities—advanced coronary atherosclerosis
◆ Global LV systolic dysfunction and reduced cardiac output

### Pericardial

◆ Pericardial effusion in 30–80% of patients: a correlation between severity of the disease is observed; thyroid function should be part of the lab work-up of any pericardial effusion
◆ Cardiac tamponade is rare, usually after many years of symptomatic disease

# Phaeochromocytoma

## Echo findings

### Myocardial

◆ Systolic LV dysfunction and dilated cardiomyopathy (norepinephrine increasing oxygen demand, apoptosis, and injury of myocytes)
◆ Echocardiographic features of Takotsubo cardiomyopathy but also transient hypo/akinesia of the basal and mid ventricular segments of LV with sparing of the apical contraction—so-called inverted Takotsubo cardiomyopathy
◆ Acute myocardial infarction or myocardial hibernation—coronary vasospasm induced by catecholamine

- Myocardial fibrosis and early diastolic dysfunction characterized by impaired relaxation

## Acromegalic cardiomyopathy

### Echo findings

- Cardiac hypertrophy: increased LV mass, thickening of intraventricular septum and both LV and RV walls. **Concentric biventricular hypertrophy is the most common feature of acromegaly (60%)**
- Diastolic dysfunction: prolonged LV diastolic relaxation
- LV systolic dysfunction at rest and heart failure with signs of dilative cardiomyopathy

### Other possible echo findings

- Valve disease: mitral or aortic valve regurgitation
- An increased diameter of the aortic root; true thoracic aortic aneurysm is rare
- Increased LV ejection fraction; hyperkinetic syndrome

# HIV disease (AIDS)

## Echo findings

- Increased LV wall thickness and elevated LV mass
- Reduction of LV ejection fraction and fractional shortening ➜ mild to severe in late disease stages

- Dilatation of all the cardiac chambers ➜ late disease stages
- LV diastolic dysfunction
- RV involvement, usually subclinical systolic and diastolic abnormalities
- Increased pulmonary systolic pressures ➜ late disease stages (HIV associated pulmonary hypertension)
- Pericardial effusion
- Valvular involvement in infective endocarditis: right-sided valves (tricuspid valve up to 90%) and left-sided (mitral and aortic 8–30%)
- Although echo findings are non-specific, precise cardiac monitoring is advisable in HIV-infected patients

## Chagas disease

### Echo findings in acute phase (over half of all infected patients)

- **Pericardial effusion: most frequent** (from moderate to severe in 40% of patients)
- LV ejection fraction is usually in normal range
- Apical or anterior wall dyskinesia (approximately 20%)
- LV dilatation is rare
- Acute myocarditis is infrequent (1–5% of patients)

### Echo findings in chronic phase

- **High rate of LV apical aneurysm (AA) with 'narrow neck'** (Fig. 17.3.19), over half of all cases, more frequently in male, and could be with mural thrombi

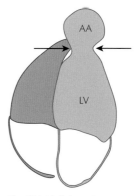

**Fig. 17.3.19** Schematic representation of a narrow-neck aneurysm, typical of Chagas disease

- RV apex could be also affected (10%)
- Segmental wall contractile abnormalities—hypokinesia of posterior wall (20–33%).
- LV but also other chambers could be dilated
- RV dysfunction secondary to LV impairment or high pulmonary pressure
- LV systolic and diastolic function is usually abnormal
- Mitral and tricuspid valve regurgitation
- In patients with normal LV ejection fraction, systolic dysfunction could be provoked by stress echocardiography ➜ biphasic response during dobutamine stress echo, predominantly at the LV posterior or inferior wall

## Suggested reading

1. Plonska E, Badano L, Lancellotti P. Echocardiography for internal medicine textbook. *Medical Tribune* Polska 2012.
2. Haque S, Gordon C, Isenberg D, et al. Risk factors for clinical coronary heart disease in systemic lupus erythematosus: the lupus and atherosclerosis evaluation of risk (LASER) study. *Rheumatol* 2010;37:322-9.
3. Ishimori ML, Martin R, Berman DS, et al. Myocardial ischemia in the absence of coronary artery disease lupus. *JACC Cardiovasc Imaging* 2011;4:27–33.
4. Nikpour M, Urowitz MB, Ibañez D, et al. Relationship between cardiac symptoms, myocardial perfusion defects and coronary angiography findings in systemic lupus. *Lupus* 2011;20:229–304.

# Index